Handbook of Spine Surgery

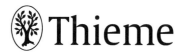

Handbook of Spine Surgery

Ali A. Baaj, MD
Instructor of Neurosurgery–Spine
Department of Neurosurgery
Johns Hopkins Hospital
Baltimore, Maryland

Praveen V. Mummaneni, MD
Associate Professor
Department of Neurosurgery
Co-Director, UCSF Spine Center
University of California–San Francisco
San Francisco, California

Juan S. Uribe, MD
Assistant Professor
Director, Spine Section
Director, Biomechanical Laboratory
Department of Neurosurgery
University of South Florida
Tampa, Florida

Alexander R. Vaccaro, MD, PhD
The Everrett J. and Marion Gordon
 Professor of Orthopaedic Surgery
Professor of Neurosurgery
Co-Director, Delaware Valley
 Spinal Cord Injury Center
Co-Chief, Spine Surgery
Co-Director, Spine Surgery
Thomas Jefferson University
The Rothman Institute
Philadelphia, Pennsylvania

Mark S. Greenberg, MD
Assistant Professor
Department of Neurological Surgery
 and Brain Repair
University of South Florida
Chief, Neurosurgery Section
James A. Haley Veterans Hospital
Tampa, Florida

Thieme
New York · Stuttgart

Thieme Medical Publishers, Inc.
333 Seventh Ave.
New York, NY 10001

Executive Editor: Kay Conerly
Editorial Assistant: Tess Timoshin
Editorial Director, Clinical Reference: Michael Wachinger
Production Editor: Kenneth L. Chumbley
International Production Director: Andreas Schabert
Senior Vice President, International Marketing and Sales: Cornelia Schulze
Vice President, Finance and Accounts: Sarah Vanderbilt
President: Brian D. Scanlan
Compositor: Prairie Papers Inc.
Printer: Sheridan Press

Library of Congress Cataloging-in-Publication Data
Handbook of spine surgery / [edited by] Ali A. Baaj . . . [et al.].
   p. ; cm.
  Includes bibliographical references and index.
  ISBN 978-1-60406-419-3 (pbk. : alk. paper)
 1. Spine—Surgery—Handbooks, manuals, etc. 2. Orthopedics—Handbooks, manuals, etc.
 I. Baaj, Ali A.
  [DNLM: 1. Spine—surgery—Handbooks. 2. Neurosurgical Procedures—methods—Handbooks. 3. Orthopedic Procedures—methods—Handbooks. 4. Spinal Cord—surgery—Handbooks. WE 39]
  RD768.H354 2012
  617.4'71—dc23
                                                             2011028108

Copyright © 2012 by Thieme Medical Publishers, Inc. This book, including all parts thereof, is legally protected by copyright. Any use, exploitation, or commercialization outside the narrow limits set by copyright legislation without the publisher's consent is illegal and liable to prosecution. This applies in particular to photostat reproduction, copying, mimeographing or duplication of any kind, translating, preparation of microfilms, and electronic data processing and storage.

Important note: Medical knowledge is ever-changing. As new research and clinical experience broaden our knowledge, changes in treatment and drug therapy may be required. The authors and editors of the material herein have consulted sources believed to be reliable in their efforts to provide information that is complete and in accord with the standards accepted at the time of publication. However, in view of the possibility of human error by the authors, editors, or publisher of the work herein or changes in medical knowledge, neither the authors, editors, nor publisher, nor any other party who has been involved in the preparation of this work, warrants that the information contained herein is in every respect accurate or complete, and they are not responsible for any errors or omissions or for the results obtained from use of such information. Readers are encouraged to confirm the information contained herein with other sources. For example, readers are advised to check the product information sheet included in the package of each drug they plan to administer to be certain that the information contained in this publication is accurate and that changes have not been made in the recommended dose or in the contraindications for administration. This recommendation is of particular importance in connection with new or infrequently used drugs.

Some of the product names, patents, and registered designs referred to in this book are in fact registered trademarks or proprietary names even though specific reference to this fact is not always made in the text. Therefore, the appearance of a name without designation as proprietary is not to be construed as a representation by the publisher that it is in the public domain.

Printed in the United States of America

5 4 3 2 1

ISBN 978-1-60406-419-3

To my parents, Abdulwahab and Hana, to my wife, Gabriela, and to my first teachers of spine surgery at the University of South Florida.

Ali A. Baaj

For my wife, Valli, and my children, Nikhita, Nikhil, and Neel, for their love and support.

Praveen V. Mummaneni

To my parents, my wife, Catalina, and my two children, Sebastian and Camila.

Juan S. Uribe

I would like to dedicate this book to my wonderful children, Alex and Juliana, whose unwavering love and support has sustained me through the most difficult of times.

Alexander R. Vaccaro

I dedicate this work to my father, Louis Greenberg, who has guided me throughout life with integrity, wisdom, and humor.

Mark S. Greenberg

Contents

Foreword
   Howard S. An xi
   Volker K. H. Sonnatag xiii
Preface xv
Contributors xvii

I   Clinical Spine Anatomy

1. Embryology of the Spine 3
   Akash J. Patel, Katherine Relyea, Daniel H. Fulkerson, and Andrew Jea

2. Craniovertebral Junction 9
   Ali A. Baaj, Edwin Ramos, and Juan S. Uribe

3. Cervical Spine 16
   Eric A. Sribnick and Sanjay S. Dhall

4. Thoracic Spine 21
   Ryan J. Halpin and Tyler R. Koski

5. Lumbar Spine 26
   Hormuzdiyar H. Dasenbrock and Ali Bydon

6. Sacral-Iliac Spine 33
   Amit R. Patel and Ravi K. Ponnappan

II   Clinical Spine Surgery

7. Physical Examination 43
   Mark S. Greenberg and Daniel Marin

8. Spinal Imaging 51
   Ishaq Y. Syed, Barrett I. Woods, and Joon Y. Lee

9. Neurophysiologic Monitoring in Spine Surgery 57
   Glen Aaron Pollock, Naomi Abel, and Fernando L. Vale

10. Pharmacology 66
    Mark S. Greenberg

11. Interventional Pain/Nonoperative Spine Procedures:
    Diagnostic and Therapeutic 71
    Daniel Marin

12. Bedside Procedures 76
    Daniel C. Lu and Praveen V. Mummaneni

13. Spinal Radiation Therapy 83
    Edward A. Monaco III and Peter Carlos Gerszten

14. Spinal Navigation 90
    Ben J. Garrido and Rick C. Sasso

15	Spinal Biologics	94
	Rafael F. Cardona-Durán and Juan S. Uribe	

III Spinal Pathology

16	Congenital Anomalies	101
	Rory R. Mayer, Katherine Relyea, and Andrew Jea	
17	Trauma	114
	Daniel K. Park and Ravi K. Ponnappan	
18	Infection	127
	William D. Long III and Peter G. Whang	
19	Tumors of the Spine	136
	Camilo A. Molina and Daniel M. Sciubba	
20	Cervical and Thoracic Spine Degenerative Disease	146
	Clinton J. Burkett and Mark S. Greenberg	
21	Degenerative Lumbar Spine Disease	154
	Michael Y. Wang	
22	Deformity	163
	David T. Anderson and Jeffrey A. Rihn	
23	Vascular Pathology of the Spine	172
	Timothy D. Uschold and Steven W. Chang	
24	Spondyloarthropathies	180
	Amir Ahmadian and Fernando L. Vale	
25	Spinal Emergencies	190
	Mohammed Eleraky and Frank D. Vrionis	

IV Surgical Techniques

26	Occipitocervical Fusion	199
	Edwin Ramos and Juan S. Uribe	
27	Chiari I Decompression	204
	Mark S. Greenberg	
28	Transoral Odontoidectomy	209
	Frank M. Phillips and Colin B. Harris	
29	C1–C2 Techniques	215
	Jau-Ching Wu and Praveen V. Mummaneni	
30	Direct Fixation of Odontoid Fractures	221
	Andrew T. Dailey and Jose Carlos Sauri-Barraza	
31	Cervical Arthroplasty	227
	Jau-Ching Wu, Ali A. Baaj, and Praveen V. Mummaneni	
32	Anterior Cervical Corpectomy	232
	Mohammad Said Shukairy and Frank M. Phillips	

33	Anterior Cervical Discectomy	238

Daniel C. Lu, Kevin T. Foley, and Praveen V. Mummaneni

34	Anterior Cervical Foraminotomy	243

Matthew J. Tormenti and Adam S. Kanter

35	Cervical Laminectomy with or without Fusion	248

Ali A. Baaj and Fernando L. Vale

36	Cervical Laminoplasty	253

Sarah I. Woodrow and Allan D. Levi

37	Posterior Cervical Foraminotomy	259

Matthias Setzer, Nam D. Tran, and Frank D. Vrionis

38	Cervical Open Reduction Techniques: Anterior and Posterior Approaches	265

Harminder Singh, George M. Ghobrial, and James Harrop

39	Resection of Pancoast Tumors	271

Jean-Paul Wolinsky and Ziya L. Gokaslan

40	Cervical-Thoracic Junction Technique	276

Matthew B. Maserati and David O. Okonkwo

41	Thoracic Pedicle Technique	285

Ryan J. Halpin and Tyler R. Koski

42	Lateral Extracavitary Approach	291

Beejal Y. Amin and Muwaffak Abdulhak

43	Transpedicular Approach	296

Frank La Marca, Paul Park, and Juan M. Valdivia

44	Costotransversectomy	300

Dean B. Kostov and Adam S. Kanter

45	Thoracoscopic Approach	304

Timothy D. Uschold and Steven W. Chang

46	Pedicle Subtraction Osteotomy/Smith Peterson Osteotomy	309

Frank La Marca, Paul Park, and Juan M. Valdivia

47	Transthoracic Approach	314

Brian Kwon and David H. Kim

48	Retroperitoneal Approaches to the Thoracolumbar Spine	318

Camilo A. Molina, Ziya L. Gokaslan, and Daniel M. Sciubba

49	Open and MIS Lumbar Microdiscectomy	325

Ali A. Baaj and Mark S. Greenberg

50	Lumbar Foraminotomy (MIS)	330

Ali A. Baaj and Juan S. Uribe

51	Lumbar Laminectomy	333

Armen Deukmedjian, Ali A. Baaj, and Juan S. Uribe

52 Posterior and Transforaminal Lumbar Interbody Fusion (PLIF/TLIF) (Open) 336
Devin Vikram Amin and Adam S. Kanter

53 Minimally Invasive Transforaminal Lumbar Interbody Fusion (MIS TLF) 341
Michael Y. Wang

54 Percutaneous Pedicle Screw Placement 348
Michael Y. Wang

55 Minimally Invasive Lateral Retroperitoneal Trans-Psoas Interbody Fusion (e.g., XLIF, DLIF) 354
Edwin Ramos, Ali A. Baaj, and Juan S. Uribe

56 Anterior Lumbar Interbody Fusion (ALIF) 359
Krzysztof B. Siemionow and Kern Singh

57 Axial Lumbar Interbody Fusion (AxiaLIF) 364
Elias Dakwar and Juan S. Uribe

58 Facet Screw Fixation/Fusion 368
Ben J. Garrido and Rick C. Sasso

59 Interspinous Process Decompression 373
Ravi Ramachandran and Peter G. Whang

60 Lumbar Arthroplasty 378
Ishaq Y. Syed, Barrett I. Woods, and Joon Y. Lee

61 Lumbosacroiliac Fixation 384
Amit R. Patel, Alexander R. Vaccaro, and Ravi K. Ponnappan

62 Sacrectomy 390
Ioannis Papanastassiou, Mohammad Eleraky, and Frank D. Vrionis

63 Vertebral Body Augmentation 398
Mohammed Eleraky and Frank D. Vrionis

64 Spinal Cord Tumor Resection 404
Michelle J. Clarke and Timothy F. Witham

65 Surgical Resection of Spinal Vascular Lesions 410
Timothy D. Uschold, Alim P. Mitha, and Steven W. Chang

Appendices

I Positioning 419
Tien V. Le, Juan S. Uribe, and Fernando L. Vale

II Selected Spinal Orthoses 423
Tien V. Le, Juan S. Uribe, and Fernando L. Vale

III Scales and Outcomes 433
Mark S. Greenberg

Index 437

Foreword

Handbook of Spine Surgery, by Ali A. Baaj, Praveen V. Mummaneni, Juan S. Uribe, Alexander R. Vaccaro, and Mark S. Greenberg, is indeed a great contribution to the field of spine surgery. The authors are to be congratulated for preparing a textbook that distills the vast amount of current information on spine surgery in an extremely well-organized and succinct manner. The authors were also fortunate to recruit prominent orthopedic and neurosurgical colleagues as well as nonsurgical experts in the field of spine today.

The book is aptly organized into sections containing spinal anatomy, clinical spinal surgery, spinal pathology, and surgical techniques, as includes useful appendices on positioning, spinal orthoses, scales, and outcomes. Each chapter is divided into appropriate subheadings such as key points, anatomy, indications, technique, complications, outcomes, frequently asked questions, and surgical pearls. The surgical pearls are an invaluable part of this book, which are not easily found in other textbooks. The illustrations are of high quality and complement the text well.

This book is written primarily for orthopedic surgeons and neurosurgeons, but is also great for residents and fellows-in-training, as well as nonoperative physicians who take care of patients with various spinal disorders. Over the past two decades, there have been great advances in the field of spine surgery, and as a result, there has been enormous information overload with countless articles, textbooks, and web content. This book serves well to digest the most current and relevant information in an outline format with appropriate figures so that the reader can assimilate information in an efficacious manner. This book should be a daily companion for practicing spine surgeons and every orthopedic and neurosurgical resident and fellow.

Howard S. An, MD
The Morton International Endowed Chair
Professor of Orthopaedic Surgery
Director of Spine Surgery and Spine Fellowship Program
Rush University Medical Center
Chicago, Illinois

Foreword

This book provides a handy and practical guide to common spinal disorders and includes nice reviews of relevant clinical and spinal anatomy; bedside techniques, type of pathology affecting the spinal column and spinal cord, and, most importantly, surgical techniques for the spine. Conveniently, each chapter begins with key points. Toward the end of the chapters, useful surgical pearls are provided, followed by common clinical questions and answers to these questions.

I congratulate the authors on providing a quick and easy reference for professionals who treat patients with spinal disorders. This book will be especially helpful for students and residents and will also provide quick reference for practicing spine surgeons.

Volker K. H. Sonntag (Retired)
Professor of Clinical Surgery
University of Arizona
Vice-Chairman, Department of Neurosurgery
Chairman, Spine Section
Director, Residency Program
Barrow Neurological Institute
Phoenix, Arizona

Preface

The discipline of spine surgery has evolved to encompass a wide range of diagnoses and procedures. The burden to efficiently review and apply these principles can be exhausting. With this in mind, we are happy to introduce the first edition of the *Handbook of Spine Surgery*, a practical handbook aimed at providing the resident, fellow, or staff with quick access to key points of common spinal diseases and management strategies.

The first of its kind in this discipline, this text has distilled a vast amount of information into key background concepts and pertinent surgical pearls. It is divided into four principal sections: Anatomy, Pathology, Clinical, and Techniques. Each chapter is in bullet-point format to make it readable and focused. Clinical pearls are emphasized, and simple board-style questions are included to highlight the salient points.

This handbook is comprehensive, yet readable and portable. It is an excellent tool for trainees not only to review spinal pathology but also to skim through surgical techniques before going into the operating room. It is equally an excellent resource for spine surgeons who choose to review the less routine procedures as described by experts in the field. This work was not meant to be a comprehensive reference book on spine surgery as such texts already exist. The strength of this handbook lies in its practicality and portability.

With the help of over sixty contributors from more than twelve academic programs representing both orthopedics and neurosurgery, we have attempted to bring a wide range of expertise to this project. *It was our intent to obtain the input of residents, fellows, and junior and senior faculty alike in compiling this work.* With the ultimate goals of advancing our field and enhancing patient care, we hope you find this handbook both practical and valuable.

Acknowledgments

The editors would like to thank all chapter contributors for making this work possible. We also thank Kay Conerly, Lauren Henry, and Tess Timoshin from Thieme Medical Publishers for their assistance in the editing and publication of this text.

Contributors

Muwaffak Abdulhak, MD, FRCS (C)
Director, Neuroscience Institute
Spine/Neurotrauma Center
Henry Ford Hospital
Detroit, Michigan

Naomi Abel, MD
Assistant Professor of Physical
   Medicine and Rehabilitation
Department of Neurosurgery
   and Brain Repair
University of South Florida
Tampa, Florida

Amir Ahmadian, MD
Resident Physician
Department of Neurosurgery
   and Brain Repair
University of South Florida
Tampa, Florida

Beejal Y. Amin, MD
Resident Physician
Department of Neurosurgery
Henry Ford Hospital
Detroit, Michigan

Devin Vikram Amin, MD, PhD
Assistant Professor
Department of Neurosurgery
Southern Illinois University
Springfield, Illinois

David T. Anderson, MD
Resident Physician
Department of Orthopaedic Surgery
Thomas Jefferson University Hospital
Philadelphia, Pennsylvania

Ali A. Baaj, MD
Instructor of Neurosurgery–Spine
Department of Neurosurgery
Johns Hopkins Hospital
Baltimore, Maryland

Clinton J. Burkett, MD
Complex and Minimally Invasive
   Spine Fellow
Department of Neurosurgery
University of South Florida
Tampa, Florida

Ali Bydon, MD
Assistant Professor
Department of Neurosurgery
Johns Hopkins University School
   of Medicine
Baltimore, Maryland

Rafael F. Cardona-Durán, MD
Director of Complex and Minimally
   Invasive Spine Surgery
Puerto Rico Neurological Spine
   Surgery, PSC
San Juan, Puerto Rico

Steve W. Chang, MD
Staff Neurosurgeon
Division of Neurological Surgery
Barrow Neurological Institute
Phoenix, Arizona

Michelle J. Clarke, MD
Assistant Professor of Neurosurgery
Department of Neurologic Surgery
Mayo Clinic
Rochester, Minnesota

Elias Dakwar, MD
Resident Physician
Department of Neurosurgery
   and Brain Repair
University of South Florida
Tampa, Florida

Andrew T. Dailey, MD
Associate Professor
Departments of Neurosurgery
   and Orthopedics
University of Utah
Salt Lake City, Utah

xviii Contributors

Hormuzdiyar H. Dasenbrock, BS
Johns Hopkins University School
 of Medicine
Baltimore, Maryland

Armen Deukmedjian, MD
Resident Physician
Department of Neurological Surgery
University of South Florida
Tampa, Florida

Sanjay S. Dhall, MD
Assistant Professor
Department of Neurosurgery
Emory University School of Medicine
Atlanta, Georgia

Mohammed Eleraky, MD
Research Associate
H. Lee Moffitt Cancer Center
 and Research Institute
NeuroOncology Program and
 Department of Neurosurgery
University of South Florida
Tampa, Florida

Kevin T. Foley, MD
Professor of Neurosurgery
Director, Spine Fellowship Program
Department of Neurosurgery
University of Tennessee Health
 Science Center
Director of Complex Spine Surgery
Semmes-Murphey Clinic
Medical Director
Medical Education and Research
 Institute
Image-Guided Surgery Research Center
Memphis, Tennessee

Daniel H. Fulkerson, MD
Assistant Professor of Neurological
 Surgery
Department of Neurosurgery
Indiana University School of Medicine
Goodman Campbell Brain and Spine
Indianapolis, Indiana

Ben J. Garrido, MD
Orthopedic Spine Surgeon
Lake Norman Orthopedic Spine Center
Mooresville, North Carolina

Peter Carlos Gerszten, MD, MPH, FACS
Peter E. Sheptak Professor
Departments of Neurological Surgery
 and Radiation Oncology
University of Pittsburgh Medical Center
Pittsburgh, Pennsylvania

George M. Ghobrial, MD
Resident Physician
Department of Neurosurgery
Thomas Jefferson University Hospital
Philadelphia, Pennsylvania

Ziya L. Gokaslan, MD, FACS
Donlin M. Long Professor
Professor of Neurosurgery, Oncology,
 and Orthopaedic Surgery
Vice-Chair
Director of Neurosurgical Spine
 Program
Department of Neurosurgery
Johns Hopkins University School
 of Medicine
Johns Hopkins Hospital
Baltimore, Maryland

Mark S. Greenberg, MD
Assistant Professor
Department of Neurological Surgery
 and Brain Repair
University of South Florida
Chief, Neurosurgery Section
James A. Haley Veterans Hospital
Tampa, Florida

Ryan J. Halpin, MD
Department of Neurological Surgery
Northwestern University Feinberg
 School of Medicine
Chicago, Illinois

Colin B. Harris, MD
Orthopedic Spine Surgeon
Syracuse Orthopedic Specialists
Syracuse, New York

James Harrop, MD, FACS
Associate Professor
Departments of Neurological and Orthopedic Surgery
Chief, Spine and Peripheral Nerve Surgery
Neurosurgery Director of Delaware SCI Center
Director, Neurosurgical Spine Fellowship
Jefferson Medical College
Philadelphia, Pennsylvania

Andrew Jea, MD
Staff Neurosurgeon
Director, Neuro-spine Program
Assistant Professor
Texas Children's Hospital Division of Neurosurgery
Baylor College of Medicine Department of Neurosurgery
Houston, Texas

Adam S. Kanter, MD
Assistant Professor of Neurological Surgery
Director, Minimally Invasive Spine Program
Department of Neurological Surgery
University of Pittsburgh Medical Center, Presbyterian
Pittsburgh, Pennsylvania

David H. Kim, MD
Associate Clinical Professor
Department of Orthopaedic Surgery
Tufts University School of Medicine
Boston, Massachusetts

Tyler R. Koski, MD
Assistant Professor of Neurological Surgery
Director of Spinal Deformity Program
Northwestern University Feinberg School of Medicine
Chicago, Illinois

Dean B. Kostov, MD
Chief Resident Physician
Department of Neurological Surgery
University of Pittsburgh Medical Center, Presbyterian
Pittsburgh, Pennsylvania

Brian Kwon, MD
Assistant Clinical Professor
Department of Orthopedic Surgery
New England Baptist Hospital
Tufts University School of Medicine
Boston, Massachusetts

Frank La Marca, MD
Associate Clinical Professor
Chief of Spine Section
Department of Neurosurgery
University of Michigan
Ann Arbor, Michigan

Tien V. Le, MD
Resident Physician
Department of Neurosurgery and Brain Repair
University of South Florida
Tampa, Florida

Joon Y. Lee, MD
Assistant Professor of Orthopaedic Surgery
Department of Orthopaedics
University of Pittsburgh Medical Center
Pittsburgh, Pennsylvania

Allan D. Levi, MD, PhD, FACS
Professor
Department of Neurosurgery
University of Miami
Miami, Florida

William D. Long III, MD
Resident Physician
Department of Orthopaedic Surgery and Rehabilitation
Yale–New Haven Hospital
Yale University School of Medicine
New Haven, Connecticut

Daniel C. Lu, MD, PhD
Assistant Professor
Department of Neurosurgery
University of California–Los Angeles
Los Angeles, California

Daniel Marin, MD
Assistant Professor
Physiatrist
Cahill Spine Institute
University of South Florida
Tampa, Florida

Matthew B. Maserati, MD
Resident Physician
Department of Neurological Surgery
University of Pittsburgh Medical Center
Pittsburgh, Pennsylvania

Rory R. Mayer, BS
Department of Neurosurgery
Baylor College of Medicine
Houston, Texas

Alim P. Mitha, MD
Cerebrovascular/Skull Base Fellow
Endovascular Fellow
Division of Neurological Surgery
Barrow Neurological Institute
Phoenix, Arizona

Camilo A. Molina, BA
Research Fellow
Howard Hughes Medical Institute
Department of Neurological Surgery
Johns Hopkins University School
  of Medicine
Baltimore, Maryland

Edward A. Monaco III, MD, PhD
Resident Physician
Department of Neurological Surgery
University of Pittsburgh Medical Center
Pittsburgh, Pennsylvania

Praveen V. Mummaneni, MD
Associate Professor
Department of Neurosurgery
Co-Director, UCSF Spine Center
University of California–San Francisco
San Francisco, California

David O. Okonkwo, MD, PhD
Associate Professor
Department of Neurological Surgery
University of Pittsburgh
Pittsburgh, Pennsylvania

Ioannis Papanastassiou, MD
Consultant
Department of Orthopaedics
Agioi Anargyroi
Athens, Greece

Daniel K. Park, MD
Attending Spine Surgeon
Department of Orthopedic Surgery
William Beaumont Hospital
Royal Oak, Michigan

Paul Park, MD
Assistant Professor
Department of Neurosurgery
University of Michigan
Ann Arbor, Michigan

Akash J. Patel, MD
Resident Physician
Department of Neurosurgery
Baylor College of Medicine
Houston, Texas

Amit R. Patel, MD
Resident Physician
Department of Orthopaedic Surgery
Hospital of the University of
  Pennsylvania
Philadelphia, Pennsylvania

Frank M. Phillips, MD
Professor
Department of Orthopaedic Surgery
Rush University Medical Center
Chicago, Illinois

Glen Aaron Pollock, MD, DVM
Resident Physician
Department of Neurosurgery
and Brain Repair
University of South Florida
Tampa, Florida

Ravi K. Ponnappan, MD
Assistant Professor
Department of Orthopaedics
Thomas Jefferson University
Philadelphia, Pennsylvania

Ravi Ramachandran, MD
Resident Physician
Department of Orthopaedic Surgery
Yale New Haven Hospital
New Haven, Connecticut

Edwin Ramos, MD
Assistant Professor of Neurosurgery
Department of Neurosurgery
University of South Florida
Tampa, Florida

Katherine Relyea, MS
Medical Illustrator
Department of Pediatric Neurosurgery
Baylor College of Medicine
Houston, Texas

Jeffrey A. Rihn, MD
Assistant Professor
Department of Orthopaedic Surgery
Thomas Jefferson University Hospital
The Rothman Institute
Philadelphia, Pennsylvania

Rick C. Sasso, MD
Professor
Chief of Spine Surgery
Clinical Orthopaedic Surgery
Indiana University School of Medicine
Indiana Spine Group
Indianapolis, Indiana

Jose Carlos Sauri-Barraza, MD
Department of Orthopaedics
Centro Médico ABC
Mexico City, Mexico

Daniel M. Sciubba, MD
Assistant Professor of Neurosurgery,
Oncology, and Orthopaedic Surgery
Director, Spine Research
Director, Minimally Invasive Spine
Surgery
Johns Hopkins University
Baltimore, Maryland

Matthias Setzer, MD
Department of Neurosurgery
Johann Wolfgang Goethe University
Frankfurt am Main, Germany

Mohammad Said Shukairy, MD
Department of Neurosurgery
Community Spine and Neurosurgery
Institute
Munster, Indiana

Krzysztof B. Siemionow, MD
Assistant Professor
Department of Orthopaedic Surgery
University of Illinois–Chicago
Weiss Memorial Hospital
Chicago, Illinois

Harminder Singh, MD
Assistant Professor
Department of Neurosurgery
Stanford University School of Medicine
Stanford, California

Kern Singh, MD
Department of Orthopaedic Surgery
Rush University Medical Center
Chicago, Illinois

Eric A. Sribnick, MD, PhD
Resident Physician
Department of Neurosurgery
Emory University
Atlanta, Georgia

Ishaq Y. Syed, MD
Assistant Professor
Department of Orthopaedics
Wake Forest Baptist Medical Center
Winston-Salem, North Carolina

Matthew J. Tormenti, MD
Neurosurgical Resident Physician
Department of Neurological Surgery
University of Pittsburgh Medical Center
Pittsburgh, Pennsylvania

Nam D. Tran, MD, PhD
Assistant Professor
H. Lee Moffitt Cancer Center
University of South Florida
Tampa, Florida

Juan S. Uribe, MD
Assistant Professor
Director, Spine Section
Director, Biomechanical Laboratory
Department of Neurosurgery
University of South Florida
Tampa, Florida

Timothy D. Uschold, MD
Neurosurgery Resident Physician
Division of Neurological Surgery
Barrow Neurological Institute
Phoenix, Arizona

Alexander R. Vaccaro, MD, PhD
The Everett J. and Marion Gordon
   Professor of Orthopaedic Surgery
Professor of Neurosurgery
Co-Director, Delaware Valley
   Spinal Cord Injury Center
Co-Chief, Spine Surgery
Co-Director, Spine Surgery
Thomas Jefferson University
The Rothman Institute
Philadelphia, Pennsylvania

Juan M. Valdivia V, MD
Clinical Lecturer
Department of Neurosurgery
University of Michigan
Chief, Neurosurgery
Ann Arbor Veteran's Affairs Health
   Care System
Ann Arbor, Michigan

Fernando L. Vale, MD
Professor and Vice-Chair
Residency Program Director
Department of Neurosurgery
University of South Florida
Tampa, Florida

Frank D. Vrionis, MD, PhD
Chief of Neurosurgery
H. Lee Moffitt Cancer Center
Professor of Neurosurgery and
   Orthopedics
University of South Florida College
   of Medicine
Tampa, Florida

Michael Y. Wang, MD, FACS
Associate Professor
Departments of Neurological Surgery
   and Rehabilitation Medicine
University of Miami Miller School
   of Medicine
Miami, Florida

Peter G. Whang, MD
Associate Professor, Spine Service
Department of Orthopaedics and
   Rehabilitation
Yale University School of Medicine
New Haven, Connecticut

Timothy F. Witham, MD, FACS
Associate Professor of Neurosurgery
Director, The Johns Hopkins Bayview
   Spine Program
Department of Neurosurgery
Johns Hopkins University
Baltimore, Maryland

Jean-Paul Wolinsky, MD
Associate Professor of Neurosurgery
   and Oncology
Clinical Director of the Johns Hopkins
   Spine Program
Johns Hopkins University
Baltimore, Maryland

Sarah I. Woodrow, MD, MEd, FRCS(C)
Department of Neurosurgery
Cooper University Hospital
Camden, New Jersey

Barrett I. Woods, MD
Resident Physician
Department of Orthopaedic Surgery
University of Pittsburgh Medical Center
Pittsburgh, Pennsylvania

Jau-Ching Wu, MD
Attending Staff
Department of Neurosurgery
Neurological Institute
Taipei Veterans General Hospital
Taipei, Taiwan

I
Clinical Spine Anatomy

1 Embryology of the Spine

Akash J. Patel, Katherine Relyea, Daniel H. Fulkerson, and Andrew Jea

I. Key Points

- The developing vertebral column is formed from somites, which develop into sclerotomes.
- Myotomes bridge the intervertebral spaces, allowing them to develop musculature that affords movement of the spine.
- The developing sclerotomes undergo chondrification and then ossification to form each vertebral unit.
- The HOX genes regulate the shape of each vertebral body.[1]
- Epiblast cells migrate to form the primitive groove, which in turn forms the notochord.
- The anterior neuropore closes on day 25 and the posterior on day 27.
- Neuroblasts form the mantle layer; the ventral portion forms the basal plates (motor) and the dorsal portion forms the alar plates (sensory).
- The caudal portion of the tube undergoes retrogressive differentiation and relative ascension of the conus.

II. Bony Anatomy

- Paraxial mesoderm forms 42 to 44 somites.
- Somites differentiate into ventromedial sclerotomes and dorsolateral dermomyotomes.
- In week 4, cells of the sclerotomes move to surround the spinal cord and notochord.[2]
- The sclerotome can be divided into a cranial area of loosely packed cells and a caudal area of densely packed cells with a "cell-free space" in between.[2]
- Sclerotomes are separated by intersegmental mesenchyme and flanked by segmental nerves, myotomes, and intersegmental arteries. Sclerotomes develop into definitive vertebrae, which causes myotomes to bridge intervertebral spaces, allowing movement of the spine.
- Between days 40 and 60, the process of chondrification begins and ossification follows, leading to the formation of each vertebral unit.

- Cells from the caudal portion of the sclerotome migrate to the cell-free space to form the annulus fibrosus of the disc, and regressing notochord forms the nucleus pulposus.
- The caudal portion of each sclerotome fuses to the cephalic portion of the adjacent sclerotome during week 6. After fusion, arteries cross vertebral bodies, with the nerves residing between them.
- Fusion of adjacent sclerotomes creates the centrum, which develops into the vertebral body.
- Cells adjacent to the neural tube form vertebral arches (or neural arches) that consist of the posterior elements.
- In general, each vertebra develops from three primary ossification centers: one for the body and one for each half of the vertebral arch.
  - There are five secondary ossification centers for subaxial vertebrae, located at the superior and inferior end plates of the body, the spinous process, and the tip of each transverse process.
  - C1 develops from the three primary ossification centers for the left and right posterior arches and for the anterior arch.
  - C2 develops from five primary ossification centers: two for the body of the dens, one for the vertebral body, and one each for the left and right neural arches.[3]
    - The tip of the dens represents a secondary ossification center.
- The shapes of different vertebral bodies are regulated by HOX genes.[1]
- The thoracic kyphosis is present during the fetal period, and the cervical and lumbar lordoses develop after birth.

III. Neural Anatomy

- By week 2, the embryo begins gastrulation and has two layers: epiblast and hypoblast. During gastrulation, epiblast cells migrate to the dorsal midline to form the primitive streak and subsequently the primitive groove.
- At the end of gastrulation there are three layers: ectoderm, mesoderm, and endoderm.
- At the edge of the primitive groove is a pit, the primitive node, where the notochordal process is formed by migrating epiblasts.
- By day 18 the primitive groove has regressed caudally and the notochord has formed.

1 Embryology of the Spine

- At three weeks' gestation, the edges of the neural plate begin to elevate to form neural folds, and their subsequent fusion in the cervical region forms the neural tube (**Fig. 1.1**).[2]
  - The anterior neuropore closes on day 25.
  - The posterior neuropore closes on day 27.
- Neural crest cells detach from the neural folds and migrate to form glia, arachnoid, pia, melanocytes, chondrocytes, chromaffin cells, osteocytes, Schwann cells, and enteric ganglia.
- The wall of the neural tube consists of neuroepithelial cells forming a pseudostratified epithelium connected by junctional complexes that differentiate into neuroblasts.[2]
- Neuroblasts form the mantle layer around the neuroepithelial layer that forms the gray matter of the spinal cord (**Fig. 1.2**).[2]
  - The ventral mantle layer forms the basal plates (motor horn), and the dorsal mantle layer forms the alar plates (sensory horn).
  - At the thoracic (T1 to T12) and upper lumbar (L1 to L2) region, the intermediate horn contains sympathetic neurons of the autonomic nervous system.
  - The boundary between the basal and alar plates is the sulcus limitans.

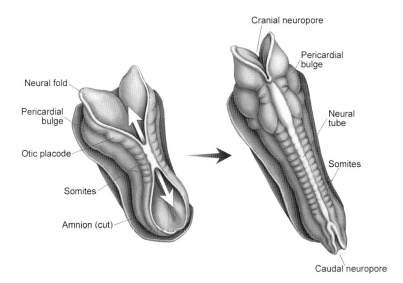

Fig. 1.1 Dorsal view of the human embryo during the third week of gestation. Note the somites on each side of the neural tube as it begins to fuse in the cervical region. The fused neural tube then continues to close both rostrally and caudally.

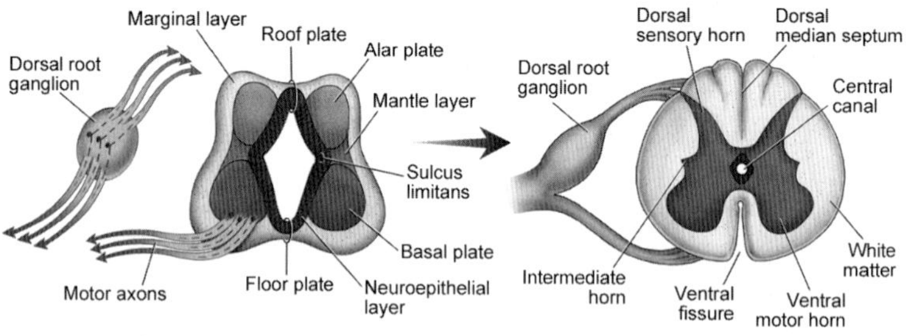

Fig. 1.2 Cross-section of the developing spinal cord demonstrates how the migrating neuroblasts from the neuroepithelial layer form dorsal and ventral mantle layers. These ultimately become the gray matter of the spinal cord. In addition, note the development of the dorsal root ganglion as well as the outward growth of the motor axons.

- The marginal layer contains nerve fibers from neuroblasts in the mantle layer that ultimately form the white matter of the spinal cord.
- The caudal tube forms during canalization (days 28 to 42).
- From day 43 to day 48, the ventriculus terminalis (a cystic structure at the caudal neural tube end) undergoes retrogressive differentiation, which is completed postnatally at 2 months.[2]
  - This results in relative ascension of the conus to its final level at L1-L2, and formation of the cauda equina and filum terminale (**Fig. 1.3**).

IV. Surgical Pearls

- Failure of the ventriculus terminalis results in a terminal myelocystocele. This cyst is lined with ependyma and communicates with the central canal.
- The sulcus limitans is the border between the sensory (dorsal) and motor (ventral) areas.
- The conus ascends to its adult level, L1-L2, by 2 months of age. It is important to keep this in mind when performing a lumbar puncture on the neonate.
- The notochord involutes and remains to develop the nucleus pulposus of the intervertebral disc
- Complete fusion of the ossification centers of C2 does not occur until age 12. Prior to this, synchondroses between ossification centers can be mistaken for fractures.

1 Embryology of the Spine

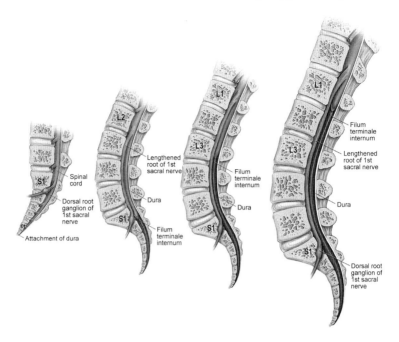

Fig. 1.3 The relative ascension of the conus and formation of the filum terminale via retrogressive differentiation.

Common Clinical Questions

1. On which day does the anterior neuropore close?
2. On which day does the posterior neuropore close?
3. The shapes of various groups of vertebral bodies are governed by which set of genes?

References

1. Wellik DM. Hox genes and vertebrate axial pattern. Curr Top Dev Biol 2009; 88:257 278
2. Sadler TW. Langman's Medical Embryology. 8th ed. Philadelphia, PA: Lippincott Williams & Wilkins; 2000
3. Greenberg MS. Handbook of Neurosurgery. 6th ed. New York: Thieme Medical Publishers; 2005

Answers to Common Clinical Questions

1. 25
2. 27
3. HOX genes

2 Craniovertebral Junction

Ali A. Baaj, Edwin Ramos, and Juan S. Uribe

I. Key Points

- The craniovertebral junction (CVJ) includes the base of the occiput (O), the occipital condyles, and vertebrae C1 and C2.
- Principal motion at O-C1 is flexion-extension and at C1-C2 axial rotation.
- The CVJ ligamentous complex is key to the stability of this region (**Fig. 2.1**).

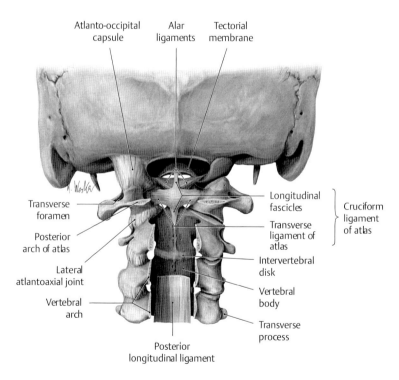

Fig. 2.1 CVJ ligamentous structures (from THIEME Atlas of Anatomy, General Anatomy and Musculoskeletal System, (c) Thieme 2005, Illustration by Karl Wesker).

II. Bony Anatomy

- CVJ refers to the base of the occiput, the atlas (C1), and the axis (C2).
- The boundaries of the foramen magnum are the basion anteriorly, the opisthion posteriorly, and the occipital condyles inferolaterally.
- C1 has no vertebral body or spinous process. It has a posterior arch and an anterior arch. It's the widest cervical vertebra, and its superior concave articular surface accommodates convex occipital condyles (**Fig. 2.2**).

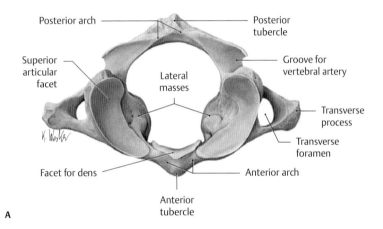

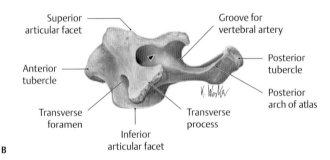

Fig. 2.2 (A) Superior and (B) lateral view of the atlas (from THIEME Atlas of Anatomy, General Anatomy and Musculoskeletal System, (c) Thieme 2005, Illustration by Karl Wesker).

- The C1 anterior tubercle (C1 "button") is the attachment site of the anterior longitudinal ligament (ALL) and the longus colli muscle.
- The vertebral artery and C1 nerve run along the superior lateral groove on C1 (sulcus arteriosus). In less than 15% of the population the groove is roofed, forming a foramen (arcuate foramen).
- C2 consists of the body, odontoid process, articulating surfaces, pedicles, pars interarticularis (note that pars and pedicles are distinct anatomical landmarks), lamina, and large, bifid spinous process (**Fig. 2.3**).[1]

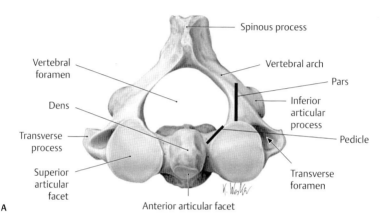

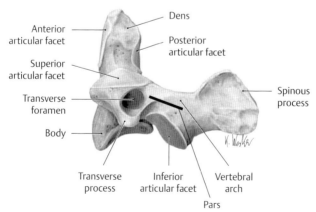

Fig. 2.3 Superior (**A**) and lateral (**B**) view of the axis (from THIEME Atlas of Anatomy, General Anatomy and Musculoskeletal System, (c) Thieme 2005, Illustration by Karl Wesker).

- The C2 odontoid (Gr. "tooth") process projects superiorly and has multiple (and overlapping) ligamentous attachments to C1 and the occiput.

III. Neural Anatomy

- Cervical nerve roots exit above their corresponding level (i.e., C2 nerve root exits above C2 pedicle).
- C1 nerve root: the posterior division (suboccipital nerve) is more prominent than the anterior division. It innervates suboccipital muscles and occasionally branches to the lesser/greater occipital nerve.
- C2 nerve root: posterior, medial (greater occipital nerve), and lateral divisions innervate suboccipital muscles and scalp from occiput to vertex.
- The lesser occipital nerve is formed by dorsal divisions of C2 and C3.

IV. Vascular Anatomy

- The vertebral artery (VA) leaves the C2 transverse foramen (becoming V3), takes a 45 degree lateral projection, and ascends (vertical portion of V3) into the C1 transverse foramen.
- The VA then courses medially (horizontal portion of V3) along the C1 sulcus arteriosus and then anteriorly through the atlantooccipital membrane, where it becomes intradural (beginning of V4 segment).
- Blood is supplied to the CVJ primarily through branches of the vertebral and occipital arteries.
- The base of the dens of C2 receives blood supply from vertebral artery branches (posterior circulation); the top is supplied by apical branch of the hypoglossal artery (anterior circulation).
- Lymphatic drainage of the CVJ is through retropharyngeal and deep cervical nodes (Grisel's syndrome: CVJ instability with concomitant retropharyngeal inflammation/infection).

V. Ligamentous and Muscular Anatomy (Table 2.1)

- Suboccipital muscles and the CVJ (**Fig. 2.4**)
  - Superior oblique: C1 transverse process laterally to occiput medially
  - Inferior oblique: C1 transverse process laterally to spinous process of C2 medially

Table 2.1 Principal CVJ Ligaments: Their Attachments and Modes of Action

Ligament	Attachments	Action
Apical	Odontoid tip (superiorly) to basion	Limits O-C2 distraction
Alar	Odontoid tip (laterally) to medial tubercle of occipital condyles and lateral masses of C1	Limits O-C2 subluxation/ hyperrotation
Cruciate	Vertical component: body of C2 to basion Transverse component: medial tubercles of C1 lateral masses to posterior dens	Prevents C1/C2 subluxation and O-C1/C2 distraction
Tectorial	Posterior aspect of vertebral bodies, dorsal to cruciate ligament (continuation of PLL)	Limits hyperflexion, distraction
ALL	Anterior aspect of vertebral bodies	Limits hyperextension, distraction
Accessory atlantoaxial	C2 body laterally to medial C1 lateral masses	Limits atlantoaxial hyperrotation
Capsular	O-C1 and C1-C2 articulating facets	Stabilizes facet joints
Anterior and posterior atlantooccipital membranes	Anterior: basion to C1 tubercle (C1 button) Posterior: opisthion to C1 posterior arch	Limit atlantooccipital distraction

Abbreviations: ALL, anterior longitudinal ligament; O, occiput; PLL, posterior longitudinal ligament.

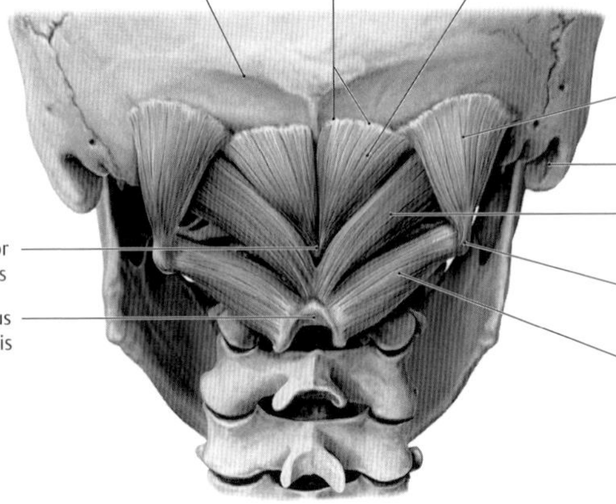

14 I Clinical Spine Anatomy

Fig. 2.4 Muscles of the suboccipital triangle (from Atlas of Anatomy, (c) Thieme 2008, Illustration by Karl Wesker).

- Rectus capitis posterior major: spinous process of C2 up to base of occiput
- Rectus capitis posterior minor: posterior tubercle of C1 up to base of occiput
- Semispinalis capitis: transverse processes of cervical vertebrae to nuchal ligament and occipital bone; superficial to suboccipital muscles
- Longissimus capitis: similar to semispinalis but runs and attaches more laterally to the occiput

VI. Surgical Pearls

- C1 nerve root, if present, can be sacrificed; though we don't routinely perform this, C2 nerve root may also be sacrificed (with minimal risk of occipital neuralgia).[2]
- Integrity of cruciate ligament must be considered before any CVJ stabilization procedure is undertaken.
- Venous plexus around C2 ganglion may cause considerable bleeding, which should not be mistaken for VA injury.
- Thin-cut CT of the CVJ and/or CT angiography (CTA) should be obtained prior to C1/C2 fixation to verify route and patency of the vertebral arteries, as well as dimensions of the pars interarticularis and/or pedicle.

Common Clinical Questions

1. What is the source of the blood supply to the odontoid process of the axis?
2. What forms the continuation of the posterior longitudinal ligament (PLL) at the CVJ?

References

1. Menezes AH, Traynelis VC. Anatomy and biomechanics of normal craniovertebral junction (a) and biomechanics of stabilization (b). Childs Nerv Syst 2008;24(10):1091–1100
2. Squires J, Molinari RW. C1 lateral mass screw placement with intentional sacrifice of the C2 ganglion: functional outcomes and morbidity in elderly patients. Eur Spine J 2010;19(8):1318–1324

Answers to Common Clinical Questions

1. Superior part: apical branch of hypoglossal artery; base: branches of the vertebral artery
2. Tectorial membrane

3 Cervical Spine

Eric A. Sribnick and Sanjay S. Dhall

I. Key Points
- The subaxial cervical spine includes C3 to C7.
- The cervical spine normally demonstrates a lordotic curvature.
- Posterior instrumentation often uses lateral mass screws because the pedicles are narrower than in the thoracic and lumbar spine, increasing the risk of neurovascular injury.
- The size and volume of lateral masses decrease from the upper to lower subaxial cervical spine.

II. Bony Anatomy
- Radiographic landmarks[1]: C3 is at the hyoid, C4 is at the thyroid cartilage, and C6 is at the cricoid cartilage.
- Palpable landmark: the anterior tubercle of the C6 transverse process (Chassaignac tubercle) is palpable.
- The width of vertebral body is usually 17 to 20 mm.
- In the coronal plane, uncovertebral joints are noted at the anterolateral aspect of the vertebral body (**Fig. 3.1**).
- The spinal canal is triangular and has a greater lateral than anteroposterior (AP) dimension.
- The AP diameter of the spinal canal decreases caudally[2]: 17 mm at C3, 15 mm at C7.

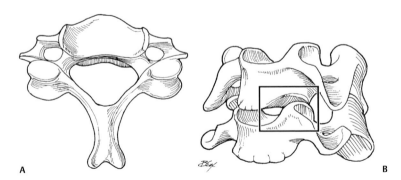

Fig. 3.1 Cervical vertebrae superior (**A**) and oblique (**B**) views.

- Lateral masses of the subaxial spine are composed of the superior and inferior articulating processes (the facet).
- A lateral mass begins lateral to where the lamina and pedicle meet.
- C7 is a transitional vertebra: the lateral mass is thinner and the pedicle is wider than in C3 to C6.
- The normal lordotic curvature of the cervical spine is 16 to 25 degrees.[3]
- Cervical disc herniation occurs most frequently at C5/6 and C6/7.
- Biomechanical studies show maximal flexion-extension at C4/5 and C5/6 and maximal lateral bending at C2/3, C3/4, and C4/5.
- The least mobile segment is C7/T1.

III. Neural Anatomy

- C3 to C7 nerve roots exit above their corresponding level (e.g., C7 exits above the C7 pedicle).
- The C8 nerve root exits above the T1 pedicle.
- The cervical spinal cord enlarges caudally and reaches a maximal cross-sectional area at C6.
- Nerve roots enter the intervertebral foramina laterally, occupy approximately one-third of the foramina, and are covered by epidural fat and venous plexus above.
- Nerve roots exit the spine at a point that is anterolateral to the superior joint facet.
- The cervical plexus is formed by the anterior rami of C1 to C4.
- The brachial plexus is formed by the anterior rami of C5 to T1.
- The cervical plexus gives rise to (1) the ansa cervicalis (supplies a branch to the hypoglossal nerve and innervates the strap muscles, except for the thyrohyoid), (2) phrenic nerve (C3 to C5, but mainly C4), and (3) cutaneous nerves of the posterior head and neck.

IV. Vascular Anatomy

- Vertebral arteries usually originate from the subclavian artery and ascend between the anterior scalene and longus colli muscles.[4]
- Vertebral arteries enter the spine at the transverse foramen of C6 (occasionally at C7).
- Vertebral artery segments: V1 (pre-foraminal), origin to transverse foramen entrance; V2 (foraminal), C6 to C2; V3, C2 to dura; V4, intradural segment to basilar artery.

- The transverse foramen is lateral to the vertebral body and anterior to the nerve root groove.
- At C3 to C5, the lateral-most aspect of the transverse foramen is often anteromedial to the midpoint of the lateral mass.
- At C6-C7, a portion of the transverse foramen is often anterior to the midpoint of the lateral mass.
- Blood supply to spinal cord includes the anterior spinal artery, the two posterior spinal arteries, and the segmental medullary arteries.
- The anterior spinal artery originates from the vertebral arteries.
- The posterior spinal arteries originate from either vertebral arteries or the posterior inferior cerebellar arteries (PICA).
- Venous drainage of the spinal cord: three anterior and three posterior longitudinally running veins.
- Spinal cord is surrounded by an anterior and a posterior venous plexus.
- The anterior venous plexus is most pronounced medial to the pedicles.

V. Ligamentous and Muscular Anatomy

- The anterior longitudinal ligament covers anterior vertebral bodies and limits extension.
- The posterior longitudinal ligament covers posterior vertebral bodies and limits flexion.
- The interspinous and supraspinous ligaments run between adjacent spinous processes and form the ligamentum nuchae.
- The ligamentum nuchae makes up the midline avascular plane.
- The carotid triangle of the neck is an important surgical landmark for anterior approaches, formed laterally by sternocleidomastoid, superiorly by dorsal portion of the digastric, and anteriorly by omohyoid.
- The carotid triangle contains the carotid sheath (common carotid, internal jugular, and vagus nerve).
- Longus colli muscles lie anterolateral to vertebral bodies and are elevated during anterior spinal procedures (**Fig. 3.2**).

3 Cervical Spine

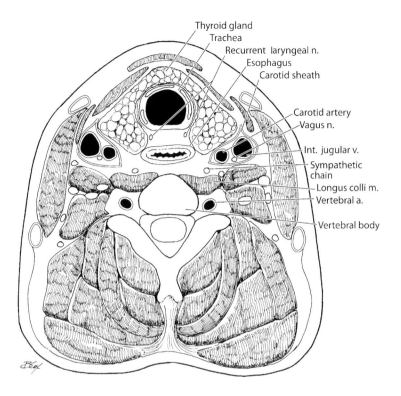

Fig. 3.2 Cross-section of the neck and spine at the C5 level.

VI. Surgical Pearls

- Uncovertebral joints provide several surgical landmarks: they define the lateral borders for corpectomy or discectomy, and they define the midline for cervical plate placement.
- The Magerl technique for lateral mass screw placement is used to avoid injuring the vertebral artery or nerve root. The drill is placed 1 mm medial to the midpoint of the lateral mass and is angled 25 degrees laterally and 30 degrees superiorly.
- During anterior procedures, instruments are most safely inserted into the lateral aspect of the canal.

- During posterior cervical procedures, the patient can be placed in a slight reverse Trendelenberg position to reduce venous engorgement.
- C7 is a transitional-level vertebra. For a posterior fusion involving C7, some surgeons advocate extending the fusion to T1 to reduce adjacent-level disease.

Common Clinical Questions

1. Where does cervical disc herniation most often occur?
2. What is the normal curvature of the cervical spine?
3. Which arteries provide the majority of blood circulation to the spinal cord?

References

1. Clark CR, Benzel EC, Currier BL, et al, eds. The Cervical Spine. 4th ed. Philadelphia, PA: Lippincott Williams & Wilkins; 2005
2. Herkowitz HN, Garfin SR, Eismont FJ, et al, eds. Rothman-Simeone: The Spine. 5th ed. Philadelphia, PA: Elsevier; 2006
3. Gore DR, Sepic SB, Gardner GM. Roentgenographic findings of the cervical spine in asymptomatic people. Spine (Phila Pa 1976) 1986;11(6):521–524
4. Ebraheim NA, Xu R, Yeasting RA. The location of the vertebral artery foramen and its relation to posterior lateral mass screw fixation. Spine (Phila Pa 1976) 1996; 21(11): 1291–1295

Answers to Common Clinical Questions

1. C5/6 and C6/7
2. The cervical spine normally has a lordotic curvature between 16 and 25 degrees.
3. The spinal cord is supplied by the anterior spinal artery (from the vertebral arteries), two posterior spinal arteries (from either the vertebral arteries or PICA), and segmental medullary arteries.

4 Thoracic Spine

Ryan J. Halpin and Tyler R. Koski

I. Key Points

- The normal thoracic spine includes 12 rib-bearing vertebral segments; anatomical variations can have 11 or 13 rib-bearing segments.
- Compared with the cervical and lumbar spine, the motion of the thoracic spine is limited due to the osteoligamentous relationship with the rib cage.
- Normal thoracic kyphosis is 10 to 40 degrees with the apex at T7.[1]

II. Bony Anatomy (Figs. 4.1 and 4.2)[2]

- The dorsal, ventral, and lateral diameters of the vertebral bodies increase from the upper to lower thoracic spine.[3]
- Thoracic kyphosis results from the wedge shape of the vertebral bodies, in which the anterior vertebral body height is less than the posterior vertebral body height.[1,3]

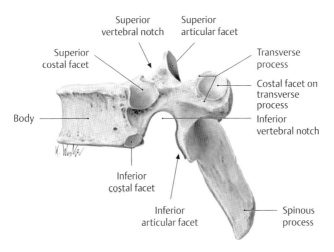

Fig. 4.1 Lateral view of thoracic vertebra (from THIEME Atlas of Anatomy, General Anatomy and Musculoskeletal System, (c) Thieme 2005, Illustration by Karl Wesker).

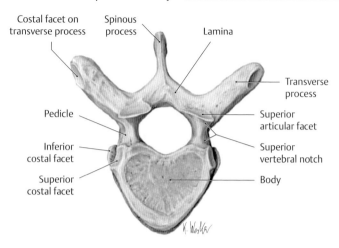

Fig. 4.2 Superior view of thoracic vertebra (from THIEME Atlas of Anatomy, General Anatomy and Musculoskeletal System, (c) Thieme 2005, Illustration by Karl Wesker).

- The ribs from T2 to T9 articulate with two vertebral bodies (at the demifacets) and the transverse costal facet of the caudal vertebral body (i.e., T2 rib articulates with T1 and T2 at the demifacets and the T2 transverse facet).
- The T1, T11, and T12 (and often T10) ribs have a full facet for articulation with the corresponding vertebrae.
- The eleventh and twelfth ribs do not articulate with the transverse process of the corresponding vertebral body.
- The thoracic facets are oriented in an intermediate plane compared with the relatively coronally oriented cervical facets and the sagittally oriented lumbar facets, and provide stability in flexion and extension.[1,3]
- Sagittal pedicle height gradually increases from the upper to lower thoracic spine.[3]
- Transverse pedicle width decreases from the upper thoracic spine to the mid-thoracic spine (T5-T6) before gradually increasing through the lumbar spine.[1,3]
- The transverse pedicle angle decreases from T1 to T12.[3]
- The diameter of the spinal canal is smaller in the thoracic than in the cervical and lumbar regions.

III. Neural Anatomy

- The thoracic nerve roots exit below the pedicle of the corresponding vertebra (i.e., T3 nerve root exits below the T3 pedicle).
- Thoracic nerves supply the trunk and abdomen. Important thoracic dermatomes include T4 at the nipple line, T6 at the base of the sternum, and T10 at the umbilicus.
- The spinal cord runs through the length of the thoracic spinal canal and ends at the conus medullaris, usually at the L1-L2 level.

IV. Vascular Anatomy

- The anterior spinal artery arises from vertebral arteries and runs in the anterior median fissure of the spinal cord.
- The paired posterior spinal arteries usually arise from the posterior inferior cerebellar arteries and travel lateral to the posterior median sulcus of the spinal cord.
- Segmental arteries from the lumbar and intercostal arteries supplement the arterial supply of the cord through six to eight radicular arteries.
- The artery of Adamkiewicz is the largest radicular artery and provides the main arterial supply to the cord from approximately T8 to the conus. It arises from the T9-L2 region in 85% and from the left side in 80% of people.[1,3]

V. Ligamentous and Muscular Anatomy (Table 4.1)

- Muscles of the thoracic spine
  - Deep layers
    - Rotatores longus and brevis, levatores costarum longus and brevis, multifidus, semispinalis thoracis, and external costal muscles
  - Intermediate layers
    - Splenius cervicis, serratus posterior superior and inferior, and erector spinae: spinalis thoracis, longissimus, iliocostalis
  - Superficial layers
    - Rhomboid, latissimus dorsi, and trapezius

VI. Surgical Pearls

- Laminectomy of the thoracic spine can increase the risk of progressive kyphosis due to the loss of the posterior tension band.
- Injury to the artery of Adamkiewicz can cause a spinal cord infarction due to the tenuous blood supply of the lower thoracic cord.

Table 4.1 Principal Thoracic Ligaments: Their Attachments and Modes of Action

Ligament	Attachments	Action
Anterior longitudinal	Ventral vertebral body and annulus	Limits extension and distraction Thickest in thoracic spine
Posterior longitudinal	Dorsal vertebral body and annulus	Limits flexion and distraction Thickest in thoracic spine
Ligamentum flavum	Lamina of adjacent vertebra	Limits flexion
Interspinous	Spinous processes of adjacent vertebra	Limits flexion and distraction
Supraspinous	Tips of spinous processes and thoracolumbar fascia	Limits flexion and distraction
Facet capsule	Superior and inferior facets of adjacent vertebra	Supports facet joint stability
Radiate	Rib and adjacent vertebral disc space and vertebral body anteriorly	Stabilizes rib attachments Contributes to limitation of thoracic flexion, extension, lateral bending, and axial rotation
Costovertebral	Rib and adjacent vertebral disc space and vertebral body dorsolaterally	
Anterior costotransverse	The rostral rib neck and the transverse process of the vertebra one level above	
Posterior costotransverse	The transverse process to the tubercle of the rib at the same level	

- Due to variable thoracic pedicle anatomy, a thin-cut computed tomography (CT) scan can be useful prior to thoracic pedicle screw placement to assist with surgical planning and avoid neural injury.
- Avoid ending spinal constructs at the thoracic kyphotic apex to prevent early instrumentation failures.

Common Clinical Questions

1. True or false: The pedicles on the concavity of a scoliotic curve tend to be larger than the pedicles on the convexity of the curve.

2. True or false: Each rib usually articulates only with its corresponding vertebral body.

3. The apex of normal kyphosis in the thoracic spine is at which level?
   A. T2-T3
   B. T5-T6
   C. T7-T8
   D. T9-T10
   E. T11-T12

References

1. Frempong-Boadu AK, Guiot BH. Thoracic spine anatomy and biomechanics. In Batjer H and Loftus C, eds. Textbook of Neurological Surgery: Principles and Practice. Philadelphia, PA: Lippincott Williams & Wilkins; 2003:1544–1551
2. Gray's Anatomy 1918 edition, public domain
3. Yoganandan N, Halliday AL, Dickman CA, Benzel E. Practical anatomy and fundamental biomechanics. In Benzel EC. Spine Surgery Techniques, Complication Avoidance, and Management. 2nd ed. Philadelphia PA: Elsevier; 2005:109–135

Answers to Common Clinical Questions

1. False: Pedicles on the concavity are usually smaller.
2. False: The majority of ribs articulate with the corresponding body as well as the body below.
3. C. Normal thoracic kyphosis is between 10 and 40 degrees and has an apex at T7-T8. Pathologic kyphosis can be centered at any level.

5 Lumbar Spine

Hormuzdiyar H. Dasenbrock and Ali Bydon

I. Key Points

- The three-column model of the spine, developed to prognosticate the stability of thoracolumbar fractures, provides a framework to categorize the relevant clinical anatomy of the lumbar spine (**Fig. 5.1**)[1]:
  • Anterior column: anterior half of the disc and vertebral body, as well as the anterior longitudinal ligament

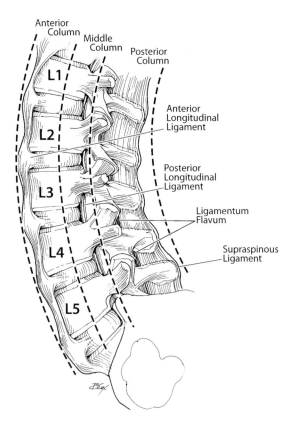

Fig. 5.1 Sagittal illustration of the lumbar spine demonstrating the three-column theory.

- Middle column: posterior half of the disc and vertebral body, as well as the posterior longitudinal ligament
- Posterior column: posterior bony arch, facet joint and its capsule, supraspinous and intraspinous ligaments, and ligamentum flavum.

II. Bony Anatomy (Tables 5.1 and 5.2)

– The intervertebral discs lie between adjacent vertebral bodies. The annulus fibrosus is the outer layer of the disc; made of rings of collagen surrounding fibrocartilaginous zones, it limits the rotation between the vertebrae. The nucleus pulposus lies in the center of the disc; primarily gelatinous, its function is to absorb compres-

Table 5.1 Bony Borders of the Vertebral Column

Bone	Column	Description	Major pathology
Vertebral body	Anterior and middle	Lumbar vertebral bodies are the largest in the spine Major weight-bearing component Anterior portion of the vertebral column	Compression or burst in trauma, osteoporosis, or tumor
Pedicle	Posterior	Short and strong Arise from the upper and posterolateral vertebral body, forming the bilateral anterolateral portions of the vertebral column Frequently, transpedicular instrumentation is placed for stabilization or fusion	May fracture in trauma, osteoporosis, or tumor
Lamina	Posterior	Short broad plates Form the bilateral posterolateral borders of the vertebral column May be removed in decompressive surgery	May fracture in trauma, osteoporosis, or tumor
Spinous process	Posterior	At the meeting point of the two laminae Forms the posterior border of the vertebral column	

Table 5.2 Borders of the Intervertebral Foramen

Anterior	Posterior borders of the adjacent vertebral bodies and discs
Superior	Inferior border of the pedicle of the superior vertebrae
Posterior	Pars interarticularis and facet joint
Inferior	Superior border of the pedicle of the inferior vertebrae

sion forces. Posterolateral herniation of the disc can compress an individual nerve root; central herniation can compress the entire cauda equina.[1]
- At the level of the pedicle, the transverse process arises. The processes of the first three lumbar vertebrae are long and slender, and those of the fourth and fifth are more pyramidal. In posterolateral lumbar fusion, the bone graft is often placed in the lateral gutter—the area lateral to the facets where the transverse processes lie.
- The pars interarticularis, also referred to as the isthmus, is a thin bone of the posterior arch of the lumbar vertebrae where the lamina and the inferior articular process join the pedicle and superior articular process. A fracture in the pars interarticularis is referred to as spondylolysis, can be found in 5 to 6% of the population, and predisposes the individual to the development of isthmic spondylolisthesis.[1]
- The facet joint is composed medially of the inferior articulating process of the superior vertebrae and laterally of the superior articulating process of the inferior vertebrae. Surrounding the facet joint is an articular capsule. Hypertrophy of the facet joint and its capsule can contribute to both spinal and foraminal stenosis.[2]

III. Neural Anatomy

- The spinal cord ends at the conus medullaris, most frequently at the level of the L1 vertebral body or the L1/L2 disc space. Inferiorly, the roots descend within the thecal sac as the cauda equina before they exit individually (**Fig. 5.2**).[3]
- The exiting nerve roots leave the vertebral column through the intervertebral foramen, closer to the superior pedicle. Far lateral disc herniations can compress the nerve root at this point (leading patients to present with radiculopathy); in such cases,

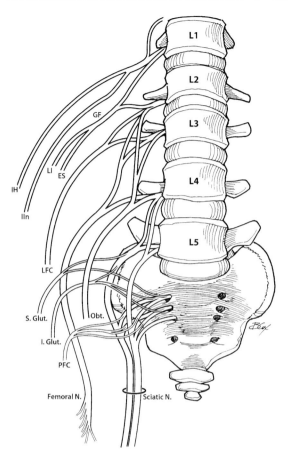

Fig. 5.2 Anterior view of the lumbar plexus.

the intervetebal disc actually compresses the nerve root of the superior level (for example, an L4/L5 disc compresses the L4 root). Far lateral herniation is much less common than posterolateral herniation of the disc. Facet hypertrophy can also lead to foraminal stenosis, which also causes radiculopathy.[1]
- Posterolateral disc herniation compresses the traversing nerve root at its lateral recess, before it reaches the intervertebral foramen. In this case, it compresses the inferior nerve root (for example, an L4/L5 disc compresses the L5 root).[1]

IV. Vascular Anatomy

- Segmental arteries arise primarily from the lumbar arteries, which in turn divide into anterior and posterior radicular arteries, which enter the intervertebral foramen along with the nerve roots. The arterial feeders of the spinal cord include branches of these radicular arteries as well as the segmental medullary arteries, which also come off of the segmental spinal arteries, with one artery coursing anteriorly and two coursing posteriorly. The cauda equina is supplied by branches of the lumbar, iliolumbar, lateral, and median sacral arteries.[3]
- Two different plexuses of veins, one external and the other internal, extend along the vertebral column. The anterior external plexus lies in front of the vertebral bodies, and the posterior external plexus lies around the posterior arch of the vertebral column. The internal vertebral plexus is a network of veins in the epidural space within the vertebral canal that are in communication with the basivertebral plexus; the veins tunnel through the cancellous tissue of the vertebral bodies. Intradural venous drainage of the spinal cord involves retrograde anterior and posterior central veins.[3]
- Approaching the lumbar spine from an anterior approach, the great vessels (the aorta and the inferior vena cava) lie directly anterior to the vertebral bodies, with the bifurcation of the vessels at the level of the L4/L5 disc space or at the level of L5. The L5/S1 disc can generally be accessed inferior to the bifurcation; to reach the L4/L5 disc, these vessels must be retracted laterally.[1]

V. Ligamentous and Muscular Anatomy (Table 5.3)

- Exposure of the lumbar spine from a posterior approach requires traversing the throracolumbar fascia. In the lumbar region, the thoracolumbar fascia is thick and is attached to the spinous processes and the supraspinous ligament. It then extends laterally, covering the erector spinae muscles.[2]
- Deep in the thoracolumbar fascia lie the erector spinae muscles, which arise from the sacrum, the spinous processes of the lumbar and thoracic vertebrae, and the iliac crest. The erector spinae muscles include the iliocostalis, longissimus, and spinalis muscles, which are important in flexion, extension, and lateral rotation of the vertebral column. Deep in the erector spinae muscles are the multifidus and rotatores muscles.[2]

Table 5.3 Ligaments of the Lumbar Spine

Ligament	Column	Attachment	Major pathology
Anterior longitudinal ligament	Anterior	Anterior margins of the vertebral bodies and intervertebral discs	May be disrupted in fracture-dislocation traumatic injuries and in spondylolisthesis
Posterior longitudinal ligament	Middle	Posterior margins of the vertebral bodies and intervertebral discs	May be disrupted in fracture-dislocation or seatbelt trauma and in spondylolisthesis
Ligamentum flavum	Posterior	Anterior border of adjacent laminae and spinous processes	May be hypertrophied in spinal stenosis
Supraspinal ligament	Posterior	Posterior borders of spinous processes	
Interspinous process ligaments	Posterior	Inferior border of superior spinous process and superior border of inferior spinous process	

VI. Surgical Pearls

- During transpedicular instrumentation placement, the landmarks used for cannulation of the pedicles are the meeting point of the pars interarticularis, the superior articulating process, and the transverse process. There is a small ridge of bone at that level called the mammillary process.
- For lumbar disc herniation, after a laminotomy is performed, feel for the inferior pedicle (L5 in an L4-L5 disc herniation). Palpate its medial wall with a Woodsen dissector. Immediately inferior is the nerve root (L5). With a nerve hook, retract the root medially and dissect superiorly until you feel a bulge (which is the herniated disc fragment).

Common Clinical Questions

1. Compression of the nerve root in the neural foramen is most often due to hypertrophy of which facet?
2. An L4/L5 far lateral herniated disc will compress which nerve root?

References

1. Greenberg MS. Handbook of Neurosurgery. 6th ed. New York: Thieme Medical Publishers; 2006
2. Drake RL, Vogl W, Mitchell AWM. Gray's Anatomy for Students. Philadelphia, PA: Elsevier; 2005
3. Netter FH. The Netter Collection of Medical Illustrations. Volume 1: Nervous System. Part 1: Anatomy and Physiology. Teterboro, NJ: Icon Learning Systems; 1983

Answers to Common Clinical Questions

1. The superior articulating facet of the lower vertebral body
2. The exiting L4 root (not the traversing L5 root)

6 Sacral-Iliac Spine

Amit R. Patel and Ravi K. Ponnappan

I. Key Points

- The sacrum is the structural link that distributes load from the lumbar spine to the pelvis through the sacroiliac joints (and vice versa).
- The bulbocavernosus reflex involves the S2 to S4 sacral nerves, and its absence or presence has prognostic significance in spinal cord trauma.
- Because of the location of the lumbosacral plexus in relation to the sacrum, sacral fractures have a high incidence of neurologic injury (up to 25%).[1]

II. Bony Anatomy

- The normal adult spine consists of five fused sacral vertebrae that form the wedge-shaped sacrum and four fused coccygeal vertebrae that form the coccyx (the skeletal remnants of a tail).
- The sacrum has four paired sacral foramina, a sacral canal, a sacral promontory (anterior projection of the S1 body), and a sacral hiatus (clinically useful for caudal epidural anesthesia)[2] (**Figs. 6.1** and **6.2**).
- The sacroiliac (SI) spine has many palpable bony landmarks, including the sacral cornu and the iliac crest. The posterior superior iliac spine may be difficult to palpate but is readily identifiable by the permanent skin dimples above the buttocks.[3]
  - An imaginary line connecting the dimples passes through the S2 spinous process and the middle of the SI joint in the anterior-posterior plane.
  - An imaginary line connecting the highest points of the iliac crest passes through the L4/L5 intervertebral disc space.
- The sacrum has multiple points of articulation:
  - The S1 body articulates with the L5 body via the L5/S1 disc to form the lumbosacral angle, which varies from 130 to 160 degrees.[3]
  - The inferior facet of L5 articulates with the superior facet of S1 and acts as a buttress to resist anterior translation.[3]
  - The apex of the sacrum articulates with the coccyx.

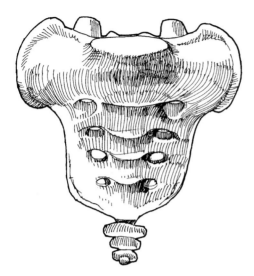

Fig. 6.1 Anterior view of the bony sacrum.

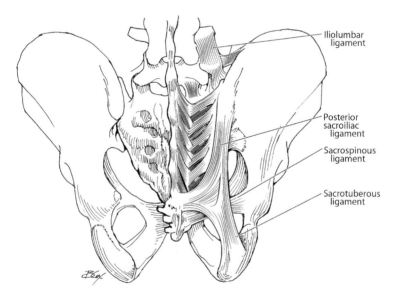

Fig. 6.2 Posterior view of bony sacrum/pelvis with the ligamentous attachments to the pelvis.

- The lateral aspects of the sacrum articulate with the two coxal (innominate) bones to form the SI joint (a true synovial diarthrodial gliding joint with limited motion). Only the anterior 25% is synovial in nature (the rest is ligamentous attachment).[1]

III. Neural Anatomy

– Ventral and dorsal branches of the sacral nerves exit the four pairs of anterior and posterior sacral foramina, respectively; the anterior foramina are larger in caliber than their posterior counterparts.[2]
  • Dermatomes are supplied by sacral nerves (**Fig. 6.3**).
– The sacral canal contains the nerve roots of the cauda equina.
– The pelvic splanchnic nerves are composed of parasympathetic fibers derived from S2 to S4 and supply autonomic innervation to various abdominal and pelvic viscera.
– The lumbosacral plexus is composed of the ventral rami from T12 to S3 and lies posterior to the psoas muscle.
– Following are major nerves that arise from this plexus[3]:
  • Sciatic nerve: composed of the ventral rami from L4 to S3, it has an anterior preaxial tibial division and a postaxial perone-

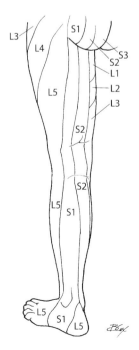

Fig. 6.3 Dermatomal map of sacral nerve roots.

al division; most commonly it exits the pelvis via the greater sciatic foramen inferior to the piriformis muscle.
- Pudendal nerve: composed of the anterior divisions of the ventral rami of S2 to S4, it supplies the perineum and external genitalia.
- Superior gluteal nerve: composed of the posterior divisions of the ventral rami of L4 to S1, it supplies the gluteus medius, gluteus minimus, and tensor fascia lata.
- Inferior gluteal nerve: composed of the posterior divisions of the ventral rami of L5 to S2, it courses with the inferior gluteal artery to supply the gluteus maximus.

IV. Vascular Anatomy

- The abdominal aorta begins at the aortic hiatus in the diaphragm at the level of T12 and bifurcates into the common iliac arteries at the level of L4.[3]
- The common iliac veins unite at the level of L5 to form the inferior vena cava.[3]
- The common iliac artery bifurcates anterior to the SI joint to form the internal iliac artery and descends posteriorly into the greater sciatic foramen to supply the pelvis, buttocks, medial thigh, and perineum.
  - The internal iliac vein sits between the SI joint and the internal iliac artery.
- The median sacral artery and vein form an unpaired vessel that originates from the posterior aspect of the abdominal aorta to supply the lower lumbar vertebrae, sacrum, and coccyx.[3]
- The lateral sacral arteries are paired and branch from the internal iliac artery and course through the anterior sacral foramina to supply the spinal meninges.[3]

V. Ligamentous and Muscular Anatomy

- The iliolumbar ligament attaches the transverse process of L5 with the ilium.[2]
    - Unstable vertical shear fractures can avulse off the L5 transverse process.
- The anterior SI, posterior SI, and interosseous ligaments suspend the sacrum between the ilia.[3]
    - The posterior SI and interosseous ligaments are thicker and limit motion.
- The sacrotuberous ligament attaches the sacrum to the ischial tuberosity; the sacrospinous ligament attaches the sacrum to the ischial spine.
    - These ligaments function to limit upward movement of the caudal portion of the sacrum and delineate the greater and lesser sciatic foramina.
- See **Table 6.1** for major muscles of the sacroiliac spine.

VI. Surgical Pearls

- Transitional vertebrae can lead to incorrect surgical localization.[2]
- Aggressive exposure of sacral ala for posterolateral fusion can endanger the L5 nerve root.[1]
- A low L5-S1 disc may not be accessible via an anterior approach due to pubic symphysis obstruction.[2]
- Anterior dissection of the superior hypogastric sympathetic plexus can result in retrograde ejaculation in males, with rates ranging from 0.42 to 5.9%.[4]

Table 6.1 Sacroiliac Muscle Anatomic Relationships

Muscle	Origin	Insertion	Innervation	Comment
Gluteus maximus	Dorsal sacrum, ilium	Gluteal tuberosity	Inferior gluteal	Extends hip, external rotates thigh
Gluteus medius	Medial ilium	Greater trochanter	Superior gluteal	Abducts thigh
Gluteus minimus	Lateral ilium	Anterior greater trochanter	Superior gluteal	Abducts thigh
Iliacus	Iliac fossa	Lesser trochanter	Femoral	Flexes hip
Psoas	T12-L5 vertebrae	Lesser trochanter	Femoral	Flexes hip, overlies lumbosacral plexus
Erector spinae	Sacrum, iliac crest, L-spinous process	T- and C-spinous process, mastoid process	Dorsal rami	Composed of iliocostalis, longissimus, and spinalis
Multifidus	C2 to S4 transverse process	Spinous process	Dorsal rami	Flex, rotate spine

Common Clinical Questions

1. Of the listed nerves, which is the most susceptible to injury during an anterior approach to the SI joint?
   A. S1 nerve root
   B. Femoral
   C. Ilioinguinal
   D. L5 nerve root
   E. Genitofemoral

References

1. Mehta S, Auerbach JD, Born CT, Chin KR. Sacral fractures. J Am Acad Orthop Surg 2006;14(12):656–665
2. Hollinshead WH. Anatomy for Surgeons: The Back and Limbs. 3rd ed. Philadelphia, PA: Harper & Row; 1982:88–92
3. Moore KL, Dalley AF. Clinically Oriented Anatomy. 4th ed. Philadelphia, PA: Lippincott; 1999:339–340, 347–355, 434–467
4. Sasso RC, Kenneth Burkus J, LeHuec JC. Retrograde ejaculation after anterior lumbar interbody fusion: transperitoneal versus retroperitoneal exposure. Spine (Phila Pa 1976) 2003;28(10):1023–1026

Answers to Common Clinical Questions

1. D. The L5 nerve root runs just anterior to the SI joint and is susceptible to injury not only in open procedures but also with percutaneous sacroiliac screw placement. It courses 2 to 3 mm medial to the SI joint.

II
Clinical Spine Surgery

7 Physical Examination

Mark S. Greenberg and Daniel Marin

I. Key Points

- There are four main components to the spinal exam: motor, sensory, reflex, and mechanical. This is in addition to the general exam, which includes observation for cutaneous and nail changes, deformity, pain behaviors, and other signs.
- Although components of a general survey nature should always be included, the physical exam is tailored to specific situations based on the history, the region of suspected involvement, and abnormal findings during the survey exam.
- No protocol can cover every contingency, and the exam must be individualized based on patient-specific factors. The order of the exam procedures must also be tailored to the situation.

II. Main Components of the Spinal-Related Exam

- Motor (strength, coordination, spasticity, muscle bulk/tone including atrophy/fasciculations)
  - Strength evaluation is usually graded using the Royal Medical Research Council of Great Britain (MRC) scale, shown in **Table 7.1**.
    - An overview of survey muscle groups to examine is shown in **Table 7.2**.
    - Further motor testing, as indicated, may include the tibialis posterior and gluteus medius (in cases of foot drop to distinguish radiculopathy from peripheral neuropathy), first lumbrical (median nerve), and abductor digiti minimi (ulnar nerve).
- Sensation (pinprick, light touch, proprioception, temperature)
  - Pinprick testing. Dermatomes and sensory distributions of peripheral nerves are shown in **Fig. 7.1**.
  - Proprioception (posterior column function) is assessed by testing joint position sense in the second toe on each foot, and/or vibratory sense with a low-frequency (128 Hz) tuning fork applied to bony prominences in the ankles.
  - Temperature sense may be crudely assessed by pressing the cool metal of a reflex hammer handle to the skin.

Table 7.1 Muscle Grading (Modified Medical Research Council System)

Grade	Strength
0	No contraction (total paralysis)
1	Flicker or trace contraction (palpable or visible)
2	Active movement through full ROM against gravity
3	Active movement against resistance
4	Active movement against resistance (subdivisions: 4−, slight resistance; 4, moderate resistance; 4+, strong resistance)
5	Normal strength (against full resistance)
NT	Not testable

Abbreviation: ROM, range of motion.

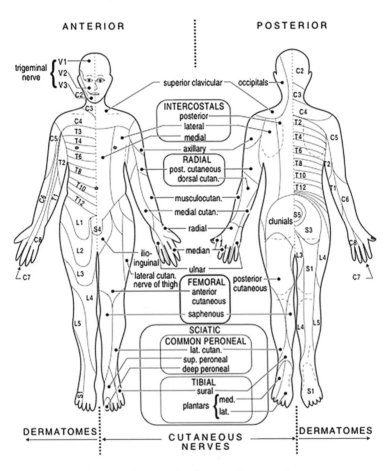

Fig. 7.1 Dermatomes and sensory distributions of peripheral nerves.

Table 7.2 Survey Muscle Groups

Muscle	Major root innervation	Peripheral nerve	Action to test
Upper extremity			
Deltoid	C5, C6	Axillary	Abduct shoulder over 90 degrees above horizontal
Biceps brachii	C5, C6	Musculocutaneous	Flexion at elbow with forearm supinated
Brachioradialis	C5, C6	Radial	Flex elbow with thumb pointing up
Extensor carpi radialis	C5, C6	Radial	Wrist extension
Triceps brachii	C7, C8		Extension at elbow
Flexor digitorum profundus I and II	C7, C8, T1	Anterior interosseus	Flex distal phalanges digits 2 and 3
Lower extremity			
Iliopsoas	L2, L3	Femoral and L1, L2, L3 roots	Thigh flexion
Quadriceps femoris	L3, L4	Femoral	Knee extension
Biceps femoris	L5, S1, S2	Sciatic	Knee flexion
Tibialis anterior	L4, L5	Deep peroneal	Ankle dorsiflexion
Extensor hallucis longus	L4, L5	Deep peroneal	Great toes extension
Gastrocnemius	S1, S2	Tibial	Ankle plantarflexion

- Reflexes (muscle stretch reflexes, pathologic reflexes, cutaneous reflexes, sacral reflexes, and priapism)
    - Muscle stretch reflexes are usually graded as shown in **Table 7.3**. The muscle stretch reflex involved is shown in **Table 7.4**.
    - Babinski sign, Hoffmann sign, and testing for ankle clonus. Assessment for long tract signs should be made in all patients to disclose unsuspected cervical or thoracic myelopathy or other causes of upper motor neuron deficit.

Table 7.3 Muscle Stretch Reflex (Deep Tendon Reflex) Grading Scale

Grade	Definition
0	No contraction (total paralysis)
0.5	Elicitable only with reinforcement*
1+	Low normal
2+	Normal
3+	More brisk than normal (hyperreflexic)
4+	Hyperreflexic with clonus
5+	Sustained clonus

*In the lower extremities, reinforcement consists of having the patient hook the tips of the fingers of the left hand into the tips of the hooked fingers of the right hand and pulling (Jendrassik maneuver). Reinforcement in the upper extremities consists of having the patient clench the teeth.

- Further reflex testing, as indicated, includes abdominal cutaneous reflexes, anal wink, and bulbocavernosus.
- Priapism may indicate spinal cord injury.
- Mechanical factors (including observation for cutaneous changes, pain behaviors, muscle bulk/tone, and provocative maneuvers)
  - Gait and station. Casual gait is assessed in all patients to check balance, weakness that compromises gait, and pain manifestations. Tandem gait and/or the Romberg test can further assess balance and posterior-column (proprioceptive) function.
  - Cervical spine
    - Cervical range of motion and specific levels of tenderness should be documented to distinguish myofascial from bone-related factors. Specific facet pain diagram patterns can be reviewed with the patient to identify problem levels.
    - The Spurling maneuver (axial loading on the vertex of the head with rotation to one side, repeated with rotation to the other side) may reproduce cervical nerve root symptoms in a patient with herniated cervical disc or foraminal stenosis.
    - Shoulder pathology can often mimic cervical spine pathology. Tenderness of the acromioclavicular joint to palpation or a positive empty-can test suggests primary shoulder pathology as a cause of shoulder pain.
  - Lumbar spine
    - Lumbar range of motion and specific levels of tenderness should be documented to distinguish myofascial from bone problems.
    - Nerve root tension signs. "Pull" on the nerve root, which can reproduce pain in situations where the nerve root is compressed.

Table 7.4 Muscle Stretch Reflexes

Nerve root involved	Corresponding muscle stretch reflex
C5	Deltoid and pectoralis*
C6	Biceps and brachioradialis
C7	Triceps
C8	Finger flexor*
L4	Patellar (knee jerk)
L5	Medial hamstrings*
S1	Achilles (ankle jerk)

*A reflex that is not widely used and may be difficult to elicit.

- Laségue sign or straight-leg raising (SLR). Supine patient raises one lower extremity (LE) at a time. Classically positive findings include pain or paresthesias in the distribution of the involved nerve root (not just back pain) at less than 60 degrees elevation. In response the patient may lift the hip on the involved side off the exam table. This procedure helps to differentiate radiculopathy from hip pathology (e.g., trochanteric bursitis). Positive in 83% of cases with nerve root compression, it is more sensitive for compression in L5 or S1 than in upper lumbar roots.
    - Femoral stretch test or reverse straight-leg raising. With patient prone, the knee is flexed on one side at a time. This test is more likely to be positive than SLR with upper lumbar nerve root compression (L2, L3, or L4).
- Hip and sacral pain. It is important to distinguish hip-mediated pathology and low back pathology.
    - Palpation over spinous processes, paraspinal muscles, greater trochanters (to assess for greater trochanteric bursitis), and SI joints (Fortin finger test) may suggest sacroiliitis.
    - FABER (acronym for flexion, abduction, external rotation, also called the Patrick test) test of the hip with the patient supine: back pain suggests musculoskeletal lower back or sacroiliac pain; groin or hip pain suggests hip pathology.
    - Shear test can help distinguish sacral pain. Patient prone, the examiner applies pressure to the sacrum while applying a traction force caudad with the corresponding limb. A test is positive if it reproduces the patient's typical pain.
    - FADIR (acronym for flexion, adduction, internal rotation) test of the hip with the patient supine can help to distinguish piriformis syndrome. Positive reponse: pain reproduc-

tion centered at half the distance between the S3 foramen and the ipsilateral greater trochanter.
- Vascular considerations: Palpation for pedal pulses to rule out vascular insufficiency.

III. Clinical Pearls

- Babinski sign or a positive Hoffmann sign: if there is no known etiology in a given patient, further investigation is required (to rule out cord compression or brain involvement).
- Cervical radiculopathy does not cause pain with shoulder abduction.
- Painless weakness in the LE is almost never due to lumbar nerve root compression. Consider diabetic neuropathy, cervical spondylotic myelopathy, or motor neuron disease, for example.

Common Clinical Questions

1. A 55-year-old male presents to your clinic with progressive lower extremity weakness and difficulty ambulating. He brings with him an MRI that shows grade 1 spondylolisthesis L5-S1 with severe central canal stenosis. Flexion/extension lumbar spine x-rays show no instability. His exam shows diffuse weakness of the LEs, diffuse reduction of pinprick sensation in the LEs, reduced Achilles reflexes, and bilateral upgoing toes. Actions that could be taken include:
   1. Decompressive laminectomy L5-S1 with attempt at reduction with bilateral pedicle screw/rod instrumentation.
   2. Lateral interbody fusion L5-S1 with lateral vertebral body plating.
   3. Anterior lumbar interbody fusion with percutaneous L5-S1 pedicle screw/rod instrumentation.
   4. MRI of the thoracic and cervical spine.

   The appropriate options to take at this time are:
   A. 1 and 3
   B. 2 and 3
   C. 1, 2, and 3
   D. 4

2. A patient presents with a 2-month history of left UE pain radiating to the thumb and index finger that has not responded to conservative therapy. He has a positive Spurling sign with the head turned to the left. Strength is normal. Reflexes are normal except for a reduction in the left biceps. An MRI of the cervical spine shows disc degeneration with protrusion into the left neural foramen at both C5-6 and C6-7. Flexion/extension cervical spine x-rays are without instability. After providing informed consent, he indicates he wishes to proceed with surgical treatment. Appropriate surgical options include the following *except*:
   A. ACDF C5-6
   B. ACDF C5-6 and C6-7
   C. ACDF C6-7
   D. Cervical disc arthroplasty C5-6

3. A 60-year-old male has diffuse weakness of the UEs with reduced reflexes, and hyperreflexia in the LEs with bilateral upgoing toes. Etiologies that could be considered include:
   1. Cervical spine stenosis.
   2. Left C5-6 foraminal herniated cervical disc.
   3. Motor neuron disease (amyotrophic lateral sclerosis).
   4. Coincident severe lumbar and cervical spinal stenosis.

   From the above list, appropriate diagnoses for this patient are:
   A. 1 and 3
   B. 2 and 4
   C. 1, 2, and 3
   D. 4

References

1. Greenberg MS. Handbook of Neurosurgery. 7th ed. New York: Thieme Medical Publishers; 2010
2. Aids to the Examination of the Peripheral Nervous System. 4th ed. Edinburgh: W.B. Saunders On Behalf Of The Guarantors of Brain; 2000
3. Malanga G, Nadler S. Musculoskeletal Physical Examination: An Evidence-Based Approach. Philadelphia, PA: Elsevier Mosby; 2006

Answers to Common Clinical Questions

1. D. Upgoing toes and diffues LE weakness and hypalgesia are never caused by compromise at L5-S1. MRI to look for cord compression above the lumbar spine is appropriate.
2. C. The sensory changes and reflex changes indicate that the C6 nerve root is involved, which implicates the disc at C5-6. Some surgeons would also treat the disc at C6-7 at the same time since it may deteriorate rapidly following fusion of C5-6, and some would perform arthroplasty at C5-6 in order to try and shield the disc at C6-7 from some of the forces that would occur with C5-6 fusion. Operating on C6-7 alone is inappropriate since this is currently not a symptomatic level.
3. A. Both cervical spinal stenosis and ALS can produce lower motor neuron findings in the UEs and lower motor neuron findings in the LEs. A unilateral foraminal herniated cervical disc will not cause this. In coincidental lumbar and spinal stenosis, the lumbar stenosis generally masks the hyperreflexia in the lower extremities.

8 Spinal Imaging

Ishaq Y. Syed, Barrett I. Woods, and Joon Y. Lee

I. Key Points

- A complete history and physical should be the initial step in evaluating a patient to formulate a preliminary clinical diagnosis and to select the appropriate imaging modality.
- Findings on imaging exams must be clinically correlated to prevent a high false-positive rate.
- Multiple imaging modalities are available to supplement evaluation of spinal pathology, to confirm diagnosis, and to guide treatment.

II. Description

- Plain radiographs
  - Convenient, universally available, and inexpensive
  - Initial imaging modality for degenerative disorders, deformity, trauma, neoplasm, and infection (for spinal deformity, consider 36 in long-cassette standing x-rays)
  - Limited ability to define subtle bony pathology and at least 30 to 40% bone loss needed for detection on plain radiographs
  - Inability to directly visualize neural structures and allow bone and soft tissue discrimination
  - Appropriately timed dynamic radiographs may help assess instability and the presence of spondylolisthesis.
    - Important in evaluation of patients in the postoperative period to assess instrumentation and successful arthrodesis
- Computed tomography (CT)
  - Provides optimal visualization of bony detail and high sensitivity in detecting fractures, with accuracy rates ranging from 72 to 91% (**Fig 8.1**)
  - Can help distinguish neural compression due to soft tissue versus bony pathology
  - CT scan alone is limited in visualization of neural structures and demonstration of intrathecal and soft tissue pathology.
  - For optimal bony detail, multiple thin cuts (1.5 to 3 mm) can be obtained with the gantry parallel to the plane of the disc.
  - Multirow detector rapid thin-slice acquisitions allow contiguous 3 mm slices to be obtained from L1 to S1 in less than 30 seconds.

- Cognizance of radiation exposure to patients is essential.
- Myelography
  - Intrathechal water-soluble contrast material mixes with cerebral spinal fluid and outlines the dural sac.
  - Diagnosis is indirectly inferrable from changes in the contour of the contrast agent–filled thecal sac.
  - Compression is demonstrated by extradural impression on the dye column and filling defects of the nerve root sleeve (**Fig. 8.2**).
  - CT myelography improves visualization of foraminal and lateral recess stenosis with axial and reconstructed images.
  - Advantageous in patients with stainless steel implants that cause significant metal artifact with MRI and patients with implantable devices (e.g., pacemaker) who cannot obtain MRI, and in evaluating fusion in postoperative patients with suspected nonunion
  - Disadvantages of myelography include invasiveness and lack of diagnostic specificity.
- Magnetic resonance imaging (MRI)[1]
  - The imaging modality of choice for the majority of spinal pathology

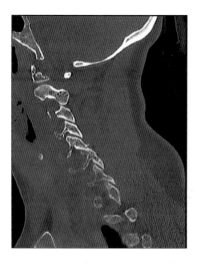

Fig. 8.1 Sagittal CT scan image demonstrates C5–6 perched fracture facet dislocation.

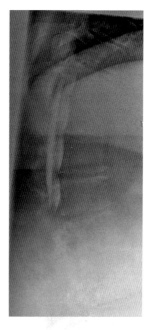

Fig. 8.2 Lateral plain radiograph after intrathecal contrast demonstrating complete block due to massive central herniated disc.

- Enhanced, noninvasive depiction of soft tissue pathology, including hematoma, infection, tumor, and ligamentous disruption, and identification of compression of neural elements (**Fig 8.3**)
- Utilizes pulsed radiofrequency (RF) and requires no radiation exposure
- T1-weighted images
  - Short repetition time (TR), 400 to 600 ms; echo time (TE), 5 to 30 ms
  - MRI findings: cortical bone, low; free water, low; adipose, high
- T2-weighted images
  - TR = 1500 to 3000 ms, TE = 50 to 120 ms
  - MRI findings: cortical bone, low; free water, high; adipose, low
- Gadolinium contrast can help distinguish postoperative scar (vascular, enhances) from recurrent disc herniation (avascular, does not enhance) on T1-weighted sequence images.
- Contrast may also be helpful in detecting tumor and infection.[2]
  - Infection: decreased signal on T1, increased signal on T2, enhancement with gadolinium, and often involves disc space
  - Tumor: intervertebral disc often spared, similar homogeneous changes present involving entire vertebral body. With metatastic disease, may show multiple noncontiguous vertebral bodies involved, indicating skip lesions and involvement of the pedicle.
- Spinal cord injury
  - Quantifies degree of spinal cord compression and injury

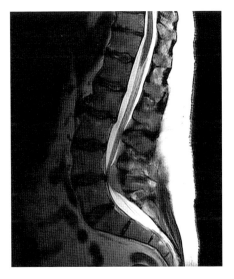

Fig. 8.3 Sagittal T2-weighted MRI image of the lumbar spine demonstrates large dorsal abscess causing severe compression of the neural elements at L4–5.

- High sensitivity in identifying ligamentous injury, including status of the posterior ligamentous complex, that may otherwise be missed on plain radiographs or CT
- Helps distinguish spinal cord edema (T1 low, T2 high) from hemorrhage (T1 high, T2 high)
- Disc degeneration
  - Advanced imaging should be reserved for patients with true radicular symptoms, with objective evidence of root irritation on examination, who have failed an appropriate course of conservative nonoperative management.
  - High-intensity zone (HIZ): radial tear of the posterior annulus, fissure extending from nucleus to the periphery, unknown clinical significance
  - Herniated disc can be found in 21% of asymptomatic individuals between the ages of 20 and 39 years.
  - Disc herniation nomenclature[3]:
    - *Protrusion:* Herniation that maintains contact with the disc of origin with a bridge as wide as or wider than the diameter of the displaced material
    - *Extruded:* Diameter of the disc material beyond the interspace is greater than the width of the bridge that may or may not connect to the disc of origin.
    - *Sequestered:* An extrusion that is no longer contiguous with the disc of origin
  - Degenerative changes in the cervical and lumbar spine are age related and equally present in asymptomatic and symptomatic individuals.
  - MRI findings must be strictly correlated with the clinical presentation.
  - Modic end plate changes[2]:
    - Type 1
      - T1 low, T2 high
      - Associated with segmental spine instability and pain
    - Type 2
      - T1 high, T2 normal
      - More common than type 1, and may be less symptomatic
    - Type 3
      - T1 low, T2 low
      - Indicative of advanced degeneration and sclerosis with less segmental instability
- Poor imaging will result from metal artifact from implants unless specific techniques are used (plastic < titanium < tantalum < stainless steel < cobalt chrome).
- Contraindications: pacemaker, inner ear implant, metal debris in the eye, ferrous metal implant in the brain

- Bone scintigraphy
  - Standard part of workup for assessing metastatic bone disease (monostotic versus polyostotic). Helps point to area for more advanced imaging and evaluation.
  - May be of value in distinguishing acute and chronic pars interarticularis fractures

III. Surgical Pearls

- Prior to obtaining any advanced imaging, a clear plan must be established for how the results will be utilized to facilitate the next line of treatment.
- A clinical diagnosis should be established based on a complete history and physical and correlated with findings on imaging prior to instituting a surgical or nonoperative treatment plan.
- Advanced imaging can be invaluable in confirming diagnosis and identifying treatment that has the best chance of clinical success.

Common Clinical Questions

1. A 57-year-old female presents with one week of intractable back pain, fever, chills, positive blood cultures, and elevated inflammatory markers. There is concern over discitis in the thoracolumbar region. MRI will likely show:
   A. Increased T1 signal and decreased T2 signal with disc space involvement
   B. Increased T1 signal, decreased T2 signal without disc space involvement
   C. Increased T2 signal and decreased T1 signal with disc space involvement
   D. Increased T2 signal and decreased T1 signal without disc space involvement
   E. Increased T2 signal and increased T1 signal with disc space involvement

2. Which of the following statements regarding spinal imaging is true?
   A. Adipose tissue causes a low-intensity signal on T1-weighted sequences and a high-intensity signal on T2-weighted images.
   B. The presence of HIZ has been correlated with the presence of symptomatic back pain.
   C. As the patient ages the sensitivity and specificity of imaging modalities such as CT and MRI improve.
   D. Spinal cord edema can be distinguished from hemorrhage via a low-intensity signal on T1-weighted images and a high-intensity signal on T2-weighted images.
   E. Benign Modic changes are characterized by a low-intensity signal on both T1- and T2-weighted images.

3. What is the best imaging modality for studying the bony anatomy preoperatively?

4. What is the appropriate initial radiographic study for spinal deformity?

References

1. Herkowitz HN, Rothman RH, Simeone FA. Rothman-Simeone: The Spine. 5th ed. Philadelphia, PA: Saunders Elsevier; 2006
2. Modic MT, Ross JS. Lumbar degenerative disk disease. Radiology 2007;245(1):43–61
3. Fardon DF, Milette PC; Combined Task Forces of the North American Spine Society, American Society of Spine Radiology, and American Society of Neuroradiology. Nomenclature and classification of lumbar disc pathology. Recommendations of the Combined Task Forces of the North American Spine Society, American Society of Spine Radiology, and American Society of Neuroradiology. Spine (Phila Pa 1976) 2001;26(5):E93–E113

Answers to Common Clinical Questions

1. C
2. D
3. Thin-slice CT of the pertinent region
4. 36 in long-cassette standing x-ray

9 Neurophysiologic Monitoring in Spine Surgery

Glen Aaron Pollock, Naomi Abel, and Fernando L. Vale

I. Key Points

- Somatosensory evoked potentials (SSEPs). Monitor the electrophysiologic integrity of the dorsal column–medial lemniscus pathway. The vascular supply of this tract in the spinal cord is predominantly from the paired posterior spinal arteries. Taken as a single modality, SSEPs monitor only the dorsal aspect of the spinal cord.
- Motor evoked potentials (MEPs). Monitor the electrophysiologic integrity of the corticospinal tract. The vascular supply of this tract in the spinal cord is from the single anterior spinal artery. MEPs monitor tracts in the ventral aspect of the spinal cord.
- Spontaneous electromyography (sEMG). The measurement of spontaneous electrical activity within a specific monitored muscle. Reflects neurotonic discharges within the muscle caused by mechanical, thermal, or metabolic irritation of the nerve or nerve root. Useful for monitoring nerve roots and peripheral nerves.
- Triggered electromyography (tEMG). The measurement of electrical activity within a specific muscle caused by electrical stimulation of the nerve, usually by stimulation of a structure in proximity to the nerve, such as the pedicle, by way of pedicle screw stimulation, to evaluate for disruption of the pedicle wall. Also allows discrimination of nervous tissue from non–nervous tissue during surgery for spinal cord tumors or the release of tethered spinal cord.

II. Essentials of Neuromonitoring

- SSEPs
  - The stimulation of mixed sensory and motor fibers caudal to the region of the spinal cord at risk, together with the recording of signals rostral to the region of spinal cord at risk. The most commonly stimulated nerves are the median and ulnar nerves for the upper extremity and the posterior tibial and peroneal nerves for the lower extremity. Responses are then monitored over the dorsal neck and scalp.

- Technique
  - Electrodes are placed over the ulnar nerve at the wrist and the posterior tibial nerve at the level of the medial malleolus.
  - One method involves a constant current of 15 to 25 mA for the ulnar nerve and 25 to 35 mA for the posterior tibial nerve, provided via a square wave pulse of around 4.7 times per second. The duration of the pulse is between 10 μs and 2 ms.[1] The intensity of stimulation is based on the maximal-amplitude response for a given patient.
  - Averaging of signals continues until a clear, reproducible waveform is identified. Supramaximal stimulation results in the activation of axons of both the dorsal column and spinothalamic pathways.
  - The largest contribution to the signal is from the dorsal column due to the presence of the A-α and A-β fibers, the largest and fastest-conducting of the sensory fibers.
  - Baseline recordings are obtained and evaluated immediately after the induction of anesthesia but prior to positioning. SSEPs are assessed again after positioning and every few minutes thereafter until completion of the surgery.
  - Alarm criteria are a 50% or greater decrease in amplitude and/or a 10% increase in latency.[2]
  - Advantage
    - Allows continuous monitoring of spinal cord integrity
  - Disadvantages
    - Delay in assessment caused by signal averaging
    - Assesses only sensory pathways (predominantly dorsal column–medial lemniscus)
    - Not sensitive to indicators of motor pathway or nerve root injury
    - Susceptible to signal degradation due to halogenated anesthetics, nitrous oxide, hypotension, and hypothermia
    - Signals undergo central amplification and can retain amplitude despite nerve root injury
- Technical pearls
  - SSEPs can be recorded from cortical or subcortical sources. Cortical sources have larger amplitude and may supply the only response when there is previous root damage; however, they are more susceptible to the effects of inhaled anesthetics.
  - Recordings at the level of the medulla reflect the nucleus gracilis and cuneatus with no intervening synapses between the sites of stimulation and recording. These recordings are more resistant to the effects of anesthetic agents.

- Detailed examination of the dorsal column pathway prior to surgery should be performed because prior deficits can affect the ability to record accurate signals. This should include assessment of two-point discrimination, vibration, and position sense.
- Alterations in anesthetic depth can affect the ability to obtain useful signals. This problem is minimized by the use of raw electroencephalography (EEG) by the anesthesia team to monitor anesthetic depth.
- MEPs
  - Involve the transcranial stimulation of the corticospinal pathway with assessment of compound motor action potential at the level of the innervated muscle
    - Technique
      - Subdermal needle electrodes or electrode discs in contact with the skin are used for transcranial electrical stimulation.
      - Multipulse electrical current of 200 to 500 V is delivered using five to nine pulses 1.1 to 4.1 ms apart with pulse trains lasting around 50 μs.[3] The resulting compound motor action potential (CMAP) at the level of the muscle is of high enough amplitude that signal averaging is not required. The resultant descending excitation of the corticospinal pathway and its generation of a CMAP is then detected via surface electrodes on the skin over the selected muscle groups or via the subdermal needle electrodes.
      - There are three types of monitoring options: recording at the muscle (CMAP), nerve (neurogenic MEP, CNAP), or direct spinal cord recording (D wave and I wave). The most frequently used monitoring utilizes electrodes at the level of specific muscle groups.
      - Interpretation of the response is based on the preliminary baseline; warning signs include a complete loss of response, a decrease in amplitude greater than 80%, an increase in threshold of greater than 100 V to elicit the CMAP response, and changes in the morphology of the response. The "all or nothing" response and the 80% decrease in amplitude are the two most commonly used methods of interpretation.[2]
    - Advantages
      - Allows assessment of corticospinal tracts
      - Allows for the option of increasing stimulation intensity to increase the size of the current field, increasing the distribution of stimulation to the cortex and subcortical

fibers. This correlates with greater axonal recruitment to overcome low signal response in patients with preexisting deficits.
- Stimulation trains can be used to increase the temporal summation at the level of the α motoneuron, thereby increasing the likelihood of achieving a response when pathologic conditions exist.
○ Disadvantages
- MEPs do not allow for continuous monitoring.
- MEPs cause muscle contraction during surgery, so the surgical team must be informed prior to each round of testing. Tongue laceration may result from forced contraction of facial muscles, requiring the placement of a bite block.
- Obtaining MEPs is more technically demanding and has a lower success rate compared with SSEPs. Preexisting motor deficits significantly reduce the likelihood of obtaining useful signals, especially from the lower extremities.
- Inhalant anesthetics decrease the pool of α motoneurons available for recruitment. Higher doses of propofol can cause suppression of α motoneurons. MEPs are affected by muscle relaxants, volatile anesthetics, and nitrous oxide. MEPs are also subject to anesthetic fade, which results in the need for increasing stimulation thresholds to achieve the same response in patients with prolonged exposure to anesthetic agents unrelated to dose effects.
- MEPs are contraindicated in patients with deep brain stimulators or cochlear implants.
- There is a slight risk of seizures with transcranial stimulation, although it has been estimated at less than 0.03%.[3]
○ Technical pearls
- Minimize the use of inhalant anesthetics by selecting intravenous anesthesia regimens. MEPs are typically obtainable when less than half the minimum alveolar concentration (MAC) of inhaled anesthetic is used.
- Alterations in anesthetic depth can affect the ability to obtain useful signals. This can be minimized by the use of bispectral index (BIS) EEG monitoring by the anesthesia team.
– Electromyography (EMG) is the measurement of electrical activity within a specific muscle.
  • In sEMG, neurotonic discharges result in electrical activity within the innervated muscle as a result of pulling, stretching,

or compression of the nerve or nerve root without any electrical stimulation by the surgeon.
- Technique
  - Electrodes are placed in muscle of interest based on the innervating nerve root.
  - Manipulation of a nerve root or peripheral nerve results in an action potential that causes depolarization of the muscle at the neuromuscular junction, resulting in a CMAP.
  - Allows for assessment of electrical discharges within the innervated muscle that indirectly monitors the nerve root at risk
  - Electrical discharges of interest manifest as spikes, bursts, or trains. Trains are of concern during sEMG because they are a continuous run of neurotonic discharges that represent continued force on the nerve or nerve root. Spikes and bursts are discharges that can alert the surgeon to close proximity to the nerve root or nerve. The surgeon should also be alerted when trains of activity are observed.
  - Increasing frequency and amplitude of discharges represent increasing recruitment of muscle fibers with an increasing chance of nerve injury. Muscles for monitoring are chosen by the corresponding nerve root to maximize coverage based on the operated spinal level. This utilizes the anatomic redundancy of muscle innervation.
- Advantages
  - Allows for continuous monitoring of the nerve root or peripheral nerve
  - Can serve as a warning of close proximity to the nerve root during retraction or manipulation when there is no direct visualization
- Disadvantages
  - sEMG is subject to interference from high-speed drills, EEG leads, cautery devices, and other equipment.
  - Underlying neurologic conditions can affect the ability to obtain useful EMG signals, especially conditions affecting the muscle directly, such as myasthenia gravis, previous botulinum toxin therapy, or muscular dystrophy.
  - sEMG discharges serve as a warning since many innocent surgical maneuvers can produce discharges of the nerve root or nerve.
  - The absence of recorded muscle activity does not guarantee nerve integrity since acute nerve transection or avulsion may result in a loss of nerve-derived signals.

- Technical pearls
  - sEMG does not allow the use of muscle relaxants or paralytics during surgery. Patient must show at least three out of four twitches for reliable monitoring.
  - To increase the ability to detect potential nerve root injury, multiple muscles with overlapping nerve root innervation are monitored for common injury levels. For example, the C5 nerve root in the cervical spine is assessed by concurrent monitoring of the deltoid and the biceps brachii muscles.
- tEMG. The measurement of electrical discharges within a given muscle as a result of electrical stimulation of the nerve root or peripheral nerve within the surgical field. A nerve root or nerve is stimulated, resulting in an action potential that causes depolarization of the muscle at the neuromuscular junction, in turn resulting in a CMAP in the innervated muscle. This is a useful technique to identify the course or location of nerves, demonstrate functional integrity, and identify tissue as nerve or not nerve.
  - Technique
    - Tissue can be stimulated directly by a probe in attempting to identify nerve versus other tissue or tumor. This technique is useful in spinal cord tumor resection as well as in surgery to relieve tethering of the spinal cord.
    - Pedicle screw stimulation is the most commonly employed technique during spinal surgery. This involves direct stimulation of a screw to identify breach of the bony cortex. This leads to indirect stimulation of the nerve root and a CMAP recorded in the corresponding muscle. An intact pedicle will have a greater electrical resistance to current, requiring greater levels of stimulation to achieve a response in the specified muscle. If the cortex of the pedicle is violated, the current will take the path of least resistance and lower levels of stimulation will be needed to result in a CMAP.
    - Lumbar spine stimulus values less than 10 to 11 mA and thoracic spine stimulus values below 6 to 8 mA are associated with pedicle cortical bone violation. Cervical stimulus values below 10 mA are associated with cortical bone violation and screw malposition.[2]
  - Advantages
    - Allows for assessment of screw placement during surgery
    - Allows for identification of lumbosacral nerve roots during surgery for tethered cord and may alter surgical strategy in up to 50% of cases[4]

- Redirection of screws often closes off the cortical breach with bony fragments, resulting in useful information when the same pedicle screw is stimulated after repositioning.
  ◦ Disadvantages
    - Subject to the same interference and signal degradation as sEMG
  ◦ Technical pearls
    - This technique does not allow the use of muscle relaxants or paralytics during surgery. The patient must display at least three out of four twitches for reliable monitoring.
    - During pedicle screw stimulation the screw itself must be stimulated as opposed to the tulip; tulips are often made of different materials, and stimulation of the tulip may lead to false-negative assessment.
    - It is not typically possible to stimulate percutaneously placed pedicle screws. The metallic screw extensions do not allow for accurate EMG thresholds. Instead, stimulation is performed on a sheathed tap (a metallic tapping instrument housed in a plastic sheath) placed into the pedicle prior to placing of the screw.

III. Practical Issues and Outcomes during Monitoring for Spinal Surgery

The goal of intraoperative monitoring of the nervous system is to prevent injury during surgical treatment of spinal disease. This is often best accomplished by the use of multiple monitoring modalities so that the most complete assessment of neurologic functional integrity of the neural tissues applicable to the specific procedure is obtained. SSEPs are used to monitor the dorsal column medial lemniscus pathway, MEPS are used to monitor the corticospinal pathway, and free-run sEMG is used for the assessment of the nerve roots and peripheral nerves. tEMG is used to assess screw placement or to guide resection of tumors or the filum terminale.

– Cervical spinal surgery. Spinal cord integrity is of major importance, so the combination of SSEPs and MEPs is used to assess for injury to the cord itself. If nerve root injury is of concern, sEMG can be added for additional safety. Although SSEPs as a single monitoring modality have a relatively low sensitivity, this is due to the fact that they do not assess the ventral cord or corticospinal tracts. Sensitivity and specificity of SSEPs have been reported as 52% and 100%, respectively, and sensitivity and specificity for MEPs were reported as 100% and 96% in the

same study,[5] suggesting that combined MEP and SSEP monitoring is the most comprehensive method of detecting neurologic injury of the spinal cord.
- Thoracic spinal surgery. Spinal cord integrity is the major concern, especially in light of the vulnerable blood supply to the mid-thoracic region. SSEPs and MEPs, when combined, provide assessment of the functional integrity of the spinal cord at this level with relatively high sensitivity and specificity.
- Lumbar spinal surgery. Below the level of the conus the nerve roots are the primary structures at risk, and sEMG and tEMG in combination with SSEPs provide assessment of the nerve root integrity. There is evidence to support multimodality monitoring with SSEPs and EMG, as this combination leads to an increase in sensitivity and specificity. One study reported a sensitivity and specificity of 28.6% and 94.7%, respectively, for SSEPs, compared with 100% and 23.7% for sEMG, in monitoring for neurologic injury during lumbosacral spinal surgery.[6]
- Surgery for tethered spinal cord. The success of detethering depends on the accurate identification of the lumbosacral nerve roots. This can be accomplished with multimodality monitoring. SSEPs have a very high specificity with the addition of sEMG and tEMG to compensate for the low sensitivity of SSEPs alone. Together, SSEPs, sEMG, and tEMG can provide near 100% specificity and sensitivity.[4] Also, the urethral and anal sphincters can be directly monitored with EMG.
- Surgery for intramedullary spinal cord tumor. As with other surgeries in the cervical or thoracic spine, spinal cord integrity is the major concern here. Multimodality monitoring with SSEPs, MEPs, and both sEMG and tEMG can be used for the highest level of safety. Muscle and D wave MEPs have been shown to have a high degree of correlation with absence versus presence of postoperative motor deficits[7] in spinal cord tumor surgery.

Common Clinical Questions

1. What neuromonitoring modalities are necessary for complete coverage of the spinal cord during surgery on thoracic levels?
2. Which neuromonitoring modality does not display a significant delay in obtaining signals?
3. Which modalities allow for continuous monitoring?

References

1. Chiappa K. Short Latency Somatosensory Evoked Potentials: Methodology. Philadelphia, PA: Lippincott-Raven; 1997
2. Gonzalez AA, Jeyanandarajan D, Hansen C, Zada G, Hsieh PC. Intraoperative neurophysiological monitoring during spine surgery: a review. Neurosurg Focus 2009;27(4):E6
3. Cros DaC K. Motor Evoked Potentials. In: Chiappa K, ed. Evoked Potentials in Clinical Medicine. 3rd ed. Philadelphia, PA: Lippincott-Raven; 1997
4. Paradiso G, Lee GY, Sarjeant R, Hoang L, Massicotte EM, Fehlings MG. Multimodality intraoperative neurophysiologic monitoring findings during surgery for adult tethered cord syndrome: analysis of a series of 44 patients with long-term follow-up. Spine (Phila Pa 1976) 2006;31(18):2095–2102
5. Kelleher MO, Tan G, Sarjeant R, Fehlings MG. Predictive value of intraoperative neurophysiological monitoring during cervical spine surgery: a prospective analysis of 1055 consecutive patients. J Neurosurg Spine 2008;8(3):215–221
6. Gunnarsson T, Krassioukov AV, Sarjeant R, Fehlings MG. Real-time continuous intraoperative electromyographic and somatosensory evoked potential recordings in spinal surgery: correlation of clinical and electrophysiologic findings in a prospective, consecutive series of 213 cases. Spine (Phila Pa 1976) 2004;29(6):677–684
7. Kothbauer KF, Deletis V, Epstein FJ. Motor-evoked potential monitoring for intramedullary spinal cord tumor surgery: correlation of clinical and neurophysiological data in a series of 100 consecutive procedures. Neurosurg Focus 1998;4(5):e1

Answers to Common Clinical Questions

1. MEPs and SSEPs are monitored to cover the dorsal aspect of the spinal cord (dorsal columns) and the ventral aspect of the spinal cord by monitoring the corticospinal tracts.
2. There is no significant delay in obtaining MEPs because they do not require signal averaging.
3. EMG and SSEPs both allow for continuous monitoring.

10 Pharmacology
Mark S. Greenberg

I. Key Points
- Treating pain early with effective doses results in overall reduction in the consumption of pain meds.
- Adjuncts to opioids for pain: NSAIDs, muscle relaxants, acetaminophen, Tramadol (not a conventional opioid), and centrally acting pain meds (e.g., gabapentin) for neuropathic pain.
- Use of steroids for spinal cord injury remains controversial, but benefits probably do not outweigh risks.
- Deep vein thrombosis (DVT) prophylaxis in spinal cord injury is critical. If prophylactic anticoagulation is contraindicated, then a vena cava interruption filter should be considered.

II. Pain Medication[1,2]
- Nonopioid analgesics
  - Acetaminophen (APAP)
    - An effective pain medication that does not inhibit peripheral cyclooxygenase activity, and is therefore not associated with altered platelet function, bronchospasm, or gastric ulceration
    - Potentiates narcotic pain medication and NSAIDs
    - The main hazard is hepatic toxicity. Use with caution with active liver disease, with chronic heavy alcohol consumption, and with glucose-6 dehydrogenase deficiency.
  - Nonsteroidal antiinflammatory drugs (NSAIDs)
    - Antiinflammatory and antipyretic
    - Single PRN doses are effective against pain even without "antiinflammatory dosing."
    - Adverse effects include reduction of renal blood flow, platelet function inhibition (permanent with aspirin, temporary with other NSAIDs), and peptic ulcers. Deleterious effect on bone healing is controversial; many surgeons hold off on NSAIDs for two weeks following fusion (a longer hiatus is not appropriate).
    - Examples of NSAIDs are naproxen (Naprosyn), diclofenac (Voltaren), and ketorolac tromethamine (Toradol). They can be given parenterally (parenteral use should not exceed 3 to 5 days). Oral dosing should be done only as continuation of parenteral dosing, not for routine use as an NSAID.

- Opioid analgesics
  - No single agent has been shown to be most effective or best tolerated as a rule, although individual differences may make certain opioids more effective in certain patients. Exception: meperidine has multiple disadvantages and has limited usefulness.
  - All produce dose-related respiratory depression. Some lower the seizure threshold. Diversion of prescribed narcotics to sale on the street for recreational use is a burgeoning problem.
  - With chronic use, tolerance develops. All may be habit forming.
  - Dosing depends more on age and prior narcotic use than on body weight.
- Weak opioids, for mild to moderate pain
  - Codeine is typically prescribed in combination with APAP. It is associated with a significant incidence of nausea and vomiting.
  - Hydrocodone is available only as a combination drug (e.g., with APAP in Vicodin and Lortab or with ibuprofen in Vicoprofen) in the United States.
- Opioids for moderate to severe pain
  - Oral: oxycodone with acetaminophen (Percocet)
  - Parenteral (intramuscular [IM] or intravenous [IV]): morphine, hydromorphone (Dilaudid). Monitor for respiratory depression. May be used for patient-controlled analgesia (PCA).

III. Anticoagulation

- Prophylactic anticoagulation
  - For patients without risk factors for blood clots, prophylactic anticoagulation for elective spine surgery is not recommended.[3]
  - For spinal cord injuries,[4] prophylaxis with either
    - Low-molecular-weight heparin (LMWH), a rotating bed, adjusted-dose heparin, or some combination of these, or
    - Low-dose (mini-dose) heparin with pneumatic compression stockings or electrical stimulation.
- Treatment for documented DVT or pulmonary embolism (PE)
  - Therapeutic anticoagulation with heparin transitioned to warfarin
  - Postoperatively: in the first week or two after spinal surgery, because of the risk of spinal hematoma, a vena cava interruption filter is preferred for DVT/PE. But for acute myocardial infarction or cardiac ischemia, therapeutic heparin may have to be used; in this case, monitor patient's neurologic signs frequently.

IV. Steroids

- Acute nerve injury
- Spinal cord injury protocol still controversial
  - The assertion: administration of methylprednisolone according to protocol within 8 hours of a spinal cord injury (SCI) (complete or incomplete) benefits sensory and motor function at 6 weeks, 6 months, and 1 year.[5,6]
  - The controversy: results could not be replicated,[7] steroid-induced myopathy might have produced a transient initial worsening that was misinterpreted as an improvement when it subsided,[8] and the risk of side effects (infectious and diabetogenic) is substantial.[9]
  - Protocol: within 8 hours of SCI, bolus with methylprednisolone 30 mg/kg IV over 15 minutes, wait 45 minutes, then start a maintenance infusion of 5.4 mg/kg/h typically maintained for 23 hours. Do not start the protocol more than 8 hours postinjury.
  - Spine tumors: for acute symptoms of spinal cord compression from metastatic tumor, decadron 10 mg IV or orally every 6 hours for 72 hours, followed by 4 to 6 mg every 6 hours.
- Epidural steroids
  - Perioperative epidural steroids after routine surgery for lumbar degenerative disease may result in a small reduction of postoperative pain and length of stay, and increased risk of not returning to work after one year,[10] but most of the evidence originates from studies not using validated outcome assessment and that favor positive results, and further study is recommended (various agents, dosages, and delivery methods were reported).
  - As part of pain management
    - Chronic low back pain: not recommended[11]; may be used to provide temporary relief in select cases
    - Acute radiculopathy: prospective studies show varying efficacy[12]
- Low back pain: oral steroids (e.g., steroid dose pack) may provide temporary improvement in symptoms; however, no difference from placebo is found at 1 week or 1 year follow-up. Use caution when combining with NSAIDs because of gastrointestinal (GI) irritation.

V. Muscle Relaxants

- Oral and IV agents used for low back pain have no activity at the neuromuscular junction. They do exhibit some centrally acting analgesic effect that appears to be independent of muscle

spasms. The most consistent effect of these drugs is drowsiness/sedation, which may help the patient rest. Tolerance develops.
- Commonly employed agents include cyclobenzaprine (Flexeril), diazepam (Valium), tizanidine (Zanaflex), and carisoprodol (Soma).

VI. Clinical Pearls
- Pain medication: early treatment with effective doses before pain becomes severe reduces the total quantity of medication needed to control the pain.

Common Clinical Questions

1. Of the following options for DVT prophylaxis in spinal cord injury,
   1. Low-dose (mini-dose) heparin alone
   2. Low-molecular-weight heparin alone
   3. Oral anticoagulation alone
   4. Low-dose heparin and pneumatic compression device

   which are recommended treatments?
   A. 1 and 3
   B. 2 and 4
   C. 1, 2, and 3
   D. 4

2. Which of the following drugs or classes of drugs causes a reduction in renal blood flow?
   A. NSAIDs
   B. Opioids
   C. Heparin
   D. Acetaminophen

3. Which of the following statements about the high-dose methylprednisolone protocol for use in spinal cord injury is false?
   A. Administration should not be undertaken more than 8 hours after the injury.
   B. The apparent benefit of methylprednisolone may have been due in part to patients recovering from steroid-induced myopathy.
   C. The number of studies that have shown a benefit from employing the protocol are almost equal to the number showing lack of benefit.
   D. Risks of high-dose methylprednisolone include sepsis, pneumonia, and deleterious effects of elevated blood glucose.

References

1. Australian and New Zealand College of Anaesthestists and Faculty of Pain Medicine. Acute Pain Management: Scientific Basis. 2nd ed. Australian and New Zealand College of Anaesthetists; 2005. Date accessed: March 4, 2010. URL: http://www.nhmrc.gov.au/_files_nhmrc/file/publications/synopses/cp104.pdf
2. Greenberg MS. Handbook of Neurosurgery. 7th ed. New York: Thieme Medical Publishers; 2010
3. Hamilton MG, Hull RD, Pineo GF. Venous thromboembolism in neurosurgery and neurology patients: a review. Neurosurgery 1994;34(2):280–296, discussion 296
4. Deep venous thrombosis and thromboembolism in patients with cervical spinal cord injuries. Neurosurgery 2002;50(3, Suppl):S73–S80
5. Bracken MB, Shepard MJ, Collins WF, et al. A randomized, controlled trial of methylprednisolone or naloxone in the treatment of acute spinal-cord injury. Results of the Second National Acute Spinal Cord Injury Study. N Engl J Med 1990;322(20):1405–1411
6. Bracken MB, Shepard MJ, Collins WF Jr, et al. Methylprednisolone or naloxone treatment after acute spinal cord injury: 1-year follow-up data. Results of the Second National Acute Spinal Cord Injury Study. J Neurosurg 1992;76(1):23–31
7. Short DJ, El Masry WS, Jones PW. High dose methylprednisolone in the management of acute spinal cord injury: a systematic review from a clinical perspective. Spinal Cord 2000;38(5):273–286
8. Qian T, Guo X, Levi AD, Vanni S, Shebert RT, Sipski ML. High-dose methylprednisolone may cause myopathy in acute spinal cord injury patients. Spinal Cord 2005;43(4):199–203
9. Hurlbert RJ. Methylprednisolone for acute spinal cord injury: an inappropriate standard of care. J Neurosurg 2000;93(1, Suppl):1–7
10. Ranguis SC, Li D, Webster AC. Perioperative epidural steroids for lumbar spine surgery in degenerative spinal disease. A review. J Neurosurg Spine 2010;13(6):745–757
11. Resnick DK, Choudhri TF, Dailey AT, et al; American Association of Neurological Surgeons/Congress of Neurological Surgeons. Guidelines for the performance of fusion procedures for degenerative disease of the lumbar spine. Part 13: injection therapies, low-back pain, and lumbar fusion. J Neurosurg Spine 2005;2(6):707–715
12. Cuckler JM, Bernini PA, Wiesel SW, Booth RE Jr, Rothman RH, Pickens GT. The use of epidural steroids in the treatment of lumbar radicular pain. A prospective, randomized, double-blind study. J Bone Joint Surg Am 1985;67(1):63–66

Answers to Common Clinical Questions

1. B
2. A
3. C. The benefit initially demonstrated could not be replicated in any other study encountered in a metaanalysis of the literature.

11 Interventional Pain/Nonoperative Spine Procedures: Diagnostic and Therapeutic

Daniel Marin

I. Key Points

This chapter focuses on nonoperative diagnostic and therapeutic spine procedures for the purpose of understanding their context, purpose, technique, and diagnostic usefulness from a perspective limited to the spine. Appropriate ordering and analysis of these procedures requires proper documentation of the severity of pain, presence of numbness, presence of weakness, and detailed distribution of pain. The chapter is not intended to be a guide or a practicum to the performance of these procedures.

II. Description

- Diagnostic procedures: disc stimulation (provocation discography)
  - Purpose: to identify pain originating from specific intervertebral discs (cervical, lumbar), typically axial in nature
  - Single-needle technique: With particular attention to sterility, and with fluoroscopic guidance, a spinal needle is inserted obliquely and advanced carefully, avoiding the ventral ramus (**Fig. 11.1,** DC), into the center of the intervertebral disc. Provocation follows using slow contrast injection attached to a line pressure transducer. Attention to disc morphology is important, and level of pain/concordance, pressure, and volume injected must continuously be monitored. Final documentation of nucleus pulposus morphology according to the Dallas discogram scale should then be made, and the patient sent for computed tomography (CT) imaging.[1]
  - Applicability: discogenic mediated pain
- Diagnostic procedures: medial branch block
  - Purpose: to block pain transmission from the medial branches of the dorsal primary rami (cervical, thoracic, lumbar) that innervate the zygapophysial joints, significant mediators of axial neck and back pain
  - Technique: With fluoroscopic guidance, a spinal needle is inserted obliquely (thoracic, lumbar), or posteriorly/laterally (cervical) and directed at the medial branch target, which is

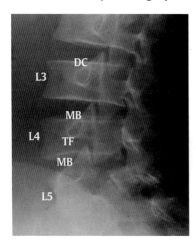

Fig. 11.1 Lumbar spine left oblique view. DC, intradiscal target; MB, medial branch target; TF, transforaminal target.

the centroid of the articular pillar in the cervical region (**Fig. 11.2**, MB), and the junction of the superior articular process and the transverse process in the thoracolumbar region[2] (**Fig. 11.1**, MB). Each joint requires a block of the superior and inferior medial branch components. Comparative local anesthetic blocks should then be performed to diagnose the correct pain level and exclude false-positives.
- Applicability: cervical spondylosis, thoracic spondylosis, lumbar spondylosis
– Diagnostic: sacroiliac joint block
  - Purpose: to inject anesthetic into the sacroiliac joint and evaluate for alleviation of pain. Corticosteroid can be added to decrease inflammation and for therapeutic effect.
  - Technique: Under the guidance of fluoroscopy, a spinal needle is inserted posteriorly and directed toward the inferior and posterior sacroiliac joint line. Confirmation of location is made with the use of contrast, and medication delivered.
  - Applicability: sacroiliac pain
– Diagnostic procedures: selective spinal nerve block
  - Purpose: to deliver a medication solution (usually anesthetic) to a spinal nerve root selectively (cervical, lumbar) in correlation with the alleviation (or absence) of a patient's symptoms
  - Technique: With fluoroscopic guidance, a spinal needle is inserted obliquely via a transforaminal approach into the neuroforamen of the spinal nerve root (cervical, thoracic, lumbar, or sacral spine). The target is the 6 o'clock position of the ped-

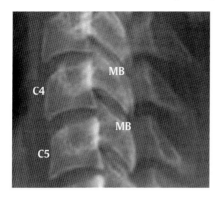

Fig. 11.2 Cervical spine lateral view. MB, medial branch target.

icle shadow of the corresponding nerve root level (**Fig. 11.1,** TF). Confirmation of location is then achieved with the use of contrast, and anesthetic delivered.
- Applicability: radiculopathy, polyradiculopathy, post-laminectomy syndrome
– Therapeutic procedures: epidural steroid injection
  - Purpose: to alleviate pain by placing corticosteroids into the epidural space in response to the symptoms of discogenic pain, spinal stenosis, radicular pain, and epidural scarring
  - Technique: With fluoroscopic guidance, a spinal needle is inserted posteriorly via a caudal, transforaminal (**Fig. 11.1,** TF), or interlaminar approach into the epidural space (cervical, thoracic, lumbar, or sacral spine). Confirmation of location is then obtained with the use of contrast, and medication delivered.
  - Applicability: discogenic mediated pain, spinal stenosis, radiculopathy, post-laminectomy syndrome
– Therapeutic procedures: percutaneous medial branch radiofrequency neurotomy
  - Purpose: to alleviate pain transmission from the medial branches of the dorsal primary rami (cervical, thoracic, lumbar) via ablation with a radiofrequency needle
  - Technique: A radiofrequency electrode needle is inserted in a manner identical to that used for the medial branch blocks mentioned earlier. Sensory and motor stimulation testing are then performed to ensure appropriate positioning and nonstimulation of a nerve root. Upon confirmation, local anesthetic is provided and medial branch nerve lesioning commenced.

- Applicability: cervical spondylosis, thoracic spondylosis, lumbar spondylosis
- Therapeutic procedures: percutaneous lead spinal cord stimulation
  - Purpose: to utilize the gate control theory[1] and block transmission of pain signals through the spinal cord by electrical stimulation over the dorsal column of the spinal cord after an appropriate percutaneous trial has been conducted
  - Technique: Place percutaneous lead(s) via an interlaminar approach, or a paddle surgical lead (typically improves coverage of axial back pain) into the epidural space (cervical or thoracic) with appropriate intraoperative testing or targeting to "cover" the patient's pain.
  - Applicability: post-laminectomy syndrome, chronic radiculopathy, peripheral neuropathy, complex regional pain syndrome
- Therapeutic procedures: trigger point injection
  - Purpose: to break up lactic acid deposit in muscles to decrease myofascial pain
  - Technique: After identification of painful taut bands in muscle, local anesthetic is applied and a small-gauge injection needle is used to pierce the skin and enter the muscle belly with the objective of breaking up the deposit.
  - Applicability: myofascial pain

III. Pearls

- Specific diagnostic spinal injections can address targeted spinal pain conditions with the goal of identifying the origin of the pain and guiding surgery.
- Epidural injections typically target canal and foraminal mediated pathology.
- Injections directed at the medial branch and dorsal primary ramus typically target posterior element sources of pain.

Common Clinical Questions

1. Which procedure(s) could be beneficial in diagnosing axial lumbar back pain?
2. What is a potential benefit of the percutaneous approach to dorsal column stimulation over the paddle lead, and vice versa?

References

1. Sachs BL, Vanharanta H, Spivey MA, et al. Dallas discogram description. A new classification of CT/discography in low-back disorders. Spine (Phila Pa 1976) 1987;12(3):287–294
2. International Spine Intervention Society. In: Bogduk N, ed. Practice Guidelines for Spinal Diagnostic and Treatment Procedures. San Francisco: International Spine Intervention Society; 2004:47–65, 112–137
3. Melzack R, Wall PD. Pain mechanisms: a new theory. Science 1965;150(699): 971–979

Answers to Common Clinical Questions

1. Medial branch blocks and epidural steroid injections could be considered in the diagnosis of axial lumbar back pain. Medial branch blocks or facet injections could be used to selectively target suspicious levels of spondylosis. Should the pain be axial and be aggravated by maneuvers increasing intradiscal pressure, discogenic pathology could be considered, as could epidural versus provocation discography. Sacroiliac pain typically will present at a point lower than will axial lumbar back pain.

2. The percutaneous approach to spinal cord stimulation allows for a testing period when the patient can "test" the system in his or her own functional environment, and have the lead removed easily if it is not found to be beneficial. The paddle (surgical) lead approach provides the benefit of better coverage of axial back pain, and would likely be the optimal choice in cases where thoracic scar tissue would impede lead passage.

12 Bedside Procedures
Daniel C. Lu and Praveen V. Mummaneni

I. Key Points
- Halo orthosis and traction: Skull fracture or severe skull osteoporosis is a contraindication for halo placement. Scalp abrasion or infection overlying the intended pin sites is also a contraindication for the procedure.
- Lumbar puncture (LP) or lumbar drain: Known or suspected intracranial mass, infection, tethered cord, or coagulopathy is a contraindication to the procedure.

II. Indications
- Halo orthosis and traction: Halo orthosis is effective at controlling abnormal motion at the C1-C2 articulation due to fracture or ligamentous injury. The purpose of the halo is to maintain normal alignment and/or immobilize the cervical spine to prevent further spinal injury and to allow for bony fusion in cases of fractures. Halo traction is utilized to limit fracture-dislocations and maintain normal alignment.[1,2]
- Lumbar puncture or lumbar drain: A lumbar puncture is indicated for collection and analysis of cerebrospinal fluid (CSF) for infection, subarachnoid hemorrhage, or elevated intracranial pressure. Additionally, intrathecal administration of medication or contrast (for myelography) can be performed via a lumbar puncture. A lumbar drain is placed if temporary CSF diversion is indicated for hydrocephalus (communicating) or wound management (pseudomeningocoele, CSF leak, etc.).

III. Technique
Halo Orthosis and Traction
- Patients should be positioned either in a sitting head-neutral position or a supine head-neutral position at the end of the bed so that the head slightly overhangs the bed. A semi-rigid collar may be used to immobilize the neck during halo application.[3]
- The appropriate-size halo ring is selected. The halo ring should accommodate the entire head circumference with clearance of approximately 1 cm.

- Halo pin sites are selected at this time, with two anterior and two posterior sites.
    - The anterior sites are centered in the groove between the supracilliary ridge and frontal prominences. Pins should be placed just superior to the lateral half of the eyebrows to avoid the supraorbital nerve and vessels. This location avoids muscular structures to diminish discomfort.
    - A posterior pin should be placed 1 cm above the apex of the pinna of each ear. A line connecting the posterior pin site with its contralateral anterior pin site should roughly bisect a line drawn between the remaining two pin sites at a right angle. This provides distribution of force for stability.
- The planned pin sites are sterilely prepared and injected with 1% lidocaine. The two pins—one front and the diagonally opposite back pin—are then finger-tightened to just touch the skin; this is repeated for the other pins. In children, multiple pins (>4) are sometimes utilized to distribute the pressure more evenly.
- A torque screwdriver (set to 6 to 8 lb of pressure) is then used to tighten the pins in diagonal pairs. The pins are now stabilized and locked down with appropriate locking nuts to the halo frame. The halo vest is then placed on the patient, the semi-rigid collar is removed, and halo and vest are stabilized with halo rods.
    - The halo vest should be adjusted so that the straps make contact with the patient's trapezius and shoulder area. There is a tendency for the vest to ride high and not touch the shoulders unless care is taken during vest application.
- For traction placement, a variety of devices are available. Gardner-Wells tongs or halo rings are the most common (**Fig. 12.1**). Pin sites for Gardner-Wells tongs are 2 to 3 finger breadths (3 to 4 cm) above the ear pinnae. The Gardner-Wells pins are spring-loaded with a force indicator; these pins are tightened until the indicator protrudes 1 mm beyond the flat surface. Pins are re-tightened daily until the indicator remains at this location for 3 days. If used, halo rings have the advantage of a compatible vest orthosis to secure the tractioned position.
- After tong or halo ring placement, the patient is transferred to a bed with a headboard attached to a pulley system with weights. With the pulley placed above the patient's head, flexion and traction can be accomplished. If the pulley is placed at the level of the pins, then straight traction forces can be applied. If the pulley is placed below the level of the patient's head, extension and traction are possible. Lateral x-rays should be obtained immediately after application of traction and after each weight

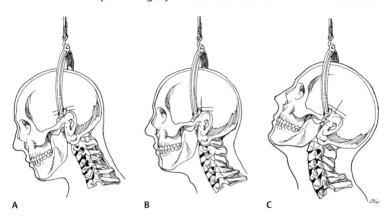

Fig. 12.1 Proper fixation points for Gardner-Wells tongs application. **(A)** Posterior placement of tongs to produce flexion of head. **(B)** Normal placement of tongs to produce straight traction. **(C)** Anterior placement of tongs to produce hyperextension of head (from Vaccaro, A. Spine Surgery: Tricks of the Trade. 2nd ed. Thieme, p. 280, Fig. 73.1A–C).

adjustment. Typically, evaluation begins with 5 lb of traction for upper C-spine injuries and 10 lb for lower C-spine injuries.
- For upper cervical injuries, evaluation of the atlanto-occipital joints is important to rule out atlanto-occipital dislocations. Such injuries should not use traction. For mid-cervical locked facets, 5 lb per level of traction weight should be applied to the injury (e.g., slowly work up to 50 lb for a C5 level facet subluxation). Prior to applying traction for cervical facet subluxation, consider MRI imaging to rule out a coincidental anterior herniated disc with cord compression. If a herniated disc is present, consider anterior operative correction instead of a trial of traction.

Lumbar Puncture or Lumbar Drain
- This bedside procedure can be performed with the patient sitting or lying down.
  - For the recumbent position, the patient is placed in a lateral decubitus posture, with neck flexed and knees brought up to the chest. This distracts the space between the spinous processes, facilitating passage of a spinal needle into the thecal sac.
  - For the sitting position, the patient should be sitting with head and arms resting on a pillow placed on a bedside stand. The back is sterilely prepared and draped.

- LP can be safely attempted at the L3 to S1 interspaces in the anatomically normal patient. The intercrestal line is identified and palpated in the midline for the L4 spinous process.
  - Initially 1% lidocaine is infiltrated subcutaneously. Subsequently, the lumbodorsal fascia is injected.
  - The spinal needle with stylet is aimed slightly rostrally to the umbilicus to approximately parallel the spinous process, and the bevel should be turned parallel to the length of the spinal column to reduce the chance of post-LP headaches.
  - The needle is advanced with a midline trajectory and a "pop" should be felt as the needle penetrates the ligamentum flavum and passes into the dura.
  - The stylet is then withdrawn to check for CSF flow; if none is seen, reinsert the stylet and advance the needle further; if no CSF flow is present, attempt another trajectory.
  - If blood is seen, wait for the blood to drain and clear, as this may represent a traumatic tap. If it does not clear, advance the needle or attempt another trajectory.
- If a lumbar drain is selected, a lumbar drain needle (14-gauge Tuohy) should be used. After entering the thecal sac with needle bevel facing laterally, the bevel is turned superiorly, and a lumbar drainage catheter with wire stylet is inserted (20 to 40 cm).
- The needle and stylet are sequentially removed, and cerebrospinal fluid (CSF) flow is confirmed by dropping the catheter below the patient.
  - A 2 × 2 gauze section is placed around the insertion site of the catheter and a Tegaderm (3M, St. Paul, MN) pad is placed on top to secure the catheter.
  - Several more Tegaderm pads are placed along the flank of the patient to secure the catheter to the patient's body.

IV. Complications

Halo Orthosis and Traction
- Pin loosening occurs in 60% of patients over a 3-month period. Pins may require retightening.
- Pin site infection (10 to 20%). Treat by placing pin at a new, adjacent site and give the patient oral antibiotics.
- Neurologic deterioration after traction may occur secondary to retropulsed disc. Consider obtaining a pre-procedure magnetic resonance image (MRI) to rule out this condition prior to traction.
- Overdistraction is another potential complication of halo/traction. This could manifest in deficits or pain and can typically be identified on the lateral x-ray.

Lumbar Puncture or Lumbar Drain
- Infection can occur in certain cases, especially those involving prolonged use of lumbar drains.
  - Superficial infection can be treated with drain removal and antibiotic treatment.
  - Epidural abscess (depending on size and neurologic compromise) may require surgical intervention (laminectomy and evacuation).
- Radicular pain can occur secondary to nerve root irritation. If persistent, consider repositioning of drain.
- Post-LP headache
  - Options include bed rest (24 hours), abdominal binder, desoxycortisone acetate, caffeine sodium benzoate, high-dose steroids, and blood patch.
  - If related to lumbar drain, consider decreasing output.
- Spinal epidural hematoma (usually in setting of coagulopathy or anticoagulation)
- Tonsillar herniation (in the presence of mass-occupying lesion)
- Intracranial subdural hygroma or hematoma
- Epidermoid tumor (increased likelihood with needle introduction without stylet). This can occur in a delayed fashion but the incidence is very low.
- Abducens palsy (often delayed 5 to 14 days post-LP and resolves without intervention in 4 to 6 weeks)

V. Post-Procedure Care

Halo Orthosis and Traction
- The pins should be retightened once a day for about 3 days at the same pressure and then retightened every week for 3 weeks.
  - A persistently loose pin may indicate migration into the inner table and should be removed, with a new one placed at different site.
  - Post-procedure radiographs are taken to verify proper head positioning with halo orthosis and traction placement.

Lumbar Puncture or Lumbar Drain
- For lumbar drain care, prophylactic antibiotics may be continued while the drain is in place, with dressings changed every three days. Drains should be removed or changed after a week.

VI. Outcomes

- Halo orthosis: Fusion rates are as high as 84% in nonelderly patients with type II odontoid fracture treated with a halo; risk factors for nonunion include advanced age and displaced odontoid fractures.
- Halo traction: Reduction of bilateral locked facets is typically easier to achieve than reduction of unilateral locked facet.
- LP: Risk of persistent or disabling complication is rated at 0.1 to 0.5%.

VII. Surgical Pearls

Halo Orthosis and Traction
- Pin tension should be uniform. Unequal pin tension will lead to migration of halo as pins migrate in the direction of the pin with the least tension.
- Adjustments during follow-up should not be limited to the halo pins. Inspection of alignment with the vest should be performed to ensure that shoulder straps are making contact with the trapezius and shoulder area. X-ray radiographs should accompany follow-up visits to ensure proper alignment.

Lumbar Puncture or Lumbar Drain
- Care must be taken in removing the Tuohy needle from the lumbar catheter to avoid shear of the catheter by the sharp bevel of the needle. The trajectory and rotation of the needle must not be altered during removal.
- Evaluation of anatomy with preoperative radiograph is essential, especially in patients with degeneration and osteophyte formation.
- If attempts at LP or drain placement are unsuccessful, placement of lumbar drain under fluoroscopic guidance may be necessary.

Common Clinical Questions

1. Frontal halo pins may compromise which nerve?
2. During retightening of halo pins during a follow-up visit, it is found that the pins can no longer be torqued to 6 lb after one complete turn. What has happened and what should be done?
3. Patient develops nausea, vomiting, and headaches 2 weeks after a workup for meningitis. What is the likely diagnosis and what is the treatment?

References

1. Chan RC, Schweigel JF, Thompson GB. Halo-thoracic brace immobilization in 188 patients with acute cervical spine injuries. J Neurosurg 1983;58(4):508–515
2. Platzer P, Thalhammer G, Sarahrudi K, et al. Nonoperative management of odontoid fractures using a halothoracic vest. Neurosurgery 2007;61(3):522–529, discussion 529–530
3. Greenberg MS. Handbook of Neurosurgery. 6th ed. New York: Thime Medical Publishers, 2006:304–306

Answers to Common Clinical Questions

1. Supracilliary nerve
2. The pin has likely breached the cortical inner table. The pin should be removed and a new pin placed at a new site.
3. The patient has likely developed post-LP headache. Treatments include bed rest, abdominal binder, hydration, and medication. If these measures fail, a blood patch is indicated.

13 Spinal Radiation Therapy

Edward A. Monaco III and Peter Carlos Gerszten

I. Key Points

- Conventional fractionated radiotherapy, defined as radiation delivered in one to two radiation beams without high precision or highly conformal techniques, is well established and widely accepted as an appropriate treatment modality for many spinal tumors.
- Stereotactic spinal radiosurgery allows for the highly conformal delivery of radiation to spinal lesions and avoids toxicity to normal tissues.
- Spinal radiosurgery has proven effective in the treatment of benign and malignant lesions along the entire length of the spine.

II. Description

Epidemiology

- Over 200,000 cases of spinal tumors are diagnosed yearly in North America.[1]
- Up to 40% of cancer patients will develop metastatic disease of the vertebrae.
- In approximately 20% of patients, spinal metastases will progress to neural element compression.
- With improved multimodality approaches for cancer treatment and greater long-term survival, the incidence and prevalence of spinal metastases are likely to increase.

Overview

- The traditional therapy for spinal tumors, primary or metastatic, includes open surgical excision, systemic chemotherapy, and conventional fractionated radiation therapy, alone or in combinations.
- In a randomized trial comparing conventional radiation therapy alone to surgery followed by radiation therapy for the treatment of spinal metastases causing spinal cord compression, Patchell and colleagues demonstrated that surgery combined with conventional radiation therapy is a superior treatment in its ability to preserve ambulation and decreases the need for both corticosteroids and opioid analgesics.[2]

- With conventional radiation therapy, one or two low-precision radiation beams are delivered to the spine over several fractions to allow for repair of the normal tissues.
- The goals of local radiation therapy have been palliation of pain, prevention of local disease progression and subsequent pathologic fractures, and halting progression of, or reversing, neurologic compromise.
- Conventional radiation therapy is limited in its effectiveness by the relative intolerance of the adjacent normal tissues (e.g., the spinal cord, nerve roots, and conus medullaris) to high radiation doses. Thus, treatment doses are limited to subtherapeutic levels, resulting in disease recurrence or progression.
- Stereotactic spinal radiosurgery is the delivery of a highly conformal, large radiation dose to a specific target, often in a single fraction (**Fig. 13.1A,B**).
- Radiosurgery offers the advantages of applying radiobiologically effective doses to a target and sparing surrounding structures.
- Intensity-modulated radiation therapy is a technology that provides the ability to vary the integrated intensities of radiation beams for the delivery of therapy. With several radiation beams all passing through multileaf collimators with different apertures, the intensity of the radiation dosing can be shaped in three-dimensional space.

Conventional Radiotherapy
- Three randomized trials have been published for spine metastases.[3]
- Approximately 70% of patients remained ambulatory after conventional radiation therapy for epidural spinal cord compression.
- Between 20 and 60% of patients regained ambulation after conventional radiotherapy.
- Pain is palliated in 50 to 70% of patients.
- The most commonly used treatment is 30 Gy delivered in 10 fractions.
- The specific dose-fractionation schedule used has not been found to have a significant impact on ambulatory status or the probability of regaining ambulation.[4]
- Local control rates for spine metastases with conventional radiotherapy are reported to be 60 to 90%.
- The effectiveness of conventional radiotherapy has been limited by the intolerance of the spinal cord to high-dose radiation.

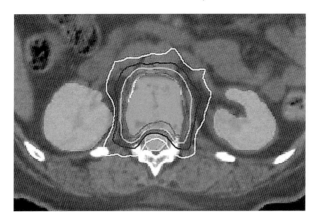

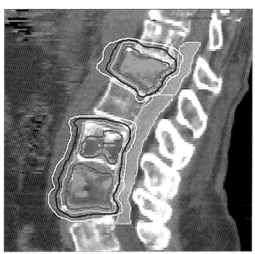

Fig. 13.1 (A,B) Case example of a 54-year-old woman with symptomatic progression on magnetic resonance image (MRI) of L1 and L4 breast metastases after prior conventional irradiation treatment. She complained of significant mechanical back pain upon ambulation. She first underwent a percutaneous cement augmentation procedure followed by radiosurgery. The prescribed dose to the planned tumor volume was 16 Gy using 9 coplanar beams (Synergy S, Elekta, Atlanta, GA). Axial and sagittal images of the treatment plan are presented.

- Certain histologies such as sarcomas, melanoma, and renal cell carcinoma are known to be relatively resistant to conventional radiotherapy doses.

Radiosurgery
- No randomized data are available to date.
- Reported outcomes demonstrate 85 to 100% of patients experiencing palliation of pain.[5]
- Use of both single fraction doses (16 to 24 Gy × 1) and hypofractionation (4 Gy × 4, 6 Gy × 5, 8 Gy × 3, 9 Gy × 3) has been reported.
- Significant toxicity does not appear to be associated with any fractionation schedule.[6]
- The majority of reported local control rates are around 90%.

Spine Radiosurgery: Two Fundamental Principles
- Target immobilization
  - Early spinal radiosurgery protocols applied an approach similar to that of cranial radiosurgery through the application of an invasive rigid frame directly to the spine.
  - Frameless techniques have become the methodology of choice because of their relative noninvasiveness.
  - Perfect static positioning cannot be accomplished using frameless methods; thus pre- and intratreatment imaging must be obtained to account for target movement due to respiration.
- Target localization
  - Frequent acquisition of localizing images during the delivery of radiation combined with adjustments to the patient's position allow for accurate targeting of the desired lesion(s).
  - Volumetric imaging allows for the detection of rotational errors in patient setup, making robust automatic registration procedures possible.
  - Cone beam imaging uses gantry-mounted kilovolt sources and detectors to acquire images during gantry rotation. The images are converted to computed tomography (CT)–like axial slices, yielding high spatial resolution and resulting in submillimeter targeting errors.

Indications for Treatment with Spinal Radiosurgery
- Pain from spinal tumors
- Primary treatment modality for newly discovered spinal metastases instead of open surgery or conventional radiation therapy
- Radiation boost for radioresistant tumors

- Progressive neurological deficit
  - May need to perform decompressive/debulking surgery for patients with progressive myelopathy (instead of using radiation treatment)
- Treatment of residual tumor after surgery
- Postsurgical tumor progression

Candidate Lesions for Spinal Radiosurgery
- Lesions associated with minimal spinal cord compromise
- Previously irradiated lesions
- Radioresistant lesions that would benefit from a radiosurgical boost
- Residual tumor following surgery
- Recurrent tumor after prior surgical resection
- Lesions requiring difficult or morbid surgical approaches
- Short life expectancy of patient, precluding open surgery
- Significant medical comorbidities precluding open surgery
- Lesions not involving overt spinal instability

III. Surgical Pearls

- Conventional radiotherapy is safe and effective, with good symptomatic response and local control of spine tumors, particularly for radiosensitive histologies, such as lymphoma, myeloma, and seminoma.
- Conventional radiotherapy is an appropriate initial therapy option for spine tumors where no contraindication exists. Contraindications include spinal instability, prior irradiation, radioresistant histology, and high-grade spinal cord compression.
  - Consider surgical decompression/debulking/instrumented stabilization procedures for cases where radiotherapy is contraindicated.
- Radiosurgery is safe and effective, with durable symptomatic response and local control for even radioresistant histologies, regardless of prior fractionated radiotherapy.
- Radiosurgery should be preferred over conventional radiotherapy for the treatment of solid-tumor spine metastases in the setting of oligometastatic disease or radioresistant histology.
- Single-fraction, highly conformal large-dose radiosurgical treatments offer excellent tumor control, symptomatic relief, and patient convenience.

Common Clinical Questions

1. What is the major factor limiting the effectiveness of conventional radiotherapy for the treatment of spine tumors?
   A. The relative resistance of the spinal cord to high-dose radiation
   B. The intolerance of the spinal cord to high-dose radiation
   C. The resistance of tumors of the spine to even high doses of radiation
   D. The instability of the spine that develops after conventional radiotherapy treatment

2. Which of the following statements is true?
   A. The most commonly used radiation dose prescription for the treatment of spine metastases is 20 Gy in 10 fractions.
   B. Randomized clinical trials have demonstrated the superiority of radiosurgery over conventional fractionated radiotherapy for the treatment of spine tumors.
   C. Certain histologies such as myeloma and lymphoma are known to be relatively resistant to radiation therapy.
   D. Reported outcomes demonstrate that 85 to 100% of patients experiencing pain from spine metastases report improvement after radiosurgery.

3. Radiosurgery should be considered as a first-line treatment for a spine tumor over conventional radiotherapy in which setting?
   A. In the setting of gross spinal instability
   B. When the lesion has already undergone treatment using fractionated radiotherapy with spinal cord tolerance doses
   C. For lymphoma, myeloma, or seminoma
   D. In the setting of widely metastatic spine disease

References

1. Posner JB. Spinal metastases, neurological complications of cancer. Philadelphia: FA Davis Company; 1995:111–142.
2. Patchell RA, Tibbs PA, Regine WF, et al. Direct decompressive surgical resection in the treatment of spinal cord compression caused by metastatic cancer: a randomised trial. Lancet 2005;366(9486):643–648
3. Gerszten PC, Mendel E, Yamada Y. Radiotherapy and radiosurgery for metastatic spine disease: what are the options, indications, and outcomes? Spine (Phila Pa 1976) 2009; 34(22, Suppl):S78–S92
4. Maranzano E, Bellavita R, Rossi R, et al. Short-course versus split-course radiotherapy in metastatic spinal cord compression: results of a phase III, randomized, multicenter trial. J Clin Oncol 2005;23(15):3358–3365
5. Gerszten PC, Burton SA, Ozhasoglu C, Welch WC. Radiosurgery for spinal metastases: clinical experience in 500 cases from a single institution. Spine (Phila Pa 1976) 2007;32(2):193–199
6. Sahgal A, Ma L, Gibbs I, et al. Spinal cord tolerance for stereotactic body radiotherapy. Int J Radiat Oncol Biol Phys 2010;77(2):548–553

Answers to Common Clinical Questions

1. B
2. D
3. B

14 Spinal Navigation

Ben J. Garrido and Rick C. Sasso

I. Key Points

- Allows intraoperative real-time navigation of instruments relative to the spinal anatomy
- Provides three-dimensional (3D) real-time anatomic information
- May increase the safety, accuracy, and efficiency of certain spine procedures
- Eliminates intraoperative radiation exposure to surgeons and accompanying staff members during procedures
- Provides a versatile array of techniques facilitating the ability to perform complex spine surgery safely

II. Description

Spinal navigation uses computer vision technology to plan and guide surgical interventions. It has evolved from a cumbersome to a more user-friendly system. Early-generation systems required a complex preregistration process through the use of either the paired-point technique or surface mapping. These techniques introduced the potential for error and were time consuming but critical in linking image data to spinal anatomy. Most of the resistance to the universal adoption of image navigation stemmed from such requirements. Newer systems combine high-precision robotics with unparalleled imaging capability, eliminating the need for preregistration. Computer-aided surgery now enables the acquisition of imaging data intraoperatively prior to incision. Current software can use either a 2D or 3D image data set acquired intraoperatively by a fluoroscopy unit or high-resolution computed tomography (CT) scanner. These images are then automatically imported into the computer workstation and used to create a 3D picture of the patient's anatomy, completing the registration process. This automatic registration process improves the anatomic localization accuracy and eliminates the need for manual point-based or surface-based registration. Subsequently, real-time tracking data are matched with previously obtained image data through the use of a fixed reference point on the patient, computer workstation, and camera system. For spine procedures, affixing the fixed reference frame/point to bone is the initial step in registration.

Components of a Navigation System

After the intraoperative image data are obtained through one of the commercial systems available, this data set is automatically uploaded to the computer workstation. A 3D image is created and linked to your working position relative to the patient's anatomy through a tracking system. There are currently two types of tracking systems that will triangulate your position in space: optical and electromagnetic (EM). Both systems allow localization of surgical instruments or implants in real time. In electromagnetic tracking an EM field is created, and changes in field are monitored to localize a tracked device. With optical tracking, cameras track instrument positions relative to the fixed reference point through an active or passive method. Active tracking entails the use of light-emitting diodes (LEDs) on the instruments and passive tracking involves the reflection of infrared light from the camera to reflective spheres on instruments. Both systems require a direct line of view between the camera and the tracked instruments to link surgical anatomy to the 3D data set in the computer workstation. The system can then triangulate the instrument's tip location, angle, and trajectory. The systems are comparable in positioning accuracy and can provide real-time, precise 3D imaging quality (**Fig. 14.1**).

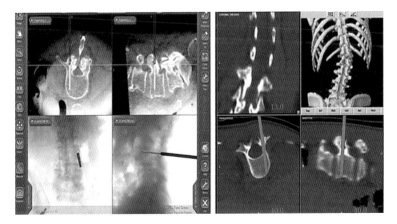

Fig. 14.1 Examples of 3D images with navigation provided by the computer workstation, with a superimposed projection of the navigated instrument or probe.

Applications and Advantages

Image navigation has improved the safety of and ability to perform complex procedures where visibility is not optimal or anatomic deformity is present. Numerous published studies have demonstrated its effectiveness in improving pedicle screw placement for complex multiplanar spinal deformities.[1] A meta-analysis of pedicle screw placement accuracy demonstrated a 95% median accuracy with navigation compared with 90% without it.[2] It is intuitive that the capability to visualize a pedicle in 3D should minimize screw insertion risks associated with pedicle asymmetry, smaller diameters, and vertebral rotation and thereby prevent nerve root or spinal cord compression. Because of the improved accuracy, operative times have also been shown to decrease with the use of image navigation.[3] Drawbacks related to increased operative time, patient registration, and data acquisition are controlled with the current real-time intraoperative data acquisition technology and software systems.[3] In addition, mean radiation exposure using image navigation has been shown to be statistically significantly lower compared with conventional fluoroscopy.[4]

Aside from pedicle screw insertion, many other versatile applications are being described for image navigation, including C1-C2 transarticular and percutaneous translaminar facet screw placement, lumbar disc arthroplasty placement, and balloon kyphoplasty. These possibilities are incorporating the advantages of image navigation and demonstrating feasibility, accuracy, and operative time reduction while reducing radiation exposure.

III. Surgical Pearls

- All staff using the system should be properly trained, to prevent errors that can lead to improper setup, inaccurate information, and surgical complications.
- The fixed referenced frame must not be inadvertently bumped, moved, or altered. This can lead to tracking and positional errors during navigation. It's important to keep the reference frame close to the surgical field for maximum accuracy.
- Spinal navigation is not a substitute for fundamental knowledge of anatomic landmarks and appropriate surgical technique. Improper use or malfunction of the system can cause navigational inaccuracies.
- Image navigation should be used to confirm anatomic landmarks and suspected locations and trajectories for hardware placement.
- The room setup plan should provide for a direct line of view between navigation components (camera, computer workstation, and reference frame).

Common Clinical Questions

1. Which of the following is not a feature of spinal image navigation?
   A. Real-time views
   B. Decreased operative time
   C. Axial views
   D. Increased radiation exposure
   E. Improved accuracy
2. Current spinal image navigation systems provide real-time tracking through what technique?
   A. Paired-point preregistration
   B. Surface mapping preregistration
   C. Continuous fluoroscopic imaging
   D. Optical or electromagnetic tracking
   E. None of the above

References

1. Kotani Y, Abumi K, Ito M, et al. Accuracy analysis of pedicle screw placement in posterior scoliosis surgery: comparison between conventional fluoroscopic and computer-assisted technique. Spine (Phila Pa 1976) 2007;32(14): 1543–1550
2. Kosmopoulos V, Schizas C. Pedicle screw placement accuracy: a meta-analysis. Spine (Phila Pa 1976) 2007;32(3):E111–E120
3. Sasso RC, Garrido BJ. Computer-assisted spinal navigation versus serial radiography and operative time for posterior spinal fusion at L5-S1. J Spinal Disord Tech 2007;20(2): 118–122
4. Smith HE, Welsch MD, Sasso RC, Vaccaro AR. Comparison of radiation exposure in lumbar pedicle screw placement with fluoroscopy vs computer-assisted image guidance with intraoperative three-dimensional imaging. J Spinal Cord Med 2008;31(5):532–537

Answers to Common Clinical Questions

1. D
2. D

15 Spinal Biologics
Rafael F. Cardona-Durán and Juan S. Uribe

I. Key Points
- Decision making for the choice of bone graft in spinal surgery is important and should be a part of all preoperative planning.
- The inherent qualities—including advantages, disadvantages, and costs—associated with each type of bone graft should be appreciated by the surgeon.
- Host bone bed preparation is key to enabling bone grafts to achieve their intended function of promoting fusion.

II. Description
Bone Graft Characteristics (Table 15.1)[1,2]
- Osteoinduction: the recruitment of mesenchymal cells and the stimulation of these cells to develop into osteoblasts and osteoclasts
- Osteogenesis: formation of new bone by host or graft mesenchymal stem cells transformed into osteoblasts
- Osteoconduction: the scaffolding provided by the graft for the proliferation of new blood vessels and bone
- Mechanical stability: the structural, anatomic, and biomechanical support provided after discectomy, corpectomy, or vertebral tumor resection

Autograft: "Gold Standard"[1–3]
- No histocompatibility or disease transmission issues
- Iliac crest (anterior or posterior) is the typical primary donor site.
- Drawbacks
  - 20% risk of long-term donor site pain
  - Increased surgical risk of blood loss and infection
    - Cancellous
      - Fulfills all bone graft criteria, except mechanical stability
    - Cortical
      - Provides superior and immediate mechanical strength
      - Diminished osteoconduction and osteoinduction
    - Corticocancellous
      - Fulfills all of the bone graft criteria
      - Example: tricortical iliac crest wedge

15 Spinal Biologics

Table 15.1 Characteristics of Bone Graft Materials[1,2,4]

Material	Osteogenesis	Osteoinduction	Osteoconduction	Mechanical stability
Cancellous autograft[a]	+++	++	++++	+/−
Cortical autograft[a]	+	+	+	+++
Vacularized autograft[b]	+++	++	+++	+++
Allograft	−	+/−	+	+
Bone marrow aspirate	+	+/−	+	−
Demineralized bone matrix	−	+	+	−
Bone morphogenic protein[c]	−	++	−	−
Collagen	−	−	−	−
Ceramics	−	−	+++	+

Notes: − = no effect; +/− = minimal effect; + = mild effect; ++ = moderate effect; +++ = strong effect; ++++ = very strong effect.
[a] Associated with donor site morbidity.
[b] Associated with high donor site morbidity and increased operative times.
[c] U.S. Food and Drug Administration approval only for anterior lumbar interbody fusion.

- Vascularized autograft
  - Technically challenging and time consuming
  - Very rarely used
  - Consider for host sites that are scarred or irradiated or that span long segments
- Autologous bone marrow
  - Source of osteoprogenitor cells and osteoinductive substances
  - Diminished donor site risks
  - Offers no osteoconduction or mechanical stability

Allograft[4]
- Eliminates risks of autograft harvesting
- Acquired through multiple organ procurement agencies
- Mainly prepared frozen or freeze-dried
- Available in various sizes and types
  - Ilium tricortical block, bicortical plug, or unicortical dowel
  - Corticocancellous matchsticks or crushed
  - Cancellous cubes, block, crushed, bone powder
  - Sections from tibia, fibula, or femur
- Drawbacks
  - Recommended for use with other types of grafts that may be osteoinductive or osteogenic
  - Minimal but present risk of disease transmission

Demineralized Bone Matrix[1,2]
- Prepared by acid extraction, reducing antigenicity but preserving osteoinductive and some osteoconductive properties
- Several formulations
- Putty, gel, chips, granules, or powder
- Primarily to be used as adjunct to other grafting material or graft extender
- Drawbacks
  - Increased cost
  - Variable efficacy between different preparations
  - No mechanical or structural properties
  - To be used with patient's own bone

Bone Morphogenetic Proteins[2–5]
- Molecules that induce the transformation of mesenchymal stem cells into osteoblasts, capable of inducing ectopic bone formation
- Approximately 20 different bone morphogenetic proteins (BMPs) from the transforming growth factor–β family
- Produced using recombinant DNA technology

- A carrier matrix is necessary to maintain the soluble factor at the graft site, keeping the BMP solution from diffusing within the adjacent tissues.
- U.S. Food and Drug Administration approval only for anterior lumbar interbody fusion (ALIF)
  - Recombinant human BMP-2 commercially available as Infuse (Medtronic, Minneapolis, MN)
- Increases fusion rates
- Drawbacks
  - Increased cost
  - Ectopic bone formation, bone resorption, or remodeling at the graft site is a potential problem if BMP is used in transforaminal lumbar interbody fusion (TLIF), posterior lumbar interbody fusion (PLIF), or corpectomy applications.
  - Hematoma, neck swelling, and painful seroma are potential problems with use in the cervical spine.

Collagen[1]
- Contributes to vascular ingrowth, mineral deposition, and growth factor binding, improving bone regeneration
- Used primarily as a carrier for other osteoinductive, osteoconductive, or osteogenic materials and as a composite with other graft extenders
- Drawbacks
  - Minimal structural support
  - Potential immunogenicity

Other Graft Extenders[2]
- Ceramics
  - Tricalcium phosphates, calcium carbonate, and hydroxyapatite
  - No risk of disease transmission
  - Engineered, biocompatible osteoconductive materials
  - Recommended for use only as bone graft extenders
  - Combined with autograft, bone marrow aspirate, BMP, or other materials

III. Surgical Pearls

- Decortication and facet joint/end plate preparation, though time consuming, are mandatory for excellent fusion.
- The costs and risks associated with pseudoarthrosis are high; therefore, achieving arthrodesis is of paramount importance.

Common Clinical Questions

1. What are the three principal properties of graft material in relation to fusion?
2. What is the "gold standard" for bone graft material (assuming no contraindications)?

References

1. Giannoudis PV, Dinopoulos H, Tsiridis E. Bone substitutes: an update. Injury 2005;36(Suppl 3):S20–S27
2. Whang PG, Wang JC. Bone graft substitutes for spinal fusion. Spine J 2003; 3(2):155–165
3. Shen FH, Samartzis D, An HS. Cell technologies for spinal fusion. Spine J 2005; 5(6, Suppl):231S–239S
4. Tumialán LM, Pan J, Rodts GE, Mummaneni PV. The safety and efficacy of anterior cervical discectomy and fusion with polyetheretherketone spacer and recombinant human bone morphogenetic protein-2: a review of 200 patients. J Neurosurg Spine 2008; 8(6):529–535
5. Vaidya R, Sethi A, Bartol S, Jacobson M, Coe C, Craig JG. Complications in the use of rhBMP-2 in PEEK cages for interbody spinal fusions. J Spinal Disord Tech 2008;21(8):557–562

Answers to Common Clinical Questions

1. Osteoinduction, osteoconduction, osteogenesis
2. Autograft (typically from iliac crest)

III
Spinal Pathology

16 Congenital Anomalies

Rory R. Mayer, Katherine Relyea, and Andrew Jea

I. Key Points

- Most developmental disorders of the spine occur in either the upper cervical or lower thoracic and lumbar regions due to defective spinal cord embryogenesis and vertebral column formation (**Fig. 16.1**). In the general workup, screen with ultrasound for antenatal diagnosis and use sagittal magnetic resonance imaging (MRI) for spinal dysraphism. Employ computed tomog-

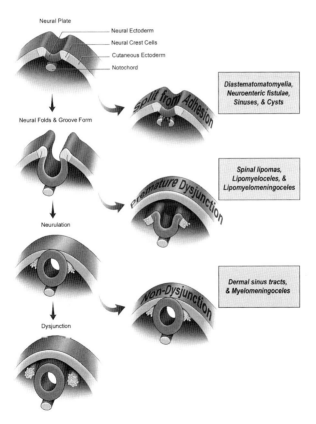

Fig. 16.1 Defects during different stages of spinal cord embryology lead to congenital anomalies of the spine.

raphy (CT) or CT myelogram to better delineate bony malformations and hydrocephalus. Use renal ultrasound to rule out pelvic kidney, unilateral agenesis, and horseshoe kidney.

II. Anomalies of Notochord Formation

Diastematomyelia
- Background
  - The spinal cord is divided vertically into two hemicords, each with its own central canal, surrounding pia, and set of anterior and posterior nerve roots.
  - May result from bifurcation of the developing notochord around an adhesion between the endoderm and ectoderm. The split notochord may influence the formation of two neural tubes and subsequent hemicords and vertebral formation. Consequently, it is common to have associated bony anomalies (spurs) at the site of diastematomyelia.
  - Accounts for 5% of congenital scoliosis and roughly 30 to 40% of myelomeningoceles
- Signs, symptoms, and physical exam
  - Most individuals have nonspecific symptoms and tethered cords requiring surgical attention.
  - The overlying skin in 66% of cases shows nevi, hypertrichosis, lipomas, dimples, hemangiomas, dermal sinus tracts, or dermoids.
- Neuroimaging
  - The conus is low lying in 75%, often with an associated thickened or fatty filum.[1]
  - The hemicords usually reunite below the cleft, enveloped in a single dura, with no spur or fibrous band found in 60% of cases (Pang Type II).[2] In contrast, the presence of two dural tubes is always associated with a fibrous or bony spur within the cleft in the remaining 40% (Pang Type I).
  - The type of spur, bony (50 to 60%) or fibrous (40 to 50%), is likely determined by the amount of trapped mesenchyme between the hemicords.
- Treatment
  - Untether the cord, coagulate and divide tethering fibrous bands extending from the dura to the spinal cord, and excise any bony spurs.
- Surgical pearls
  - Remove the spur before untethering the cord to prevent retraction of the cord against the bony septum.

- Remove dural cuff and arachnoid covering the bony spur to prevent regeneration of spur.

Split Notochord Syndrome
- Background
  - Deviation or splitting of the notochord secondary to a retained link between the endoderm and ectoderm. The most severe form, a dorsal enteric fistula, is a communication between the bowel and the dorsal skin. Dorsal enteric fistulae traverse the prevertebral soft tissues, vertebral bodies, the spinal canal, and its posterior elements. Any portion of the tract may involute or fibrose, leaving fistulae or cysts.
  - Dorsal enteric sinuses open on the skin surface
  - Dorsal enteric cysts are found in the intraspinal or paraspinal compartments.
- Signs, symptoms, and physical exam
  - Dorsal enteric fistula present in newborn with a bowel ostium on the back.
  - Intraspinal enteric cysts usually present between 20 and 40 years of age as episodic local or radicular pain that may progress to myelopathy.
- Workup
  - Cyst incision, drainage, and pathologic examination to rule out infectious processes
- Neuroimaging
  - Radiography will help determine the presence and degree of vertebral clefting.
  - Follow with CT/MR imaging to define the degree of fistulation or cyst involvement.
- Treatment
  - Complete surgical excision is the best treatment. Chemical arachnoiditis resulting from cystic material often produces dense adhesions that make later operations more difficult.

III. Anomalies of Dysjunction

Spinal Lipomas[3]
- Background
  - Fat and connective tissue masses attached to the spinal cord and meninges
  - Lipomyelomeningoceles and lipomyeloceles (84%) and intradural lipomas (4%) may arise from premature separation of the neuroectoderm from the cutaneous ectoderm, provid-

ing space for mesenchymal tissue to invade the canal of the neural tube and promote fat formation. However, the exact cell lineage and subsequent pattern of differentiation to adipocytes have not yet been undetermined. Fibrolipomas of the filum terminale (12%) probably result from an abnormality of retrogressive differentiation.
- Signs, symptoms, and physical exam
  - Multiple cutaneous anomalies including midline/paraspinal mass, focal hirsutism, dermal sinus, rudimentary tail, atretic meningocoele, and/or capillary hemangioma. Neurologic deficits affect 60 to 70% of patients, but younger children more often have a cutaneous sign caused by tethering or by the lipoma mass.
  - Pain, an unusual finding in infants, is often the most common presenting symptom in older children and adults. It often becomes worse with activity and is rarely radicular in nature.
  - Lipomyelomeningoceles and lipomyeloceles
    - Typically present before 6 months of age with bladder dysfunction common in 50% and half presenting without neurologic compromise
    - Neuroorthopedic syndrome (33 to 50%): lower-extremity deformities such as clubfoot, length discrepancies, scoliosis, trophic ulcers, and hip subluxations
  - Intradural lipomas may present with an ascending monoparesis or paraparesis, spasticity, cutaneous sensory loss, or defective deep sensation.
- Neuroimaging
  - Use MRI for surgical planning and to detect associated malformations (split cord, arachnoid cysts, meningoceles, and syringomyelia). T1-weighted MRI helps visualize lipomas and T2-weighted MRI is useful for meningoceles and syringomyelia. A low-lying conus is found in many patients and suggests tethering in those with small filum lipomas.
  - CT myelography is less informative and more invasive but may be used if MR is contraindicated. CT may also be utilized to assess for bony anomalies.
- Treatment
  - Surgically debulk/resect lipomatous mass and untether if symptomatic, or do so when the conus medullaris is low lying in conjunction with a terminal filum lipoma.[4]
  - Asymptomatic cases: there is debate over conservative treatment versus prophylactic surgery.

- No significant difference in risk of neurological deterioration
- For subdural lipomas, the goal is decompression, not detethering or complete excision.
- If considerable lipoma is found within the central canal, debulk to reduce pressure on neural tissue but avoid full resection, for which a myelotomy may be needed.
  - Surgical pearls
    - When the neural placode is positioned dorsal to the open spinal canal, consider the use of an ultrasonic aspirator or laser to carefully debulk the lipoma.

Dorsal Dermal Sinuses[5]
- Background
  - Thin, squamous, epithelia-lined channels associated with (epi)dermoid tumors
  - Due to a focal incomplete separation of neuroectoderm from cutaneous ectoderm
- Signs, symptoms, and physical exam
  - History of recurrent meningitis despite antibiotics due to bacterial passage along the tract or from chemical irritation if the cyst (e.g., cholesterol crystals) ruptures
  - A patent sinus tract may leak cerebrospinal fluid (CSF).
  - A hairy nevus or hyperpigmented skin may be seen.
- Neuroimaging
  - T1- or T2-weighted MRI usually reveals the dermal sinus tract running at an oblique angle through the underlying tissues, and diffusion MRI can define its margins.
  - Anomalies of the bone may range from absent to focal or multilevel spina bifida.
- Treatment
  - Treat early with excision of the dimple, tract, and any intradural connections or masses.

Myelocele and Myelomeningocele[6]
- Background
  - A failure of closure of the neural tube linked to folate deficiency in pregnancy. The neural and cutaneous areas of ectoderm remain contiguous, forcing mesenchymal tissue that normally forms the posterior elements to become displaced laterally.
- Signs, symptoms, and physical exam
  - Newborn with an exposed, raw, red tissue placode positioned in the midline

- Level determines severity of neurologic deficits, with the most common being lumbosacral or thoracolumbar. Hydrocephalus is common secondary to Chiari II malformation.
- Workup
  - Maternal serum a-fetoprotein (MSAFP) levels may be used to screen at 16 to 18 weeks gestation. Use amniocentesis if MSAFP and ultrasound suggest an abnormality.
- Neuroimaging
  - Associated anomalies include syringohydromyelia, diastematomyelia, lipoma, arachnoid cyst, dermoid/epidermoid, and vertebral anomalies (e.g., hemivertebrae).
  - Chiari II observed to varying degree in all patients with myelomeningoceles.
    - The posterior neuropore may remain open too long, decompressing the ventricular system and allowing the posterior fossa to close when premature and small.
    - Hydrocephalus usually results within 48 hours of myelomeningocele closure.
  - The spine is rarely imaged prior to closure/repair, whereas postoperative neurologic deterioration requires imaging. Symptomatic retethering is a diagnosis of exclusion. If the spine is normal, image the brain to rule out hydrocephalus or shunt malfunction.
- Treatment
  - Surgically close within 48 hours to stabilize neurologic deficits and prevent infection
  - Manage postoperative complications: CSF leak, retethering, and/or hydrocephalus
- Surgical pearls (**Fig. 16.2**)
  - Reconstruct the neural tube and close the pia, dura, thoracolumbar fascia, and skin to prevent meningitis and to protect functional tissue in the neural placode

IV. Anomalies of Caudal Cell Mass

Tight Filum Terminale Syndrome
- Background
  - Incomplete retrogressive differentiation is the suspected etiology.
- Signs, symptoms, and physical exam
  - Possibilities are bladder dysfunction, sensory changes, orthopedic deformities (e.g., clubfoot), radiculopathy, and scoliosis associated with a short, thick filum and low-lying conus.

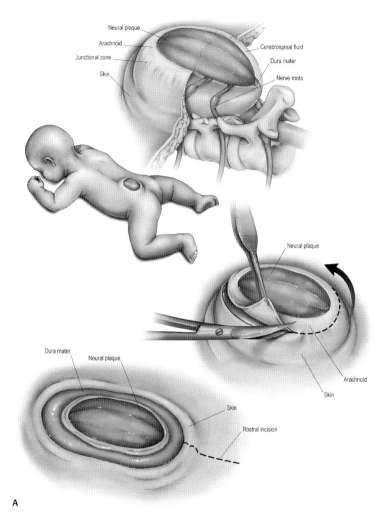

Fig. 16.2 **(A)** The multilayer closure begins with an initial circumferential incision following the arachnoid-skin junction to isolate the neural plaque and spinal cord. The skin incision is continued rostrally in the midline to observe the caudal-most intact lamina and the dura beneath it. *(Continued on page 106)*

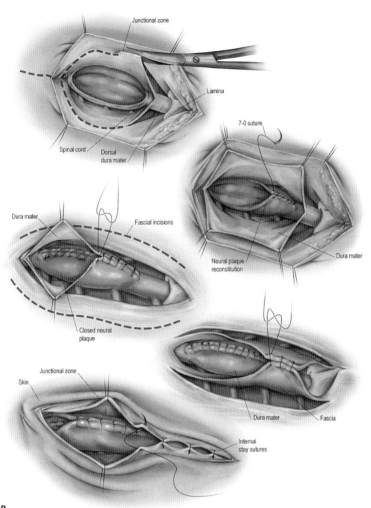

B

Fig. 16.2 *(Continued)* **(B)** An inferior and lateral dissection toward the caudal edge of the defect isolates the dura. The caudal defect is extended and the residual dura dissected. In the midline, the dura is then approximated following that of the lateral arachnoid. The lumbosacral fascia is identified and incised bilaterally with dissection from the posterior iliac crest and sacrospinalis muscle, with care taken to not disrupt the sacral fascial attachments. The lateral edges of the fascial flaps are then folded toward the midline and sutured in place over the dorsal surface of the dura. The subcutaneous tissue, if present, is closed. The placement of sutures in the area where the dura joins the dermis will provide for tight internal sutures that will reduce tension during later skin closure.

- Neuroimaging
    - Utilize T1-weighted MRI. Roughly half of patients have a thick, fibrotic filum with tethered cord syndrome, and 23% have small fibrolipomas. The conus is usually low lying, and 25% have a small hydromyelia within the conus that resolves after untethering.
- Treatment
    - Resect the filum when clinical criteria for tethered cord syndrome are satisfied.
- Surgical pearls
    - Ensure that there are no nerve roots adherent to the undersurface of the filum.

Fibrolipomas of the Filum Terminale
- Background
    - Fibrolipomas result from aberrations of filum terminale development.
    - A long and fibrous filum projects from the conus and penetrates through the subarachnoid space and dura, connecting dorsally to the first coccygeal segment.
- Signs, symptoms, and physical exam
    - Often asymptomatic, patients may not present with symptoms until late adulthood.
    - Following presentation, monitor patient for signs of tethering.
- Neuroimaging
    - May be found in conjunction with a tight filum terminale
- Treatment
    - Resect lipomas of the filum to untether the spinal cord to prevent progressive orthopedic deformity and neurologic deficit and to preserve sphincter function

Syndrome of Caudal Regression
- Background
    - Likely caused by a disruption of the caudal mesoderm before the fourth week of gestation, resulting in an abnormal distal spinal cord and vertebrae
    - Approximately one-sixth of patients have diabetic mothers.
- Signs, symptoms, and physical exam
    - Spectrum includes lower extremity fusion (sirenomelia), lumbosacral agenesis, anal atresia, malformed external genitalia, bilateral renal aplasia, and pulmonary hypoplasia with Potter facies. The vast majority of patients present with a neurogenic bladder.

- Neuroimaging
  - The spinal canal is very stenotic above the last intact vertebra.
  - MRI may demonstrate a wedge-shaped cord terminus, which is characteristic.
  - Lipomas or a lipomyelomeningocele may cause tethering.
- Treatment
  - A large proportion of patients have a tethered cord that may require untethering.

V. Anomalies of Segmentation

Klippel-Feil Syndrome[7]
- Background
  - Congenital fusion of two or more cervical vertebrae. Spectrum runs from vertebral body fusion (congenital block vertebrae) to fusion of the entire vertebrae.
  - Due to a failure, during 3 to 8 weeks of gestation, of normal segmentation of prospective somatic mesoderm into discrete cervical somites. This failure may involve disordered notch signaling and the PAX gene family.
  - Type I: fusions at C1 with or without associated caudal fusions, most often with other congenital anomalies. Type II: fusions no higher than C2-C3. Type III: fusions caudal to C2-C3. Type IV: synonymous with Wildervanck syndrome.
- Signs, symptoms, and physical exam
  - Often asymptomatic, although the classic triad (occurring in less than 50%) involves a short neck, low posterior hairline, and limited neck motion best elicited with flexion-extension or lateral bending. C1-C2 fusions often present with pain in childhood, whereas lower cervical fusions may present in the second or third decade when symptomatic junctional degeneration occurs.
  - May occur in association with basilar impression or atlantooccipital fusion
  - Associated with scoliosis, facial asymmetry, torticollis or neck webbing, Sprengel deformity (congenital elevation of the scapula), synkinesia, or cervical ribs
  - Systemic congenital anomalies: deafness (in 30%), unilateral renal agenesis, cardiopulmonary (ventricular septal defect most common), and a variety of central nervous system findings

- Symptoms rarely relate directly to vertebral fusion, but may result from adjacent hypermobile nonfused segments leading to degenerative arthritic changes or instability.
- Workup
  - Electrocardiogam, chest x-ray, and renal ultrasound. Audiology testing may contribute to workup.
- Neuroimaging
  - Initial studies to visualize fusion should include anteroposterior, lateral, and open-mouth odontoid views followed by serial lateral flexion-extension C-spine radiography to evaluate for instability of the atlanto-occipital, atlantoaxial, and subaxial joints.
  - Image the thoracic and lumbar spine to rule out scoliosis and other abnormalities.
  - Flexion-extension MRI is indicated if preliminary studies suggest instability.
- Treatment
  - Consider activity modification, bracing, and/or traction to reduce symptoms, delay surgery, and prevent major neurologic deficits that may occur, even after minor trauma.
  - Operate in case of progressive symptomatic segmental instability or neurologic deficits.
- Surgical pearls
  - At the risk of further limitations in mobility, occasional fusion of adjacent unstable nonfused segments may be needed.
  - Sublaminar wires should be used with caution in cases of posterior instrumented fusion because they carry an unacceptably high risk of neurologic injury and may not be applicable in children with anomalous vertebrae.

Common Clinical Questions

1. Myelomeningoceles result from:
   A. An anomoly of notochord formation.
   B. Premature dysjunction.
   C. Nondysjunction.
   D. Regression of the caudal cell mass.

2. The majority of spinal lipomas result from:
   A. An anomoly of notochord formation.
   B. Premature dysjunction.
   C. Nondysjunction.
   D. Regression of the caudal cell mass.

3. A tight filum terminale results from:
   A. An anomoly of notochord formation.
   B. Premature dysjunction.
   C. Nondysjunction.
   D. Regression of the caudal cell mass.

References

1. Gan YC, Sgouros S, Walsh AR, Hockley AD. Diastematomyelia in children: treatment outcome and natural history of associated syringomyelia. Childs Nerv Syst 2007;23(5): 515–519
2. Pang D, Dias MS, Ahab-Barmada M. Split cord malformation: Part I: A unified theory of embryogenesis for double spinal cord malformations. Neurosurgery 1992;31(3):451–480
3. Finn MA, Walker ML. Spinal lipomas: clinical spectrum, embryology, and treatment. Neurosurg Focus 2007;23(2):E10
4. Pang D, Zovickian J, Oviedo A. Long-term outcome of total and near-total resection of spinal cord lipomas and radical reconstruction of the neural placode, part II: outcome analysis and preoperative profiling. Neurosurgery 2010;66(2):253–272, discussion 272–273
5. Elton S, Oakes WJ. Dermal sinus tracts of the spine. Neurosurg Focus 2001; 10(1):e4
6. McLone DG, Knepper PA. The cause of Chiari II malformation: a unified theory. Pediatr Neurosci 1989;15(1):1–12
7. Tracy MR, Dormans JP, Kusumi K. Klippel-Feil syndrome: clinical features and current understanding of etiology. Clin Orthop Relat Res 2004; 424(424):183–190

Answers to Common Clinical Questions

1. C. Myelomeningoceles result from a localized failure of neural tube closure, with the neural folds remaining in continuity with the overlying cutaneous ectoderm.

2. B. Intradural spinal lipomas, lipomyeloceles, and lipomyelomeningoceles probably result from the premature separation of the neuroectoderm from the cutaneous ectoderm, allowing mesenchyme to enter the ependyma-lined canal of the neural tube, inducing fat formation.

3. D. The suspected etiology involves an abnormality of regression and differentiation of the caudal cell mass.

17 Trauma

Daniel K. Park and Ravi K. Ponnappan

I. Key Points

- The thoracolumbar spine (T11–L1) is the most common site of spinal injury.
- Surgical treatment is indicated for progressive neurologic impairment, patient mobilization, mechanical instability, and intractable pain.
- Recognition is key to management and prevention of secondary injury.

II. General Principles

- Field management
  - A, **a**irway; B, **b**reathing; C, **c**irculation
  - Spinal immobilization
    - Rigid cervical collar, lateral bolsters, rigid backboard
    - Pediatric patients require recessed head board or pediatric board.
- Emergency room management
  - Repeat ABCs; add **d**isability and **e**xposure
  - Standard imaging
  - Neurogenic shock
    - Hypotension in the presence of bradycardia
    - Management with vasopressors and modest fluid resuscitation
- Classification
  - American Spinal Injury Association (ASIA) scoring scale (**Table 17.1**)
    - Complete: no motor or sensory function below zone of injury
    - Incomplete: partial motor or sensory function below zone of injury (**Table 17.2**)
  - Ten to 15% of patients have noncontiguous spinal fractures.
  - Orthogonal radiographs (anteroposterior [AP]/lateral C, T, and LS spine)
  - Computed tomography (CT)
    - Useful for visualizing occipital-cervical and cervicothoracic junctions
    - Must include sagittal and coronal reconstructions if plain x-ray not utilized
    - Not as useful for ligamentous injury assessment

Table 17.1 ASIA Neurological Scoring System

Grade	Description
A	Complete: No motor or sensory function is preserved in the sacral segments
B	Incomplete: Sensory but not motor function is preserved below the neurologic level and includes the sacral segments
C	Incomplete: Motor function is preserved below the neurologic level, and more than half of the key muscles below the level have a muscle grade <3
D	Incomplete: Motor function is preserved below the neurologic level, and at least half of the key muscle groups below the level have a muscle grade >3
E	Normal

Note: The caudal-most normal level is the neurologic level.

Table 17.2 Incomplete Spinal Cord Injury Patterns

Syndrome	Prognosis	Description
Central cord	Fair	Due usually to hyperextension injury with greater upper extremity involvement and more proximal than distal muscle groups
Anterior cord	Poor	Due to injury of anterior spinal artery; loss of pain, temperature, and motor
Brown-Sequard	Best	Due to hemi-transection of cord or lateral injury; ipsilateral motor loss, vibration, and position sense and contralateral pain and temperature
Posterior cord	Fair	Loss of vibration and position sense

- Magnetic resonance imaging (MRI)
  - Required in all cases with neurologic impairment or deficit.
  - Ligamentous structures visualized on T1.
  - Edema visualized on T2 with short tau inversion recovery (STIR).
- Steroid management
  - Controversial, should be based on institutional protocol (see Chapter 10).
- Surgical timing[1]
  - Early decompression (<72 h) may improve neurologic outcomes.
  - Early decompression (<24 h) may result in better clinical outcomes.

III. Cervical Trauma

Atlanto-occipital Dissociation (Fig. 17.1)
- Background
  - Clinical suspicion paramount
  - Mechanism: high-energy rotational or flexion-extension force
- Signs, symptoms, and physical exam
  - Often fatal; neurologic presentation can range from no deficits to quadraparesis[2]
  - Derangements in cardiorespiratory parameters common
- Neuroimaging
  - Powers ratio: ratio of distance from basion to C1 lamina divided by distance from opisthion to anterior ring of C1
    - Identifies anterior subluxation if ratio >1
    - May miss posterior subluxation
  - Wackenheim line
    - Line from posterior surface of clivus—normally its inferior extension should barely touch posterior aspect of odontoid tip
    - If line runs behind odontoid, there is posterior dissociation.
    - If line runs in front, there is anterior dissociation.
  - Atlanto-occipital condyle distance
    - Should be less than 5 mm
- Treatment
  - Closed reduction with halo-vest application or occipitocervical fusion

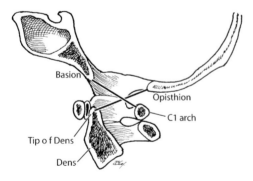

Fig. 17.1 Powers ratio for assessing craniovertebral stability.

- Traction should generally be avoided (10% risk of neurologic deterioration).
  - Surgical pearls
    - Obtain a CT angiogram (CTA) or MR angiogram (MRA) to assess vertebral artery integrity as part of the preoperative planning.
    - Use of MRI for assessing integrity of ligaments may help with decision to fuse occiput to C1, C2, or a more caudal spot.

Atlas (C1) Fracture
- Background
  - Neurologic injury is rare due to large space available for the spinal cord.
  - Can occur anterior, posterior, or combined (Jefferson)
  - Status of transverse atlantal ligament (TAL) is critical to surgical decision making.
  - Mechanism is axial loading.
- Signs, symptoms, and physical exam
  - Typically does not lead to neurologic deficits
  - With severe fractures, complete and incomplete injuries are possible, including medullary dysfunction.
- Neuroimaging
  - Open-mouth odontoid view to assess the relationship of lateral mass of C1 on C2
  - Spence rule (>7 mm composite overhang is unstable)
  - CT scan with coronal and sagittal reconstruction
  - CTA to rule out vertebral artery dissection/occlusion
  - MRI to assess TAL integrity
- Treatment
  - Rigid cervical orthosis or halo for 3 months if TAL intact
  - C1-C2 fusion if nonunion or TAL incompetent
- Surgical pearls
  - Obtain a CTA or MRA to assess vertebral artery integrity as part of the preoperative planning.

Axis (C2) Fracture and Traumatic Spondylolithesis of C2 (Hangman's Fracture)
- Background
  - Associated with high-velocity trauma
  - C2 fractures among the most common spinal fractures in the elderly
  - Mechanism is a combination of hyperextension, compression, and rebound flexion (**Fig. 17.2**).

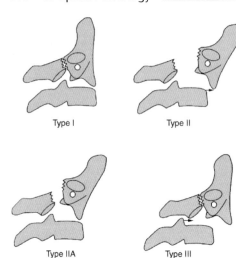

Fig. 17.2 The Levine and Edwards classification of traumatic spondylolistheseis of the axis (hangman's fracture). (From Feliciano DV, Mattox KL, Moore EE. Trauma, 6th Edition; http://www.accesssurgery.com.) Copyright © The McGraw-Hill Companies, Inc. All rights reserved.

- Signs, symptoms, and physical exam
  - Patients are typically asymptomatic with nonangulated, nondisplaced fractures.
  - Complete or incomplete injuries are possible with severe fractures.
  - Cerebellar findings (nausea/vomiting, asymmetric exam, ataxia) may suggest vertebral artery injury.
- Neuroimaging
  - CT scan with reconstructions
  - CTA to rule out vertebral artery dissection/occlusion
- Classification/treatment
  - Type I: minimal displacement (<3 mm) and halo for 12 weeks
  - Type II: significant displacement (>3 mm) and angulation >11 degrees
    - Cervical traction to reduce and halo for 10 to 12 weeks
  - Type IIa: minimal displacement (<3 mm) but angulation >11 degrees
    - Reduction in extension followed by halo; avoid traction
  - Type III: associated facet dislocation—anterior C2-C3 or posterior C1-C3 fusion
- Surgical pearls
  - Obtain a CTA or MRA to assess vertebral artery integrity as part of the preoperative planning

Dens Fracture (C2)
- Background
  - Among the most common spinal fracture injuries in the elderly after falls
  - Sometimes associated with simultaneous C1 fractures
  - Mechanism: hyperflexion or hyperextension (**Fig. 17.3**)
- Signs, symptoms, and physical exam
  - Neck pain and tenderness on palpation typical
  - Usually does not cause neurologic deficits (due to the width of the canal in this region)
  - Severe angulated fractures may cause complete or incomplete injuries
- Neuroimaging
  - CT scan with reconstructions recommended even if fracture is evident on plain radiograph
  - MRI may be helpful for assessing integrity of cruciate ligament (surgical implications)
- Treatment[3]
  - Type 1: avulsion fracture at tip—rigid collar
  - Type II: at the waist/base (**Fig. 17.1**)—rigid collar versus halo versus early fixation
    - Anterior odontoid screw or posterior C1-C2 instrumented fusion

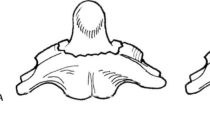
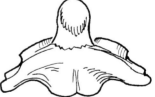
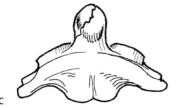

Fig. 17.3 (A–C) Anderson D'Alonzo classification of dens fractures. (A) Type III fracture, (B) Type II fracture, (C) Type I fracture.

- Type III: within the body—halo or rigid collar, based on displacement
- Posterior fixation options include wiring, transarticular, pedicle/pars, intralaminar
- Surgical pearls
  - Ensure that the anterior cruciate ligament is intact before attempting an anterior odontoid screw fixation.

Subaxial Spine (C3-C7)
- Background
  - Particularly common in high-speed motor crashes and diving accidents
  - Allen-Ferguson classification system, based on mechanism
    - Flexion compression: blunting at anterosuperior margin → loss of anterior height → teardrop fragment → <3 mm of displacement of posterior body into canal → more severe displacement of posterior body into canal
    - Vertical compression: central cupping of one end plate → disruption of both end plates
    - Flexion distraction: failure of posterior ligamentous complex with facet subluxation only in flexion → unilateral facet dislocation → bilateral facet dislocation → bilateral facet dislocation with at least 100% vertebral body displacement
    - Extension compression: unilateral posterior arch fracture → bilaminar fractures → circumferential disruption
    - Extension distraction: failure of anterior ligamentous complex → involves posterior ligamentous complex
  - Lateral flexion: ipsilateral fractures of the centrum and posterior arch → fracture of body with contralateral bony or ligamentous failure in tension
- Signs, symptoms, and physical exam
  - Mild compression fractures or nondisplaced facet fractures may not cause deficits.
  - Significant fractures (either in anterior or posterior columns) may cause devastating deficits and/or radiculopathies.
- Neuroimaging
  - CT and MRI typically necessary to appreciate the extent of injury.
  - CTA recommended if any fracture involves the transverse foramen.
- Treatment
  - Based on stability and neurologic injury
  - Considerations
    - Is there mechanical instability?

- Is there neurologic compromise necessitating direct or indirect decompression?
- Are there patient factors (e.g., multitrauma)?
• Stable: nonoperative, rigid cervical orthosis
• Unstable: surgical fusion via anterior versus posterior versus combined approach
– Surgical pearls
• Ending a fixation construct at C7 posteriorly may lead to delayed cervical-thoracic junction kyphosis.
• Ensure the posterior elements are intact when an anterior cervical vertebral body fracture is present. Posterior element involvement may indicate a highly unstable, three-column injury.

Thoracolumbar Fractures
– Background
• Most common region is the thoracolumbar junction (T11-L2).
• Due to transition from fixed thoracic spine to mobile lumbar spine
• Thoracolumbar injury classification and severity score (TLIC-SS) proposes that operative treatment be based upon three factors[4,5]:
- Morphology of fracture
- Posterior ligamentous complex
- Neurologic status
• Compressive flexion (**Fig. 17.4**)
- Instability factors: >50% height loss, >30 degrees angulation, >30 degrees of focal kyphosis
• Flexion-distraction injury (Chance fracture/seatbelt injury)
- Bony fracture without subluxation or dislocation
  - Treat with hyperextension body brace or cast
- Ligamentous injury
  - Posterior instrumented fusion to restore tension band
• Torsional flexion (fracture-dislocation)
• Vertical compression (burst fractures)
- Anterior approach allows better decompression of retropulsed fragment.
- Posterior approach allows restoration of the tension band and reduction.
- Combined approach allows for optimal decompression and reconstruction.
– Signs, symptoms, and physical exam
• Significant fractures at the level of the conus may cause bowel/bladder dysfunction as well as significant lower extremity weakness.

- Tenderness on palpation with or without neurologic deficits after high-velocity accidents should raise suspicion of a spinal fracture.
- Neuroimaging
  - CT with coronal and sagittal reconstructions best for evaluation of middle column
  - MRI best for spinal cord and disc evaluation
- Treatment
  - Stable: nonoperative management—brace
  - Unstable: operative reconstruction ± decompression
    ◦ Neurologic injury considered unstable injury

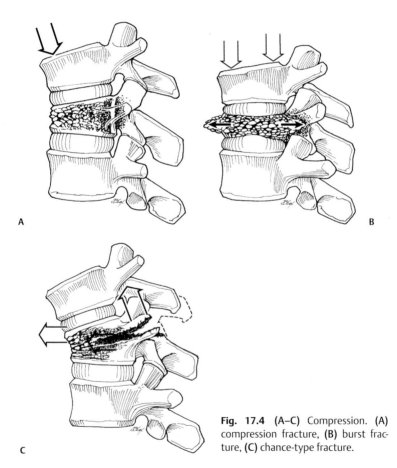

Fig. 17.4 (A–C) Compression. (A) compression fracture, (B) burst fracture, (C) chance-type fracture.

- Approach
  - Anterior approach optimal for decompression
  - Posterior ligamentous complex injury requires tension band reconstruction.
- Timing[1,6]
  - Urgent medical/critical care stabilization/optimization
  - Surgical intervention when medically optimized
  - Early treatment may provide better outcomes and fewer complications.
  - Definition of "early" is controversial.
- Surgical pearls
  - Progressive neurologic deficits (due to expanding hematoma, for example) are atypical but require urgent surgical intervention.
  - Short-segment and long-segment posterior fixation, as well as anterior reconstruction, have all been shown to be effective biomechanically. Choice of approach must be tailored to type, location, and severity of fracture.

Sacral Fractures
- Background
  - Classification (**Fig. 17.5**)
    - Zone 1: across the ala and can affect L5 nerve root
      - <10% have neurological injury
    - Zone 2: through the neuroforamina, causing unilateral symptoms
    - Zone 3: through the body and highest incidence (~56% with neurologic injury)
    - Others
      - Transverse (may miss on plain radiograph)
      - U-shaped fractures
      - Results from axial load
  - Central fractures (zone 3) have the highest incidence of neurologic injury.
  - L5 most common nerve root affected
  - Mechanism: fall from height or associated pelvic ring fracture
- Signs, symptoms, and physical exam
  - Depending on zone involved, sacral fractures can result in significant deficits from L5 root to lower sacral roots.
  - Ankle dorsiflexion/plantar flexion affected with L5/S1 involvement
  - Bowel/bladder function affected with sacral root involvement

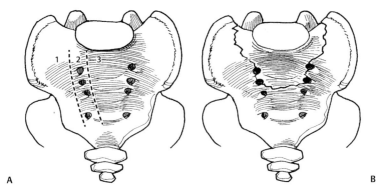

Fig. 17.5 (A–B) Sacral fractures. (A) Zones 1, 2, and 3. (B) U-shaped fracture.

- Neuroimaging
  - Transverse fractures may be missed on pelvic CT and AP radiographs.
  - Best seen on lateral radiograph of the sacrum or CT reconstructions
- Treatment
  - Minimally displaced impacted fractures are stable and may be treated nonoperatively.
  - Displaced fractures require reduction and fixation.
  - Iliopelvic reconstruction/fusion may be required to restore weight-bearing biomechanics.
- Surgical pearls
  - Fully threaded screws should be used to avoid overcompression for sacral fractures.

Common Clinical Questions

1. List these incomplete spinal cord injuries in the order of best prognosis to worst.
   A. Brown-Sequard, anterior cord, central cord
   B. Central cord, Brown-Sequard, anterior cord
   C. Brown-Sequard, central cord, anterior cord
   D. Anterior cord, central cord, Brown-Sequard

2. A patient presents with a ligamentous flexion distraction injury of the thoracolumbar junction. The patient has focal 40 degrees of kyphosis and a normal neurologic examination. Patient management should include:
   A. Hyperextension brace
   B. Posterior tension band reconstruction
   C. Anterior spinal fusion
   D. Physical therapy

3. A polytrauma patient is intubated with an unknown neurologic injury. What is the best modality for assessing acute spinal cord injury?
   A. CT scan
   B. T1-weighted MRI
   C. T2-weighted MRI
   D. Flexion and extension cervical radiographs

References

1. Fehlings MG, Perrin RG. The timing of surgical intervention in the treatment of spinal cord injury: a systematic review of recent clinical evidence. Spine (Phila Pa 1976) 2006; 31(11, Suppl):S28–S35, discussion S36
2. Harmanli O, Koyfman Y. Traumatic atlanto-occipital dislocation with survival: a case report and review of the literature. Surg Neurol 1993;39(4):324–330
3. Maak TG, Grauer JN. The contemporary treatment of odontoid injuries. Spine (Phila Pa 1976) 2006; 31(11, Suppl):S53–S60, discussion S61
4. Vaccaro AR, Baron EM, Sanfilippo J, et al. Reliability of a novel classification system for thoracolumbar injuries: the Thoracolumbar Injury Severity Score. Spine (Phila Pa 1976) 2006; 31(11, Suppl):S62–S69, discussion S104
5. Vaccaro AR, Lehman RA Jr, Hurlbert RJ, et al. A new classification of thoracolumbar injuries: the importance of injury morphology, the integrity of the posterior ligamentous complex, and neurologic status. Spine (Phila Pa 1976) 2005;30(20):2325–2333
6. Rutges JP, Oner FC, Leenen LP. Timing of thoracic and lumbar fracture fixation in spinal injuries: a systematic review of neurological and clinical outcome. Eur Spine J 2007;16(5):579–587

Answers to Common Clinical Questions

1. C
2. B
3. C

18 Infection

William D. Long III and Peter G. Whang

I. Key Points

- Swift and accurate diagnosis of spinal infections is necessary to prevent structural instability or neurologic compromise.
- Hematogenous spinal infections develop from the seeding of the cartilaginous end plates, which allows pathogens to propagate within the avascular disc space before spreading to the adjacent vertebral bodies.
- Granulomatous infections may be caused by one of several fungal, bacterial, and spirochete pathogens that generally give rise to an indolent clinical course.
- Postoperative infections most often develop secondary to direct inoculation of the wound with skin flora and are characterized by pain and tenderness at the surgical site.

II. Pyogenic Vertebral Osteomyelitis and Discitis[1–4]

- Background
  - Vertebral osteomyelitis accounts for about 1% of all skeletal infections.
  - Discitis typically arises as a result of hematogenous spread such that the pathogens emanate from the vascular end plates into the avascular disc space before disseminating to the adjacent vertebral bodies.
  - Pyogenic infections most frequently involve the lumbar spine (58%), followed by the thoracic (30%) and cervical (11%) regions.
  - Gram-positive organisms such as *Staphylococcus aureus* and *Streptococcus* species are the most commonly isolated organisms (67 and 24% of cases, respectively).
- Signs, symptoms, and physical examination
  - The most prevalent signs and symptoms are axial pain (86%) and fever (60%).
  - Neurologic changes such as radicular numbness and muscle weakness may be present in as many as one-third of patients.
  - Patients should be questioned regarding any ongoing constitutional symptoms, travel history, or recent procedures that may be suggestive of a diagnosis of infection.

- Workup
  - White blood cell count (WBC) may be increased in these patients, although in many this value will be normal.
  - Erythrocyte sedimentation rate (ESR) is more sensitive but is relatively nonspecific for infection.
  - C-reactive protein (CRP) is elevated in at least 90% of patients with spinal infections and is a reliable indicator of the disease course because it tends to rise acutely with the onset of an infection but returns to baseline rapidly as it resolves.
  - Blood cultures may be useful because they have been shown to reveal the causative pathogen in up to 58% of hematogenous spinal infections.
  - Urinalysis and culture with sensitivities should also be obtained to rule out an infection of the urinary tract, which may spread to the spine.
- Neuroimaging
  - Plain radiographs are the standard form of initial imaging study for suspected cases of spinal infections and will frequently exhibit abnormalities (89% of cases).
  - Computed tomography (CT) may display early pathologic changes within the spinal column as well as any fluid collections in the surrounding soft tissues.
  - Magnetic resonance imaging (MRI) is the ideal diagnostic modality for identifying pyogenic discitis.
    - Edema and fluid may be evident within the discs and adjacent tissues on T2-weighted images.
    - Addition of gadolinium contrast can enhance the visualization of paraspinal and epidural enhancement suggestive of active infection.
  - Technetium-99m/gallium-76 citrate bone scans or indium-111 tagged WBC studies are extremely sensitive for diagnosing spinal infection but are less specific.
- Treatment
  - First-line treatment for pyogenic infections is administration of broad-spectrum intravenous (IV) antibiotics for at least 6 to 8 weeks until culture-specific regimens may be initiated.
    - Identify the pathogen with biopsy, blood, or tissue cultures prior to treatment initiation.
  - Immobilization may be beneficial for reducing pain and stabilizing the spine.
  - Surgery may be warranted if appropriate medical management fails or if the patient develops neurologic deterioration or spinal instability/deformity.

- The goals of surgery include debridement of the infected tissue, decompression of the neural structures, and stabilization of the spine.
- Surgical pearls
  - Vertebral osteomyelitis and discitis frequently affect the spinal column and may require an anterior procedure (**Fig. 18.1**).
  - Posterior stabilization may also be necessary in instances where there is significant instability or deformity.
    - Avoid stainless steel implants in these cases as there is a tendency for bacteria to form a biofilm on them.
    - Titanium implants are preferred because they don't promote bacterial biofilm colonization.
  - Autogenous bone is an excellent graft material for fusion in an infected surgical field, although allograft and metal may also be reasonable options for select cases.

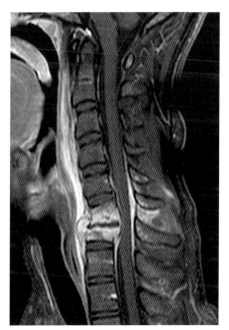

Fig. 18.1 Cervical discitis/epidural abscess with end plate involvement, relative sparing of the vertebral body, and epidural collection compromising the cervical canal.

III. Granulomatous Infections[1,2,4,5]

- Background
  - Granulomatous infections caused by certain bacteria, fungi, and spirochetes are far less common than pyogenic infections in the United States (US).
  - Spinal inoculation generally is done within the peridiscal metaphysis of the vertebral body adjacent to the end plate.
    - An inflammatory response produces a granuloma with a caseous abscess.
    - The infection propagates along the anterior longitudinal ligament to encompass contiguous levels.
  - The most common pathogen is *Mycobacterium tuberculosis*, an atypical bacteria that is more prevalent in underdeveloped nations but is becoming more common in the US.
    - Pott described the first surgical drainage of a tuberculous abscess in 1779, and his name has become synonymous with spinal disease.
    - Neurologic deficits may be observed in up to 47% of affected individuals.
    - The spine is the most common site of skeletal involvement (1% of all patients and nearly 50% of those with musculoskeletal manifestations).
  - Fungal species (e.g., *Aspergillus, Blastomyces, Coccidioides, Cryptococcus,* and *Histoplasma*), spirochetes (e.g., *Actinomyces israelii* and *Treponema pallidum*), and parasites are more unusual causes of granulomatous spinal infections.
- Signs, symptoms, and physical examination
  - Granulomatous spinal infections are characterized by a prolonged duration (i.e., months to years) of symptoms, including back pain and constitutional complaints.
  - The thoracic spine is the most common region of the spine for infection, which may give rise to significant kyphotic deformities.
  - Neurologic compromise and paraplegia may develop more frequently with tuberculous infections than with pyogenic osteomyelitis due to their predilection for the posterior elements.
- Workup
  - All patients should be assessed with a tuberculin purified protein derivative (PPD) skin test.
  - ESR, CRP, WBC, and blood cultures may be less informative in these cases.

- Sputum should be acquired for acid-fast bacilli (AFB) and fungal cultures.
- Neuroimaging
  - Individuals suspected of having tuberculous infections should be assessed with a chest x-ray, which may demonstrate pulmonary disease as well as any extensive bony lesions or focal kyphosis.
  - MRI is the imaging modality of choice and will often show destruction of the vertebral bodies with relative sparing of the intervertebral discs.
- Treatment
  - Pathogen-directed antimicrobial therapy
    - Six to 12 months of a multidrug treatment, including isoniazid, rifampin, pyrazinamide, and streptomycin or ethambutol is the standard regimen for *Mycobacterium tuberculosis.*
    - Antifungals such as amphotericin B or ketoconazole are employed for culture-documented fungal disease.
  - Surgical intervention is not routinely performed for these infections unless there is a failure of pharmacotherapy, progression of deformity, instability, or neurologic decline.
- Surgical pearls
  - These types of infections may bring about considerable destruction of the vertebral bodies, which may require reconstruction of the anterior column.
  - Supplementary posterior fixation may also be indicated to minimize the risk of developing a postoperative deformity.
  - Colonization of metallic implants rarely occurs with granulomatous infections.
    - Avoid stainless steel implants
    - Postoperative imaging with CT and MRI is easier with titanium implants (decreased artifact compared with stainless steel implants).

IV. Epidural Infections

- Background
  - Abscesses most often arise from adjacent vertebral osteomyelitis/discitis but may also develop from hematogenous extension or direct inoculation from spinal procedures.
  - *Staphylococcus aureus* is the most common pathologic organism.
  - Epidural infections usually affect the thoracic and lumbar spines, where they typically exist in the posterior epidural

space; in the cervical spine they are normally located anterior to the thecal sac.
- Signs, symptoms, and physical examination
  - Patients regularly complain of axial pain but symptoms may be more subtle with less virulent organisms.
  - Larger lesions may compress the neural elements and give rise to neurologic deficits.
- Workup
  - Standard infection laboratories (e.g., WBC, ESR, and CRP) with blood cultures
  - Identification of a specific pathogen may require a needle or open biopsy to acquire tissue for culture.
- Neuroimaging
  - MRI is the most sensitive and specific imaging study because it clearly demonstrates any fluid collection in the epidural space.
- Treatment
  - Patients who are neurologically intact may be candidates for nonsurgical treatment consisting of long-term antibiotic therapy.
  - Surgical decompression ± stabilization is generally indicated for individuals who have failed medical management or who present with neurologic deterioration.
- Surgical pearls
  - Operative approach is largely influenced by the location of the infection.
  - While a laminectomy may be sufficient to address posterior abscesses, an anterior procedure may also need to be performed in the setting of vertebral osteomyelitis or ventral abscess.
  - Concomitant arthrodesis may be warranted in cases where spinal instability has been caused by the infection or any subsequent decompression.

V. Postoperative Infections[1,2,4,6]

- Background
  - Surgical site infection (SSI) has been reported in up to 12% of adults undergoing spinal operations.
  - SSI is associated with longer hospital stays, higher complication rates, and increased mortality.
  - Risk factors for SSI include increased age, obesity, diabetes, tobacco use, poor nutritional status, greater intraoperative blood loss, prolonged surgical time, complete neurologic inju-

ries, revision surgery, placement of instrumentation, disseminated cancer, and a posterior operative approach.
- Postoperative SSI ordinarily arises following direct inoculation of the wound with normal skin flora.
- Signs, symptoms, and physical examination
  - The typical SSI is clinically evident and associated with obvious erythema, edema, and drainage from the incision, although subfascial lesions may yield few external signs of infection.
  - Patients may or may not complain of pain or exhibit constitutional symptoms.
- Workup
  - WBC, ESR, and CRP are frequently elevated and may be used as serial markers to confirm the resolution of a SSI.
  - Wound cultures are essential for directing antimicrobial therapy.
    - Sampling of deep wound collections is preferable since superficial drainage is prone to contamination with skin flora.
    - Intraoperative cultures represent the ideal method for identifying the causative organism.
- Neuroimaging
  - CT may reveal pathologic changes such as an abscess or hematoma, but these findings may be difficult to differentiate from nonspecific postoperative changes.
  - MRI is ideal for identifying fluid collections, but in many cases there will be an increased signal on T2-weighted images and contrast enhancement in the surgical field regardless of whether a SSI is present.
- Treatment
  - Prophylactic antibiotics administered 60 minutes before a spinal procedure have been shown to reduce the incidence of SSI by up to 60%.
  - Additional doses of intraoperative antiobiotics should be dispensed for prolonged surgical procedures with significant blood loss or gross contamination.
  - Definitive therapy for established SSI is open irrigation and debridement.
  - IV antibiotics are typically continued for a minimum of 6 weeks, at which time patients may be switched over to oral medications depending on clinical course and laboratory profile.
- Surgical pearls
  - Deep wound cultures should be obtained intraoperatively prior to the delivery of antibiotics and irrigation of the tissues.

- Metallic hardware is frequently left in place to maintain stability, but any loose bone graft should be removed to prevent the formation of a nidus of bacteria.
- Following open irrigation and debridement, the wound may be closed primarily over drains, covered with a vacuum dressing, or left open.

Common Clinical Questions

1. Which laboratory test is best for following the resolution of a spinal infection?
   A. White blood cell count
   B. Erythrocyte sedimentation rate
   C. C-reactive protein
   D. Platelet count

2. What are the most common organisms that are isolated in cases of vertebral osteomyelitis and discitis?
   A. Gram-positive cocci
   B. Gram-negative rods
   C. *Mycobacterium tuberculosis*
   D. Fungi

3. Surgical intervention is most clearly indicated for which of these conditions?
   A. L3-L4 discitis associated with low back pain
   B. Incisional drainage following a recent discectomy
   C. Granulomatous infection involving the T6-T7 vertebral bodies with no obvious deformity or compression of the neural elements
   D. C5-C6 epidural fluid collection resulting in progressive weakness and numbness

References

1. Whang PG, Grauer JN. Infections of the spine. In Lieberman JR, ed. AAOS Comprehensive Orthopaedic Review. Rosemont, IL: American Academy of Orthopaedic Surgeons; 2009:727–734
2. Tsiodras S, Falagas ME. Clinical assessment and medical treatment of spine infections. Clin Orthop Relat Res 2006;444:38–50
3. Mylona E, Samarkos M, Kakalou E, Fanourgiakis P, Skoutelis A. Pyogenic vertebral osteomyelitis: a systematic review of clinical characteristics. Semin Arthritis Rheum 2009;39(1):10–17
4. An HS, Seldomridge JA. Spinal infections: diagnostic tests and imaging studies. Clin Orthop Relat Res 2006;444:27–33
5. Swanson AN, Pappou IP, Cammisa FP, Girardi FP. Chronic infections of the spine: surgical indications and treatments. Clin Orthop Relat Res 2006;444: 100–106
6. Pull ter Gunne AF, Cohen DB. Incidence, prevalence, and analysis of risk factors for surgical site infection following adult spinal surgery. Spine (Phila Pa 1976) 2009; 34(13):1422–1428

Answers to Common Clinical Questions

1. C
2. A
3. D

19 Tumors of the Spine
Camilo A. Molina and Daniel M. Sciubba

I. Key Points
- Spine tumors are broadly organized into three general categories depending on the spine compartment invaded by the neoplasm: extradural, intradural extramedullary, and intradural intramedullary (**Fig. 19.1**).
- Overall, magnetic resonance imaging (MRI) is the best modality for viewing neoplasms in and around the spine and thus best for determining the localizing compartment of a neoplasm.
- Determining which compartment is affected is essential to every aspect of managing the patient. The crucial information yielded includes the primary differential diagnosis (**Fig. 19.1**), the pathophysiologic mechanism connecting the presence of the tumor to the clinical syndrome, and the appropriate surgical strategy.

II. Metastatic Epidural Spine Tumors
- Background
  - Metastatic spine tumors are more prevalent than primary spine tumors.[1,2]
  - Out of 1.5 million annually incident cancer cases, 10% result in symptomatic secondary metastases, and the bony spine is the third most common site of metastases. The thoracic spine is the most commonly afflicted.[1]
  - Peak incidence: fourth to sixth decade. Men are more likely to be afflicted.[1]
  - The two most likely origins of spinal metastasis are breast and lung cancer.[1]
  - The two most common mechanisms of spread to the spine are hematogenous spread and direct extension.[1]
- Signs, symptoms, and physical exam
  - Presentation is a factor of systemic tumor spread, amount of bony destruction, extent of neural compression, and tumor growth rate.[1,3]
  - Physical examination is crucial to elicit appropriate signs of neurologic dysfunction, pain, and palpable masses. A thorough history is essential to elicit risk factors (e.g., cigarette smoking).

19 Tumors of the Spine

Extradural

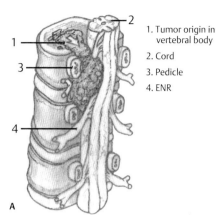

1. Tumor origin in vertebral body
2. Cord
3. Pedicle
4. ENR

Intradural-Extramedullary

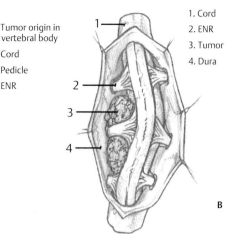

1. Cord
2. ENR
3. Tumor
4. Dura

Intramedullary

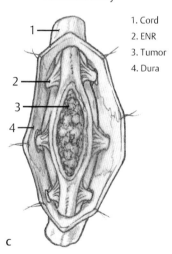

1. Cord
2. ENR
3. Tumor
4. Dura

Fig. 19.1 (A–C) Artistic rendition demonstrating the structural relationship of differently compartmentalized neoplasms to the spinal cord and adjacent structures. Differential diagnosis based on compartmentalization of the neoplasm (from Khanna AJ, ed. Magnetic Resonance Imaging for Orthopaedic Surgeons. Thieme; Pg. 318, Fig. 12.1; pg. 329, Fig. 12.17; pg. 332, Fig 12.22).

- Pain is the most common initial complaint and can be categorized as radicular (radicular compression or foraminal stenosis), mechanical (spinal instability due to compromised vertebral bodies and adjacent structures), or local pain.
- Motor and autonomic dysfunctions are the second most common signs of metastatic epidural spinal cord compression (MESCC).[1]

- Sensory dysfunction signs such as anesthesia, hyperesthesia, and paresthesias are the next most common. When signs are of myelopathic origin, patients describe symptoms as being distributed in a bandlike fashion.
- Compromise of bowel or bladder function and loss of the ability to ambulate are crucial prognosticators.
- Other important signs include those of systemic neoplastic disease, such as marked weight loss.

– Workup and neuroimaging
  - Diagnostic blood work should include prostate-specific antigen assays, blood chemistry, and blood cell counts.
  - The gold standard for imaging of metastatic spine disease is MRI without and with contrast because of the quality of visualization of the bone–soft tissue interface, elucidating compression or invasion of osseous, neural, and paraspinal structures. T2-weighted images and T1 contrast-enhanced images have the highest yield.[1,3]
  - Computed tomography (CT) is useful for detailed rendition of osseous anatomy, myelography studies (in cases of MRI contraindication), evaluation of vascular supply, and whole body scans to detect the tumor of origin.
  - Plain radiographs are relatively insensitive but can be useful to screen for pathologic fractures, spinal deformities, sclerotic lesions, lytic lesions, and large masses.

– Treatment
  - For the most part, treatment goals are therapeutic, as curative treatment is possible only in select cases (i.e., solitary renal cell carcinoma). Therapeutic goals include preserving neurologic function, mechanical stabilization, and pain relief.
  - Surgical candidacy factors include functional status (the most prognostic factor of postoperative neurologic function),[1] age, and life expectancy (with 3 months considered a minimum). Objective scales are available for patient selection.[3]
  - Surgical goals should be achieving optimal resection, decompression, and stabilization (i.e., vertebral body reconstruction and pedicle instrumentation).
  - Nonsurgical candidates can be managed via minimally invasive means such as vertebroplasty or kyphoplasty.
  - Adjuvant treatments include pharmacotherapy (tumoricidal and palliative) as well as radiation therapy (conventional radiotherapy or stereotactic radiosurgery).[1]

- Surgical pearls
  - Although surgical exposure is always of utmost importance, these patients often have poor healing capabilities due to systemic cancer spread, previous use of corticosteroids, and radiation exposure to the surgical field. For this reason, surgical exposure and wound closure should be done with plastic surgery as needed to avoid postoperative wound complications.

III. Primary Epidural Spine Tumors

- Background
  - Ten percent of the tumors that affect the bony spine are primary epidural spine tumors, and they occur more frequently in men than in women.[2]
  - The most frequently encountered primary spine tumors are chordomas, chondrosarcomas, osteosarcomas, and Ewing sarcoma.[2,4] Chordomas are slow-growing tumors and represent 1% of primary spine tumors.[5] Chondrosarcomas are responsible for 7 to 12% of primary spine tumors.[2] Osteosarcomas are less common but are the most common malignant tumor of *osseous* origin. Predisposing factors include adolescence, a family history of retinoblastoma, and previous exposure to ionizing radiation.[2]
  - Among children, eosinophilic granulomas and Ewing sarcoma are the most common benign and malignant tumors, respectively.[2]
  - Hemangiomas are the most common benign and plasmacytomas the most common malignant primary epidural spine tumors in adults.[2]
  - Other, rare tumors include giant cell tumors, aneurysmal bone cysts, osteoid osteomas, and osteoblastomas.[2,4]
- Signs, symptoms, and physical exam
  - Chordomas: The most common symptoms are back and neck pain. Nearly a third of patients will demonstrate signs of neurologic deficit, and physical exam may identify a palpable mass.[2,5]
  - Chondrosarcomas: Signs and symptoms of radiculopathy, myelopathy, cauda equina syndrome, and nocturnally exacerbated focal pain are common.[2,4]
  - Osteosarcomas: The most common presentation is an insidious development of back pain that is exacerbated nocturnally.[2,4]

- Ewing sarcoma: Patients most commonly present with symptoms of pain and local inflammation, and this is frequently misdiagnosed as infection. Signs and symptoms of systemic illness such as weight loss and fever are also common.[2,4]
- Plasmacytomas: In addition to symptoms of pain and neurologic deficit, patients commonly present with diffuse osteoporosis, bone fractures, and osteolytic bone lesions.[2,4]

– Workup and neuroimaging
  - Histopathological analysis of the lesion is crucial for selecting appropriate intervention in respect to each tumor origin (i.e., prognosis and sensitivity to pharmacotherapy or radiotherapy).[3]
  - MRI is the gold standard for chordomas and chondrosarcomas, which are both hyperintense under T2 weighting.[2,5] However, chondrosarcomas can be differentiated from chordomas and other tumors via gadolinium enhancement, which yields a characteristic ring-and-arc pattern.[4]
  - The gold standard for imaging osteosarcomas is positron emission tomography (PET) scanning due to its ability to measure bone turnover. Highly mineralized tumors are hyperintense on T1-weighted MRI. Tumors with low mineralization are hyperintense on T2-weighted imaging.[2]
  - Ewing sarcoma lesions can be detected via conventional radiography because they have a mottled, moth-eaten appearance. The possibility of distant metastases should be ruled out via a whole-body CT scan.[2]
  - In case of suspicion of multiple myeloma, blood cell counts, blood chemistries, and serum/urine electrophoresis should be obtained. These studies may show evidence of renal failure, infections, hypercalcemia, anemia, or Bence-Jones proteins. Diagnostic bone marrow biopsies are also appropriate. The lesions can be imaged via CT or MRI (T2-weighted) and are usually not hot (i.e., no increased uptake) on a bone scan.[2,4]

– Treatment of primary epidural spine tumors
  - The most important prognostic factors for primary spine tumor include tumor identity, location or spread, size, and histologic grade.
  - Ideally, the neoplasms should be completely excised via en bloc resection with wide surgical margins and avoidance of tumor breach. Breach is correlated with a high local recurrence rate.[2]
  - Local recurrence of the neoplasm can be avoided with concomitant adjuvant therapy such as chemotherapy and radio-

therapy (note, however, that osteosarcomas and chondrosarcomas are radioresistant).
- Ewing sarcoma can be managed with chemotherapy, in particular a combination of four drugs: doxorubicin, cyclophosphamide, vincristine, and dactinomycin. In addition, Ewing sarcoma is radiosensitive and can be treated via conventional radiotherapy.[2]
- Plasmacytomas do not need surgical intervention. They can be managed with pharmacotherapy (i.e., chemotherapy and adjuvant bisphosphonates) and radiotherapy. Surgical intervention is reserved for cases of marked spinal instability.[2]

– Surgical pearls
- Primary epidural tumors: En bloc spondylectomy is the gold standard for radio-insensitive tumors (chordoma, chondrosarcoma, etc.). Such techniques should be attempted by surgeons experienced in such procedures, often in conjunction with thoracic surgery, orthopedic surgery, general surgery, vascular surgery, and plastic surgery.

IV. Intradural Extramedullary Spinal Cord Tumors

– Background
- Intradural extramedullary tumors are the second most common tumor type in the spine.[6]
- Primary lesions in this compartment arise from perineural coverings of nerve roots or from the meninges; thus meningiomas, schwannomas, neurofibromas, and paragangliomas account for the majority of tumors in this compartment.[6]
- Although the majority of tumors are benign, they can result in significant neurologic dysfunction.

– Signs, symptoms, and physical exam
- Symptomatology is usually of insidious onset. The most common complaint is localized or radicular (and thus not pathognomonic) pain. Other signs and symptoms include gait problems, weakness, paresthesia, impotence, and autonomic dysfunction.[6]
- The presence of an acute headache should raise suspicion of subarachnoid hemorrhage.
- Physical examination findings include Brown-Sequard syndrome and signs of long tract involvement, such as Babinski sign, clonus, and hyperreflexia.
- Extramedullary tumors can sometimes be distinguished from intramedullary tumors by the fact that intramedullary tumors

spare dorsal tracts whereas extramedullary tumors normally affect all sensory modalities.[6]

- Workup and neuroimaging
  - Imaging is essential to identifying the tumor compartment (i.e., intramedullary versus extramedullary).
  - MRI is the gold standard, but when it is contraindicated, CT myelography is the imaging of choice.
  - Meningiomas, schwannomas, neurofibromas, and paragangliomas are all hyperintense on MRI T2-weighted images. They are all iso- or hypointense in T1-weighted images.[6]
  - Schwannomas can be distinguished from meningiomas because schwannomas may demonstrate cystic changes within the tumor and appear as focal areas of increased signal in T2-weighted images. In contrast, meningiomas rarely develop cystic changes. Schwannomas are also often dumbbell shaped.[6]
  - Paragangliomas demonstrate strong enhancement upon administration of gadolinium contrast.
  - Metastatic lesions should be suspected in a patient with a previous history of cancer, and in such a case imaging should include a whole-body scan to assess systemic spread of the metastatic neoplasm.[1]
- Treatment
  - Complete microsurgical excision of intradural extramedullary tumors is optimal but not always possible due to factors that dictate surgical approach (i.e., anterior or posterior cord location) and the degree to which neural structures are involved by the neoplasm. For example, neurofibromas normally grow from the central root as an enlargement of the nerve itself, making complete surgical resection very challenging. This is in contrast to schwannomas, which typically involve only one fascicle of a nerve root, making it possible to completely dissect the mass and preserve the remainder of the nerve root function.[6]
  - When complete resection is not possible without neurologic compromise, partial resection that avoids neurologic compromise is at times appropriate. This decision is individualized to patient, and factors to consider are patient age, neurologic status at presentation, tumor histopathology and size, and factors predisposing to local recurrence, such as a medical history of neurofibromatosis.
  - The risk of local recurrence can be reduced postoperatively with adjuvant chemotherapy and radiotherapy for sensitive tumors.

- Radiosurgery can be considered in cases of recurrence, multiple lesions, and an absence of compressive myelopathy.
- Surgical pearls
    - Careful attention should be given to removing such tumors from the spinal cord rather than attempting to initially dissect the tumor–spinal cord interface. Often this requires initial internal tumor debulking. In this way, the spinal cord is not manipulated in its most compressed state.

V. Intramedullary Spinal Cord Tumors

- Background
    - Intramedullary spinal cord tumors make up roughly 6 to 8% of all tumors of the central nervous system.[6]
    - The two most common intramedullary spinal cord tumors are low- or high-grade astrocytomas and ependymomas.[6]
    - Low-grade astrocytomas are more common in children whereas ependymomas are more prevalent in adults.[6]
    - High-grade astrocytomas often have a poor prognosis because they are highly infiltrative and have a high rate of recurrence.[6]
- Signs, symptoms, and physical exam
    - Intramedullary spine tumors have a nonspecific presentation. Initial signs and symptoms can be of insidious onset or follow a trivial injury.
    - Presenting signs and symptoms include radicular pain, localized pain, dysesthesia, paresthesia, spasticity, torticollis, extremity weakness, Brown-Sequard syndrome, and autonomic dysfunction.[6]
    - In children, these tumors can present as a failure to achieve developmental milestones.[6]
    - Intramedullary tumors that localize to the cervical spine may also be accompanied by hydrocephalus.[2]
- Workup and neuroimaging
    - MRI is the gold standard for imaging intramedullary spinal cord tumors.
    - T1-weighted images reveal the solid tumor component when performed before and after administration of gadolinium contrast.
    - T2-weighted images allow visualization of cystic elements and the cerebrospinal fluid.
    - When viewed axially, astrocytomas are located eccentrically in the spinal cord and may display heterogeneous enhancement under T1 weighting. In contrast, ependymomas are visualized most often in the center of the spinal cord when

imaged axially. In addition, ependymomas most often exhibit homogeneous enhancement.[6]
- Plain radiographs may be useful preoperatively as a baseline reference for managing spinal deformity, as in the case of scoliosis patients.
- A CT myelography study is acceptable when MRI is contraindicated.
- Treatment
  - Histologic grade and preoperative neurologic function are the most significant prognostic factors for surgical management of intramedullary spinal cord tumors. High-grade astrocytomas have approximately an 80% mortality rate within the first 6 months of diagnoses. Conversely, it is possible to completely surgically resect and cure ependymomas.[6]
  - The approach to surgical resection varies with tumor type and tumor characteristics.
  - Astrocytomas have a grayish yellow, glassy appearance. They should be resected beginning at the midpoint of the neoplasm and moving in an inside-to-outside fashion. The tumor should be debulked until the border between the spinal cord and tumor can be reasonably demarcated.[6]
  - Ependymomas have a red or dark gray appearance and display a characteristic visible boundary in relation to the spinal cord. Ependymomas can be resected en bloc and separation at the tumor–spinal cord boundary can be achieved by applying a microsurgical laser or plated bayonet in the axial direction.
  - Electrophysiologic monitoring can be used to assess the patient's neurologic status throughout the procedure. This includes somatosensory evoked potentials (SSEPs) and motor evoked potentials (MEPs).[6]
- Surgical pearls
  - Often these tumors can be easily suctioned off of the normal parenchyma of the spinal cord when they are necrotic (high-grade astrocytoma) or when a good plane is noted between the tumor and cord (ependymoma or low-grade astrocytoma). Extreme care should be taken to avoid dissecting the plane between tumor and cord with instruments as these maneuvers contuse and stretch the cord; rather, suction should be used for debulking and sharp dissection in locations where the tumor is focally tethered to the cord.

Common Clinical Questions

1. The *least* common histology of metastatic tumor arising in the spine is:
   A. Breast adenocarcinoma
   B. Prostate adenocarcinoma
   C. Non-small cell lung adenocarcinoma
   D. Transitional cell carcinoma of the bladder

2. Classic initial presentations of metastatic epidural spinal cord compression include all of the following except:
   A. Abdominal pain
   B. Bladder retention
   C. Localized back pain
   D. Gait imbalance

3. The most important predictor of survival in patients with spine tumor is:
   A. Presence of metastases in the liver
   B. Histopathology of the lesion
   C. Number of spinal levels involved
   D. Local invasion into paraspinal tissues

References

1. Sciubba DM, Gokaslan ZL. Diagnosis and management of metastatic spine disease. Surg Oncol 2006;15(3):141–151
2. Sundaresan N, Rosen G, Boriani S. Primary malignant tumors of the spine. Orthop Clin North Am 2009;40(1):21–36
3. Donthineni R. Diagnosis and staging of spine tumors. Orthop Clin North Am 2009; 40(1):1–7
4. Knoeller SM, Uhl M, Gahr N, Adler CP, Herget GW. Differential diagnosis of primary malignant bone tumors in the spine and sacrum. The radiological and clinical spectrum: minireview. Neoplasma 2008;55(1):16–22
5. Sciubba DM, Chi JH, Rhines LD, Gokaslan ZL. Chordoma of the spinal column. Neurosurg Clin N Am 2008;19(1):5–15
6. Abul Kasim K, Thurnher MM, McKeever P, Sundgren PC. Intradural spinal tumors: current classification and MRI features. Neuroradiology 2008; 50(4):301–314

Answers to Common Clinical Questions

1. D
2. A
3. B

20 Cervical and Thoracic Spine Degenerative Disease

Clinton J. Burkett and Mark S. Greenberg

I. Key Points
- Cervical and thoracic degenerative disease is a chronic condition but can present as acute.
- Magnetic resonance imaging (MRI) is usually the imaging modality of choice for diagnosis.
- Radicular and axial pain may be treated conservatively, but myelopathy or worsening neurologic function generally requires surgical intervention.

II. Cervical Disc Herniation
- Background
  - Dehydration and fragmentation of the nucleus pulposus of cervical discs with age are natural processes.[1]
  - The annulus and often the posterior longitudinal ligament tear, allowing the nucleus to herniate into the spinal canal, where it may compress the cord or the adjacent root at its foramen.[1]
  - Acute disc rupture occurs more often laterally in the spinal canal due to the relative weakness of the posterior longitudinal ligament in that area; as a result, root compression occurs more often than cord compression.[1]
  - Infarction of the cord and root may occur if compression and ischemia are severe, although it is rare.[1]
- Signs, symptoms, and physical exam
  - Lateral disc herniations cause pain that radiates from the neck to the shoulder/arm and into the hand; the disc usually impinges on a nerve exiting from the neural foramen at the level of the herniation (e.g, a C6-C7 disc is associated with C7 radiculopathy).
  - C5 symptoms: shoulder abduction (deltoid) weakness, shoulder paresthesias, deltoid and pectoralis reflexes diminished[2]
  - C6 symptoms: forearm flexion (biceps) weakness; upper arm, thumb, and radial forearm sensory alteration; biceps and brachioradialis reflexes diminished[2]
  - C7 symptoms: elbow extension (triceps) weakness; second and third digit sensory alteration; triceps reflex diminished[2]

- C8 symptoms: hand intrinsic muscle weakness; fourth and fifth digit sensory alteration; finger jerk reflex diminished[2]
- Central disc herniation can cause myelopathy and central cord syndrome.
– Workup
- Complete history and physical
- Basic laboratory studies
– Neuroimaging
- Based on localization of signs and symptoms
- MRI is the imaging modality of choice for visualizing soft tissue and the spinal cord/nerve roots.
- Computed tomography (CT) myelogram: when MRI cannot be done or when better bone imaging is needed
- Plain CT: good for bone imaging
- Plain x-rays: good for bone imaging, anteroposterior (AP)/lateral views useful for visualizing alignment, flexion/extension views useful to assess subluxation/instability
– Treatment
- Over 90% of patients with acute cervical radiculopathy due to cervical disc herniation can improve without surgery.[2]
- Surgery is indicated for those who fail to improve or those with progressive neurologic deficit who are undergoing nonsurgical management.
- Anterior surgical options: anterior cervical discectomy with or without fusion, plating, or artificial disc (arthroplasty), anterior cervical foraminotomy
- Posterior surgical options: posterior cervical laminectomy/foraminotomy with or without fusion, keyhole laminectomy (for lateral "soft disc" herniation)
– Surgical pearls
- Partial or complete corpectomy may be required if herniated disc is sequestered posterior to vertebral body and is not accessible by discectomy.

III. Cervical Spondylotic Myelopathy

– Background
- Caused by the reduction in the sagittal diameter of the cervical spinal canal as a result of congenital and degenerative changes[3]
- Often due to degeneration of the intervertebral disc producing a focal stenosis due to a "cervical bar," which is usually a combination of osteophytic spurs and/or protrusion of disc material[2]

- Most common type of spinal cord dysfunction in patients over the age of 55 years[2]
- Cord injury likely occurs as the result of several interrelated factors: direct compression of the cord, microtrauma associated with neck flexion and extension, and vascular injury.[4]
- Risk factors include cigarette smoking, frequent lifting, and diving.
- Signs and symptoms may overlap with those of amyotrophic lateral sclerosis (motor neuron disease).[2]

– Signs, symptoms, and physical exam
  - Gait disturbance, often with lower extremity weakness or stiffness, is a common early finding.[4]
  - Cervical pain and mechanical signs are uncommon in cases of pure myelopathy.
  - Typical earliest motor findings are weakness in the triceps and hand intrinsic muscles.
  - Clumsiness with fine motor skills (writing, buttoning buttons)[4]
  - Glove distribution sensory loss in the hands or several levels below the area of cord compression
  - Reflexes are hyperactive at a varying distance below the level of stenosis; pathologic reflexes may be present (e.g., Hoffmann, Babinski, clonus).
  - Central cord syndrome, in which motor and sensory deficits affect the upper extremities more than the lower extremities, may occur acutely after trauma with hyperextension in those with cervical stenosis.

– Workup
  - Complete history and physical
  - Basic laboratory studies

– Neuroimaging
  - Based on localization of signs and symptoms
  - MRI is the imaging modality of choice for visualizing soft tissue and the spinal cord and nerve roots, but cannot distinguish between disc and bone (**Fig. 20.1**).
  - CT myelogram: when MRI cannot be done or when better bone imaging is needed. Can still visualize spinal cord and nerve roots, but does not provide information about changes within the spinal cord parenchyma. Risks of lumbar puncture and/or intrathecal contrast injection need to be considered.
    ○ Plain CT: good for bone imaging and may demonstrate narrow canal, but does not provide adequate information regarding soft tissues.

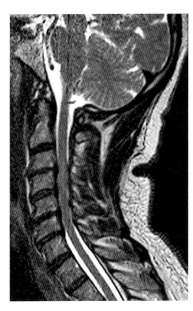

Fig. 20.1 Sagittal T2-weighted MRI of the cervical spine demonstrating multilevel degenerative disc disease, canal stenosis, and signal change in the cord.

- Plain x-ray: good for bone imaging, may demonstrate narrow canal (posterior vertebral line to spinolaminar line <12 mm). Flexion/extension view may demonstrate dynamic instability.
- Treatment
  - Nonoperative management (prolonged immobilization with rigid cervical bracing, eliminating "high-risk" activities, bed rest, and antiinflammatory medications) may be considered for mild myelopathy.
  - More severe myelopathy should be treated with surgical decompression.
  - Surgical approaches
    - Posterior—not ideal for correction of kyphotic deformity
      - Laminectomy alone (higher incidence of late kyphotic deformity)
      - Laminectomy + instrumentation/fusion (lateral mass screws, etc.)
      - Laminoplasty (if patient has myelopathic symptoms without axial neck pain)

- Anterior—ideal for correction of kyphotic deformities
  - Anterior cervical discectomy and fusion (ACDF)
  - Corpectomy and fusion: when compression extends beyond region of disc space
  - Combination of ACDF + corpectomy and fusion
  - Anterior procedures that include more than three disc levels will need posterior instrumentation/fusion in addition for stability.
- Surgical pearls
  - Bone imaging (CT or x-ray) is important for detecting ossified posterior longitudinal ligament (OPLL) when suspected based on MRI. If present, may influence approach (posterior instead of anterior) or procedure (corpectomy instead of ACDF) to prevent intraoperative durotomy.

IV. Thoracic Disc Herniation

- Background
  - Incidence of clinically significant herniation is 1 patient per 1 million people.[5]
  - 0.25% of all herniated discs[2]
  - <4% of operations for all herniated discs[5]
  - 75% occur below T8; most common at T11/T12[2]
- Signs, symptoms, and physical exam
  - Axial pain may be mechanical. Can sometimes be confused with cardiac, pulmonary, or abdominal pathology.
  - Lateral or centrolateral herniations can present with radicular pain around chest wall along the path of an intercostal nerve in a dermatomal pattern.
  - Central herniations are associated with a high incidence of spinal cord compression and long tract signs (lower extremity hyperreflexia, Romberg sign, Babinksi reflex, clonus, ataxic gait, loss of rectal tone, and decreased perianal sensation).
  - In severe cases, the lesion may cause loss of bowel or bladder function and progress rapidly to incomplete or total flaccid paraplegia.
- Workup
  - Complete history and physical
  - Basic laboratory studies
- Neuroimaging
  - Based on localization of signs and symptoms
  - MRI is the imaging modality of choice for visualizing soft tissue and the spinal cord and nerve roots, but it cannot distin-

guish between disc and bone; scout film with MRI of entire spine needed to localize level precisely.
- CT myelogram: when MRI cannot be done, or when better bone imaging is needed along with ability to still visualize spinal cord and nerve roots; does not provide information about changes within the spinal cord parenchyma; can show calcification in disc (occurs in 30 to 70% of symptomatic thoracic discs); risks of intrathecal contrast injection need to be considered
  - Plain CT: good for bone imaging but does not provide adequate information regarding soft tissues
  - Plain x-ray: good for bone imaging and essential as an intraoperative reference to determine correct level
  - Intraoperative fluoroscopy: it is often easier to count vertebrae upward from the sacrum or to use the ribs as a reference than to count down from C1. Use AP to localize since lateral is difficult to obtain, especially in upper/mid-thoracic spine. If doubt persists, intraoperative myelography can be performed to identify the correct level, but risks of intrathecal contrast injection need to be considered.
- Treatment
  - Asymptomatic thoracic disc herniations without evidence of spinal cord compression require no treatment.
  - Symptomatic thoracic disc herniations without evidence of spinal cord compression should initially be treated nonoperatively (at least 4 to 6 weeks).
    - Acute herniations resulting in axial pain
      - Activity modification
      - Nonsteroidal antiinflammatory drugs (NSAIDs)
      - Physical therapy
    - Radicular pain/paresthesias
      - Oral corticosteroids
      - Epidural steroid injections
    - Surgery may be considered for unrelenting symptoms despite nonoperative treatment.
  - Symptomatic thoracic disc herniations causing spinal cord compression should be treated surgically.
    - Approaches
      - Anterior—good for midline or broad-based herniations or densely calcified disc herniations
        - Transsternal or via resection of medial aspect of clavicle (for upper thoracic lesions)

- Anterolateral—good for midline or broad-based herniations or densely calcified disc herniations
  - Transthoracic transpleural via thoracotomy (usually right-sided to avoid heart)
  - Video-assisted thoracoscopic (VATS)—not widely used
  - Minimally invasive transthoracic transpleural or retropleural
- Posterolateral—good for lateral or soft disc herniation
  - Transpedicular
  - Costotransversectomy
  - Lateral extracavitary
- Posterior (laminectomy)—not recommended due to high incidence of neurologic injury

- Surgical pearls
  - The anatomy involved in surgery for thoracic herniated discs is not often encountered by the spine surgeon, who must understand this anatomy thoroughly before taking a patient to the operating room.
  - Calcified discs are difficult to treat via posterolateral approaches, so consider an anterior or anterolateral approach for these lesions.
  - Ensure that the disc level is precisely localized by intraoperative fluoroscopy before proceeding with bone removal and discectomy.
  - Posterolateral approaches may require instrumentation, especially if performed bilaterally.
  - Consider somatosensory evoked potentials (SSEPs) and motor evoked potentials (MEPs) intraoperatively, especially if myelopathy is present.

Common Clinical Questions

1. A C6/C7 lateral disc herniation will compress which nerve root and cause what physical exam findings?
2. On lateral C-spine x-ray, what spinal canal diameter is considered to be stenotic?
3. Is laminectomy the best approach for excising a herniated thoracic disc?

References

1. Hoff JT, Papadopoulos SM. Cervical disc disease and cervical spondylosis. In Wilkins RH, Rengachary SS, eds. Neurosurgery. New York: McGraw-Hill; 1996:3765–3774
2. Greenberg MS. Handbook of Neurosurgery. 7th ed. New York: Thieme Medical Publishers; 2010
3. Placide RJ, Krishnaney AA, Steinmetz MP, Benzel EC. Surgical management of cervical spondylotic myelopathy. In Schmidek HH, Roberts DW, eds. Schmidek & Sweet Operative Neurosurgical Techniques: Indications, Methods, and Results. Philadelphia, PA: Elsevier; 2006:1865–1878
4. Kumar VGR, Madden C, Rea GL. Cervical spondylotic myelopathy. In Winn HR, ed. Youman's Neurological Surgery. Philadelphia, PA: Saunders; 2004: 4447–4458
5. Deckey JE. Thoracic disc herniation. In Devlin VJ, ed. Spine Secrets. Philadelphia, PA: Hanley & Belfus; 2003:264–266

Answers to Common Clinical Questions

1. C7 nerve root is compressed, causing triceps weakness, second and third digit paresthesias and/or sensory loss, and diminished triceps reflex.
2. <12 mm
3. No. Laminectomy is not recommended because of the high rate of neurologic injury associated with this approach.

21 Degenerative Lumbar Spine Disease
Michael Y. Wang

I. Key Points
- Degenerative disease of the spine is a ubiquitous problem and part of the natural aging process. Treatment, surgical or otherwise, is directed at specific symptoms, pathologies, and syndromes.
- Skeletoligamentous disorders are typically the result of intervertebral disc disease, facet disease, or both. Sacroiliac and hip joint pain can also be contributors to back pain.
- Determining the "pain generator" is not always straightforward and requires a synthesis of data from the medical history, physical exam, provocative testing, and imaging.

II. Background
- Degeneration of the lumbar spine is the result of natural aging, environmental insults, and genetic predisposition.
- Degenerative changes may be asymptomatic.[3]
- Specific disease states, such as rheumatoid arthritis and ankylosing spondylitis, can accelerate or alter the pathology and clinical presentations.
- Changes that develop over time include loss of water volume within the nucleus pulposus with loss of disc height, disc bulging, facet joint degeneration, and osteophyte formation across the joints (both the intervertebral discs and facet joints). Eventual loss of motion occurs.

III. Specific Conditions
Radicular Pain
- Signs, symptoms and physical exam
  - Diagnosis requires a correlation between the pain distribution and the compressed nerve root identified on imaging.
  - Sharp, shooting pain in a given dermatome, but it may be dull or aching as well
  - Pain, paresthesias, weakness, and diminished reflexes can be found on exam.

- Workup and neuroimaging
  - Diagnostic testing includes magnetic resonance imaging (MRI), computed tomography (CT) scan (if the offending pathology is suspected to be osseous), or in some cases CT myelogram.
  - If there is doubt as to the level or location of the pathology, a test nerve root injection with anesthetic may be diagnostically helpful.
  - Classic pathology is a paracentral disc herniation; other possibilities include compression due to foraminal collapse, facet joint overgrowth, or a far lateral disc herniation.
- Treatment
  - Treatment of radiculopathy is directed at nerve decompression. This can be done with a laminectomy, laminoforaminotomy, or microdiscetomy.
  - In cases where compression is from foraminal collapse due to loss of spinal alignment (e.g., spondylolisthesis or degenerative scoliosis) a fusion with intervertebral height restoration may be indicated.
- Surgical pearls
  - During a laminectomy, laminoforaminotomy, or microdiscectomy, care must be taken to avoid excessive facet joint removal. These joints are critical to the stability of the spine, and no more than half of a joint should be removed in a unilateral approach.
  - Following surgical decompression scar formation can result in radiculitis or, rarely, arachnoiditis. Minimizing manipulation and nerve root retraction may be helpful.

Neurogenic Claudication
- Signs, symptoms, and physical exam
  - Diagnosis is highly dependent on the history. Patients typically complain of unilateral or bilateral leg pain, numbness, and weakness that can be precipitated by standing or walking.
  - The ability to walk farther when bending forward (as when pushing a shopping cart) is classic.
  - Vascular claudication is suggested when relief occurs with rest without the need to flex at the waist, and must be ruled out by evaluating peripheral pulses (for suspected cases an ankle-brachial index [ABI] may be useful).
- Workup
  - Diagnostic testing includes an MRI or CT myelogram to evaluate the size of the lumbar spinal canal and neuroforamina.

- Neuroimaging
  - Compression may be due to congenital stenosis, disc bulging, ligamentum flavum hypertrophy, facet joint overgrowth, spondylolisthesis, or any combination.
- Treatment
  - Surgical intervention is directed at patients who have failed conservative measures, such as epidural injections, and includes decompression with the possibility of an adjunct fusion.
  - Standard treatment involves the use of a midline laminectomy with foraminotomies.
  - Indirect decompression can be achieved with an interspinous spacer device, which causes focal flexion and stretching of the ligamentum flavum and facet joints.
  - Unilateral hemilaminotomy for bilateral decompression is another, less invasive option that preserves more of the skeletoligamentous structures.
- Surgical pearls
  - Curved Kerrison rongeurs can be useful to reach out to the distal foramina and should be placed on the caudal and dorsal aspect of the foramen, as this is the least likely location for the exiting nerve root.
  - In performing a hemilaminotomy for bilateral decompression, care should be taken to preserve the ipsilateral ligamentum flavum, which will displace the dura ventrally. This reduces the risk of dural injury while work is being performed on the contralateral nerve roots. Ipsilateral decompression can be performed after the opposite side has been decompressed.

Axial Back Pain from Intervertebral Disc Disease (without Deformity)

- Signs, symptoms, and physical exam
  - The most classic disc-related mechanical pain syndromes present as pain that worsens with activity and lessens with rest.
  - Anterior thigh pain can also be associated with low back pain, as the symptoms may follow a somatotopic pattern.
  - Physical examination may reveal pain relief with extension maneuvers and provocation with flexion, although these findings are not universal.
  - It is important to eliminate other insidious causes of axial pain, such as infection or malignancies.
- Workup
  - MRI to examine the disc and neighboring structures
  - CT myelogram when MRI is contraindicated

- Flexion-extension films to rule out spondylolisthesis
- Neuroimaging
    - The disc nucleus progressively loses the high signal on T2 (so-called "black disc") and loss of disc height will also occur.
    - Adjacent bony end plates may exhibit high T2 signal, classified as Modic changes.
    - Plain x-rays may also reveal degeneration, but dynamic flexion and extension views may be more effective in revealing any instability.
    - CT scans may demonstrate osteophytes and are less useful. In marginal cases a provocative discogram can be used to assess the disc's internal morphology, ability to tolerate the injectate's pressure, and any symptoms associated with injection.[1]
- Treatment
    - Treatment of disc-related pain remains controversial and requires that patients have failed conservative treatment measures.
    - For patients who have intractable symptoms and demonstrable pathology, treatment may be directed at disc removal or the elimination of motion.
    - This can be performed with a posterolateral instrumented fusion; anterior, posterior, or transforaminal lumbar interbody fusion (ALIF, PLIF, TLIF); lateral interbody fusion; extreme lateral interbody fusion (XLIF), or total disc arthroplasty.
- Surgical pearls
    - It is generally believed that if surgical treatment of disc-related pain is warranted, then an interbody fusion is preferable to posterolateral fusion.
    - For patients who will undergo disc arthroplasty, care must be taken to exclude those with facet disease, as the posterior joints must continue to function after the operation.

Axial Back Pain from Facet Joint Disease
- Signs, symptoms, and physical exam
    - The zygapophyseal joint (facet joint) is a synovial joint that is prone to arthritic changes and is a possible pain generator.
    - Pain that worsens with provocative maneuvers such as back extension may be a simple diagnostic clue.
    - Facet pain can radiate into the lower extremity, mimicking a painful radiculopathy.
- Workup
    - MRI, flexion-extension films, and single-photon emission computed tomography (SPECT) bone scan helpful

- The definitive diagnostic test is an anesthetic or steroid injection (controversy surrounds the relative efficacy of intraarticular versus periarticular joint injections).
- Hip or sacroiliac joint pathology must also be considered as a possible source of "back pain."
- Neuroimaging
  - High T2 signal in the joint as well as increased focal uptake on SPECT bone scans can be valuable predictors.[4]
- Treatment
  - Interventional treatment of isolated facet joint disease is with anesthetic/steroid injections or dorsal ramus rhizolysis.
  - In addition, physical therapy and antiinflammatory medications are often helpful.
- Surgical pearls
  - Obtain dynamic films to rule out spondylolisthesis.
  - Fusion/fixation of the facet joint remains controversial.

Spondylolisthesis
- Signs, symptoms, and physical exam
  - Spondylolisthesis may be the result of congenital, traumatic, degenerative, or iatrogenic etiologies.
  - A degenerative spondylolisthesis typically affects the L4/L5 level, although any level may become involved.
  - A fatigue fracture of the pars followed by progression of slippage may also be classified as a form of degeneration due to chronic mechanical load.
  - The clinical syndrome may cause leg pain, back pain, or both.
- Workup
  - MRI and flexion-extension films are mandatory.
- Neuroimaging
  - Diagnostic testing can include MRI imaging to evaluate neural entrapment. Flexion-extension x-rays are mandatory to assess the gross stability of the level, which affects treatment decisions (**Fig. 21.1**).
- Treatment
  - Typically involves decompression and fusion. A common approach is laminectomy for decompression followed by instrumented fusion.
  - Controversy exists over the utility of correcting the slippage.
  - The use of interbody fusion increases the rate of arthrodesis but poses the threat of higher complication rates.
- Surgical pearls
  - High-grade slips where realignment is desired can often be treated more effectively by instrumenting the level above (L4-

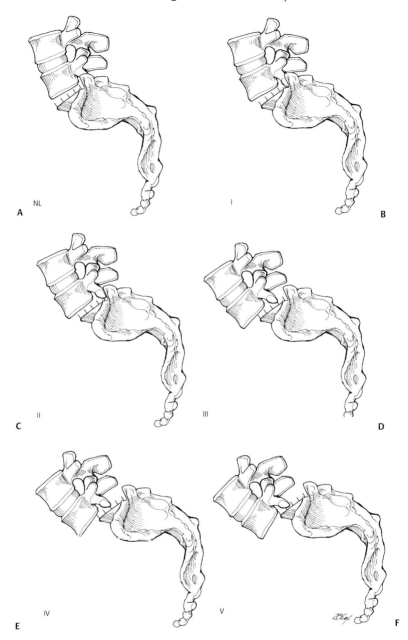

Fig. 21.1 (A–F) Meyerding classification of spondylolisthesis: Normal, Grade I, 0 to 25%; Grade II, 26 to 50%; Grade III, 51 to 75%; Grade IV, 76 to 100%; Grade V, >100% (spondyloptosis).

S1 in a L5/S1 slip) to bring the middle intermediary screw up to a rod connecting the two end screws.
- The exiting nerve root at the slip level is displaced ventrally. Aggressive correction of a high-grade slip can result in foot drop. Close electromyographic (EMG) monitoring for nerve root irritation may allow assessment of the stretch/tension on this structure.

Degenerative Scoliosis and Kyphosis
- Signs, symptoms, and physical exam
  - Evaluation of patients with spinal deformity requires not only a standard physical examination but also an assessment of the patient's standing and lying postures.
  - Any progression of deformity should also be evaluated with serial imaging. The frequent coincidence of hip and sacroiliac joint arthritis and leg length discrepancies needs to be assessed.
  - Because this disease entity typically affects older females, an evaluation of bone density may be warranted and the appropriate measures to augment bone density undertaken.
  - In addition, assessment of any contributing hip flexion contractures may be necessary.
- Workup
  - Diagnostic imaging requires an assessment of neural element integrity (MRI or myelography), disc and facet joint disease, as well as local and global spinal alignment.
- Neuroimaging
  - MRI, dynamic x-rays, and CT scanning are essential for preoperative planning.
  - Thirty-six inch standing x-rays are mandatory to determine coronal alignment (Cobb angle) and loss of sagittal balance.
- Treatment
  - The treatment of this patient population is complicated, requiring significant investment in preoperative planning, surgical intervention, and postoperative care. Critical decision-making factors include:
    - Source and nature of complaints (pain, reduced activities of daily living (ADLs), neurologic symptoms, abnormal postures, cosmetic concerns)
    - The degree of deformity and its relative contribution to the patient's symptoms

- The extent (levels and amount of correction) of the deformity that needs to be treated
- The amount (quality and number of levels) of fixation needed
- The surgical technique necessary to achieve correction
- Need for fusion adjuncts (osteobiologics, bracing, and bone stimulation)
- Anesthetic considerations and risks
- Nutrition and metabolic concerns
- The extent to which rehabilitation will be necessary after surgery

– Surgical pearls
  • Careful preoperative planning, including measurements of preop sagittal/coronal imbalance, is essential to achieving good clinical and surgical outcomes.

Common Clinical Questions

1. Lumbar facet joint pain is best treated with:
   A. Massage therapy
   B. Electrostimulation
   C. Joint injections
   D. Surgical fusion

2. Causes of spondylolisthesis include all of the following *except*:
   A. Neoplastic
   B. Degenerative
   C. Traumatic
   D. Iatrogenic

3. Studies critical to the evaluation of a spinal deformity include:
   A. Blood tests for rheumatoid arthritis
   B. Genetic assessment of predilections for deformity
   C. SPECT nuclear medicine bone scan
   D. 36 inch standing x-rays

References

1. Carragee EJ, Chen Y, Tanner CM, Truong T, Lau E, Brito JL. Provocative discography in patients after limited lumbar discectomy: a controlled, randomized study of pain response in symptomatic and asymptomatic subjects. Spine (Phila Pa 1976) 2000;25(23):3065–3071
2. Fujiwara A, Tamai K, Yamato M, et al. The relationship between facet joint osteoarthritis and disc degeneration of the lumbar spine: an MRI study. Eur Spine J 1999;8(5):396–401
3. Jensen MC, Brant-Zawadzki MN, Obuchowski N, Modic MT, Malkasian D, Ross JS. Magnetic resonance imaging of the lumbar spine in people without back pain. N Engl J Med 1994;331(2):69–73
4. Kim KY, Wang MY. Magnetic resonance image-based morphological predictors of single photon emission computed tomography-positive facet arthropathy in patients with axial back pain. Neurosurgery 2006;59(1):147–156

Answers to Common Clinical Questions

1. C
2. A
3. D

22 Deformity

David T. Anderson and Jeffrey A. Rihn

I. Key Points

- The scoliotic spine has, in addition to a coronal curve, a rotational deformity in which the apical vertebra rotates. The three-dimensional nature of the disease process must be taken into account in planning surgery.
- A magnetic resonance image (MRI) should be obtained in the workup of adolescent idiopathic scoliosis when there are neurologic abnormalities, midline cutaneous findings, a left thoracic curve, rapid curve progression, or a hyperkyphotic thoracic alignment.
- In planning surgery for adolescent idiopathic scoliosis, all major curves and structural minor curves should be included in the fusion levels.[1]
- In younger patients treated with posterior-only fusion, subsequent growth anteriorly can create a crankshaft phenomenon.
- Scheuermann kyphosis must be differentiated from postural kyphosis, which reduces on hyperextension lateral radiographs. Additionally, postural kyphosis does not exhibit the accentuated hump on the Adam forward bending test that is seen with Scheuermann kyphosis.

II. Adolescent Idiopathic Scoliosis

- Background
  - Scoliosis is defined as an abnormal curvature of the spine in the coronal plane greater than 10 degrees.
  - Etiologies include idiopathic, which makes up 80% of all cases, as well as congenital, neuromuscular, and syndrome-related.
  - Idiopathic scoliosis is classified based on age at diagnosis: infantile, 0 to 3 years; juvenile, 4 to 10 years; adolescent, 11 to 17 years; and adult, 18 years and older.
  - Curves may be classified as major or minor. The major curve is of the greatest magnitude and is considered the first to develop (**Fig. 22.1**).[1]
  - Minor, or compensatory, curves develop later and basically serve to balance the head and trunk over the pelvis.

Type	Proximal Thoracic	Main Thoracic	Thoracolumbar / Lumbar	Curve Type
1	Non-Structural	Structural (Major*)	Non-Structural	Main Thoracic (MT)
2	Structural	Structural (Major*)	Non-Structural	Double Thoracic (DT)
3	Non-Structural	Structural (Major*)	Structural	Double Major (DM)
4	Structural	Structural (Major*)	Structural	Triple Major (TM)
5	Non-Structural	Non-Structural	Structural (Major*)	Thoracolumbar / Lumbar (TL/L)
6	Non-Structural	Structural	Structural (Major*)	Thoracolumbar / Lumbar - Main Thoracic (TL/L - MT)

*Major = Largest Cobb Measurement, always structural
Minor = all other curves with structural criteria applied

STRUCTURAL CRITERIA
(Minor Curves)
Proximal Thoracic: - Side Bending Cobb ≥ 25°
- T2 - T5 Kyphosis ≥ +20°

Main Thoracic: - Side Bending Cobb ≥ 25°
- T10 - L2 Kyphosis ≥ +20°

Thoracolumbar / Lumbar: - Side Bending Cobb ≥ 25°
- T10 - L2 Kyphosis ≥ +20°

LOCATION OF APEX
(SRS definition)

CURVE	APEX
THORACIC	T2 - T11-12 DISC
THORACOLUMBAR	T12 - L1
LUMBAR	L1-2 DISC - L4

Modifiers

Lumbar Spine Modifier	CSVL to Lumbar Apex
A	CSVL Between Pedicles
B	CSVL Touches Apical Body(ies)
C	CSVL Completely Medial

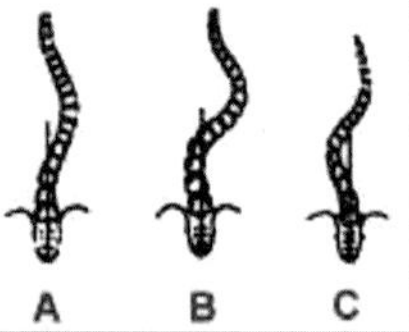

Thoracic Sagittal Profile T5 - T12		
−	(Hypo)	< 10°
N	(Normal)	10°- 40°
+	(Hyper)	> 40°

Curve Type (1-6) + Lumbar Spine Modifier (A, B, or C) + Thoracic Sagittal Modifier (-, N, or +)
Classification (e.g. 1B+): _____

Fig 22.1 Developed in 2001, the Lenke classification provides treatment recommendations for various AIS deformities. Major and structural minor curves are included in the instrumented fusion and the nonstructural curves are excluded. (From Clements DH et al. "Did the Lenke Classification Change Scoliosis Treatment?" Spine 36(14):1142–1145.)

- Structural curves are rigid and cannot be corrected to less than 25 degrees with lateral bending. Nonstructural curves are less rigid and can be corrected.[1]
- The normal spine has a thoracic kyphosis between 20 and 40 degrees and a lumbar lordosis between 40 and 70 degrees, and is straight in the coronal plane without rotation.
- The scoliotic spine not only has a coronal curve, but also has a rotational deformity where the apical vertebra rotates. Most progressive AIS is convex right in the thoracic spine. Any left thoracic curve should be worked up with MRI for underlying abnormalities.
- Scoliosis causes changes in the physiology of the discs and vertebrae due to compressive forces on the concave side of the curve. Increased pressure reduces growth, causes wedging of discs, and changes the remodeling of the bone. All this

contributes to continued asymmetric growth, worsens the deformity, and perpetuates the process.
- Signs, symptoms, and physical exam
  - The physician should include questions about the patient's recent growth, physical signs of puberty, onset of menses, and axillary/pubic hair.
  - Family history of scoliosis should be obtained.
  - A thorough review of systems can shed light on other conditions associated with scoliosis.
  - Important findings in the history include severe back pain, presence of neurologic symptoms, age at onset of scoliosis, and rate of progression.
  - Severe back pain with radicular or myelopathic symptoms requires further imaging with MRI to rule out any specific underlying etiology such as syringomyelia, Chiari malformation, tethered cord, diastematomyelia, or intraspinal tumors.
  - Neurologic history should include questions about difficulties with writing, grasping, balance, walking, or climbing stairs; loss of bowel or bladder function; weakness; or numbness and tingling.
  - Trunk shape and balance should be assessed. The posterior torso should be examined with the patient standing. Look for shoulder, trapezial, scapular, and trunk or flank asymmetry.
  - A plumb line dropped from the C7 spinous process should fall in line with the gluteal cleft.
  - The lateral aspects of the rib cage should be aligned with the ipsilateral iliac crest. Often patients perceive a curve in the spine as a hip or pelvis problem.
  - The Adam forward bending test should be performed. With the knees straight and palms together, the patient is asked to bend forward at the waist. The examiner observes the patient from behind to assess lumbar and midthoracic rotation, from the front to assess upper thoracic rotation, and from the side to assess kyphosis.
  - A scoliometer may be used to measure the angle of trunk rotation (ATR). An ATR of 5 to 7 degrees is associated with a Cobb angle of 15 to 20. The rib hump deformity can also be measured in centimeters.
  - Pelvic tilt due to leg length inequality can be assessed by examining the patient from behind and placing blocks under the short leg to equalize the lengths.
  - Skin should be inspected for abnormalities such as café-au-lait spots or axillary freckling, both associated with neurofibromatosis. Dimpling of the skin, hair tufts, or any midline

cutaneous abnormality may indicate spina bifida and should be further explored. In addition, any skin laxity may indicate Marfan or Ehlers-Danlos syndrome.
- The neurologic exam should include assessment of the patient's balance, sensation, and motor strength. Patient's gait and ability to heel-toe walk should be assessed. Abdominal reflexes, deep tendon reflexes, Hoffman and Babinski signs, and clonus should all be included in the test.
– Neuroimaging
  • Standing posteroanterior (PA) plain radiographs of the entire spine down to the pelvis on a single 3-foot cassette should be obtained. Skeletal maturity can be assessed based on the iliac apophysis (Risser method). The Cobb angle measures the coronal plane curvature and is determined by the angle between the line parallel to the superior end plate of the most tilted cephalad vertebra and the line parallel to the inferior end plate of the most tilted caudal vertebra (**Fig. 22.2**).

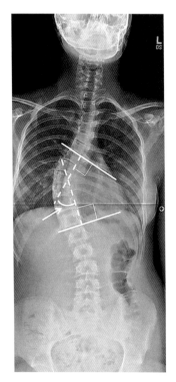

Fig. 22.2 A full-length standing PA radiograph of a 16-year-old female with adolescent idiopathic scoliosis. This patient has a right thoracic curve. The Cobb method of curve measurement is depicted. To perform a Cobb measurement, lines are first drawn parallel to the superior end plate of the most tilted cephalad vertebra and the inferior end plate of the most tilted caudal vertebra. Lines are then drawn perpendicular to the end plate lines. The angle between these perpendicular lines is the Cobb angle.

- Full-length standing lateral plain radiographs are obtained at initial screening if there is back pain, or if there is an obvious sagittal or coronal deformity. Also, lateral lumbar films are obtained to evaluate for spondylolysis or spondylolisthesis.
- PA bending plain radiographs are obtained when surgery is being contemplated. Bending films assess the flexibility of the curve(s) and aid in operative planning. Again, if a curve corrects to less than 25 degrees with lateral bending, it is considered non-structural.
- MRI is not routinely obtained in adolescent idiopathic scoliosis (AIS). Neurologic abnormalities, midline cutaneous findings, left thoracic curves, rapid curve progression, or hyperkyphotic thoracic alignment warrants MRI.

– Treatment
- Curves less than 20 degrees should be monitored with radiographs and clinical exam every 6 to 12 months. Patients growing rapidly should be seen more frequently.
- Curves 20 to 40 degrees are generally treated with a brace. The effectiveness of bracing depends on the remaining spinal growth. The Milwaukee brace has fallen out of favor (because of the neck piece) and has given way to the more cosmetically favorable and comfortable underarm braces like the Boston and Wilmington braces. These should be worn full-time (23 hours a day). The Charleston brace is worn only at night.
- Patients with curves that progress to 45 to 50 degrees are usually candidates for surgery. Factors to consider include clinical deformity, risk of progression, level of skeletal maturity, and pattern of curve.[2]
- According to Lenke and colleagues, all major curves and structural minor curves should be included in the fusion levels.[1]
- Posterior spinal fusion using instrumentation such as hooks, pedicle screws, wires, or hybrid constructs is the mainstay of surgical correction. Pedicle screws give an ability to apply three-dimensional corrective forces that hooks cannot.
- Complications of operative treatment include neurologic injury, blood loss, and implant failure. Spinal cord monitoring is routinely used to decrease the risk of neurologic injury.
- In younger patients treated with posterior-only fusion, subsequent growth anteriorly can create a crankshaft phenomenon.

– Surgical pearls
- Large curves that measure over 70 degrees may be rigid and technically difficult to correct. Combined anterior and posterior fusion has been recommended by some surgeons. Removing the disc and releasing the anterior longitudinal ligament

(ALL) anteriorly allows increased flexibility of the curve along with greater curve correction, and enables the surgeon to fuse the anterior vertebral column, minimizing the risk of developing a crankshaft phenomenon.

III. Scheuermann Kyphosis

- Background
  - Originally described by Holger Werfel Scheuermann, this is a rigid sagittal deformity of the thoracic spine that cannot be actively corrected.[3]
  - The vertebral bodies are wedged anteriorly at three consecutive levels.
  - There are three types of Scheuermann kyphosis (SK). Type I is the classic deformity with the apex between T7 and T9; type II is thoracolumbar in nature, with the apex between T10 and T12; and type III is a lumbar lordosis.
  - The etiology of SK remains unknown; however, several theories have been proposed, including an avascular necrosis of the vertebral ring apophysis, end plate deterioration and collapse as a result of the herniation of disk material into the vertebra, simple wedging caused by mechanical forces, and endocrine and genetic factors.[4]
  - Histology studies have revealed significant end plate irregularities, including Schmorl nodes, which are essentially disk herniations into the vertebral body.
- Signs, symptoms, and physical exam
  - SK is typically idiopathic in nature but can be associated with Turner syndrome and cystic fibrosis.
  - A complete history and physical exam are important to distinguish SK from postural kyphosis.
  - The typical patient presents around puberty and relays a history of a progressive thoracic kyphosis. Often a compensatory lumbar lordosis can be appreciated on exam. Hamstring tightness is often found.[5]
  - Patients may have pain at the apex of the curvature. Pain is more common in athletes.
  - A complete physical exam noting the sagittal and coronal alignment is important.
  - Often a compensatory lumbar lordosis can be established. This is associated with increased pelvic tilt, which leads to hamstring tightness or contractures. Therefore, a straight-leg raise test should routinely be performed.
  - Patients may present with a stiff-legged, short-stride gait.

- As with suspicion of any deformity, a forward bending test should be performed to rule out a concurrent scoliosis, which is present in up to one-third of patients with SK.
- With forward bending, the SK patient will display a sharp (often 90 degrees) hump, as opposed to the rounded back seen in postural kyphosis.
- Flexibility testing and a complete neurologic exam should be performed.
- Neuroimaging
  - Standing full-length PA and lateral views should be obtained. Diagnosis is made based on the lateral radiograph (**Fig. 22.3**). Sorenson defined SK as a thoracic kyphosis greater than 45 degrees with anterior vertebral body wedging greater than 5 degrees at three or more consecutive levels. Normal thoracic kyphosis is between 20 and 40 degrees.
  - Postural kyphosis corrects on hyperextension lateral radiographs.
  - Although Schmorl nodes are common in SK, they are not pathognomonic.
  - MRI should be obtained only if a patient presents with neurologic symptoms.

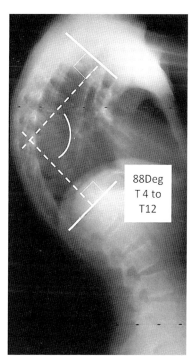

Fig. 22.3 A full-length standing lateral radiograph of a 17-year-old male with Scheuermann kyphosis. This figure demonstrates the technique for measuring the degree of thoracic kyphosis, which in this patient is 88 degrees.

- Treatment
    - The severity of the deformity (greater or less than 50 degrees), the age of the patient, skeletal maturity, and associated symptoms should all be considered in contemplating treatment.
    - Nonoperative treatment ranges from observation with serial radiographs to postural exercises to bracing.
    - Bracing is usually utilized in skeletally immature patients with a kyphosis of 50 to 75 degrees with an apex between T6 and T9. Studies have shown that bracing can achieve a 50% reduction in the kyphosis when worn full-time (>22 hours a day) for 12 to 18 months, followed by part-time (>12 hours a day) use until skeletal maturity is reached.
    - Operative treatment should be considered in patients with kyphosis greater than 70 degrees, adults with residual deformity and intractable pain, a patient with progressive neurologic deficit, and skeletally immature patients who are poor candidates for bracing.[4]
    - A posterior-only approach is indicated in patients with a kyphosis greater than 70 degrees that is correctable to 50 degrees. This approach avoids a thoracotomy, is technically less demanding, and decreases surgical time. Drawbacks are possible hardware failure and loss of 5 degrees of correction in long-term follow up.
- Surgical pearls
    - Rigid curves that are not correctable to 50 degrees or less on the hyperextension lateral radiograph may require an anterior release prior to posterior fusion. Often these procedures are staged and entail longer hospital stay, higher blood loss, and the morbidity of a thoracotomy. Anteriorly, the ALL and the discs are removed at multiple levels to increase flexibility.

Common Clinical Questions

1. When is a MRI warranted in the workup of a patient with idiopathic scoliosis?
2. When planning for surgery in adolescent idiopathic scoliosis, what levels should be included in the fusion?
3. What are the main differences between postural kyphosis and Scheuermann kyphosis?

References

1. Lenke LG, Betz RR, Harms J, et al. Adolescent idiopathic scoliosis: a new classification to determine extent of spinal arthrodesis. J Bone Joint Surg Am 2001;83-A(8):1169–1181
2. Harrington PR. Treatment of scoliosis. Correction and internal fixation by spine instrumentation. J Bone Joint Surg Am 1962;44-A:591–610
3. Scheuermann HW. The classic: kyphosis dorsalis juvenilis. Clin Orthop Relat Res 1977; 128(128):5–7
4. Wenger DR, Frick SL. Scheuermann kyphosis. Spine (Phila Pa 1976) 1999; 24(24):2630–2639
5. Murray PM, Weinstein SL, Spratt KF. The natural history and long-term follow-up of Scheuermann kyphosis. J Bone Joint Surg Am 1993;75(2):236–248

Answers to Common Clinical Questions

1. In the presence of neurologic abnormalities, midline cutaneous findings, left thoracic curves, rapid curve progression, or hyperkyphotic thoracic alignment
2. According to Lenke and colleagues, all major curves and structural minor curves should be included in the fusion levels.
3. Postural kyphosis reduces on hyperextension lateral radiographs. Additionally, postural kyphosis does not exhibit the accentuated hump on the Adam forward bending test that is seen with Scheuermann kyphosis.

23 Vascular Pathology of the Spine

Timothy D. Uschold and Steven W. Chang

I. Key Points

- The Spetzler et al nomenclature for spinal vascular lesions classifies arteriovenous malformations (AVMs) and arteriovenous fistulas (AVFs) according to anatomic location. Lesion classification does not rigidly dictate optimal treatment strategy but may provide a useful framework to guide decision making.[1]
- Spinal angiography is the gold standard and is warranted for all arteriovenous lesions.
- Thorough understanding of spinal angiographic anatomy, surgical vascular anatomy, and segmental variability is essential for decision making.
- A high index of suspicion should be maintained in the presence of spinal vascular lesions. Protean clinical findings, imaging appearance, and low incidence often result in diagnostic delay.

II. Cavernous Malformations

- Background
  - Cavernous malformations are benign vascular neoplasms that may occur in sporadic or familial forms. Spinal cavernomas favor thoracic over cervical locations, with lumbar next in frequency.
  - Intramedullary is the most common location, although intramedullary exophytic, intradural extramedullary, and extradural locations have been reported.
  - Peak incidence of symptomatic hemorrhage is reported in the fourth decade.
- Signs, symptoms and physical examination
  - Acute: due to large hemorrhage, may result in long-tract dysfunction or radicular symptoms (including pain) depending on location; acute meningeal signs are rare.
  - Progressive decline or stepwise deterioration: due to repeated hemorrhages and/or hemosiderin toxicity; improvement between events is usually incomplete.
  - Estimated bleed rates have been reported at 1.4 to 4.5% per patient-year. The rate of subsequent hemorrhage may approach 66% per patient-year.

- Workup
  - Magnetic resonance imaging (MRI) with gradient-recalled echo (GRE) sequences
  - Detailed family history, MRI of the brain, and possible familial screening should be considered. As many as 50% of patients may harbor intracranial cavernomas as well.[2]
- Neuroimaging
  - MRI is the modality of choice. Cavernomas are angiographically occult.
  - MRI appearance: T1 and T2 "popcorn" heterogeneity reflects vascular sinusoids containing blood products of different ages. Surrounding T1 and T2 hypointensity reflects the rim of hemosiderin-stained parenchyma. Hypointense "blooming" notable on GRE sequences, with absence of flow voids.[3]
- Treatment
  - Gross total excision is the treatment goal and is protective against future hemorrhage.
  - Conservative management is a consideration for small asymptomatic lesions, especially deep-seated lesions that fail to reach the pial surface on axial images.[2,4]
- Surgical pearls (see also Chapter 64)
  - Appropriate zones of entry from a posterior or posterolateral approach include midline myelotomy, dorsal lateral sulcus, or laterally between the dentate ligaments.
  - Whenever possible, sharp dissection is preferred. Piecemeal excision is common.
  - Care is necessary to preserve hemosiderin-stained parenchyma surrounding the cavernoma. The developmental venous anomaly should be preserved whenever possible.[2,4]

III. Arteriovenous Lesion

- Background
  - Intradural-dorsal AVF
    - Considered an acquired lesion, attributed to venous outflow dysfunction
    - Low-flow fistula involves radiculomedullary artery as it pierces the dural root sleeve, resulting in arterialized coronal venous plexus. Type B lesions recruit feeders from adjacent levels, but a single fistulous point is always present.
    - Accounts for 60 to 80% of spinal vascular lesions. Typically affects males more than females, ages 40 to 60, and has predilection for the thoracolumbar spine.

- Intradural ventral
  - High-flow anastomosis between anterior spinal artery (ASA) and ventral venous plexus. Varix formation, flow rate, complexity, and multiplicity of feeding pedicles increase with types A to C.
  - Occurs in younger patients (20 to 60 years) and favors the thoracolumbar spine
- Extradural
  - High-flow direct anastomosis between epidural artery and vein, may receive multisegmental arterial contributions[1]
  - Sporadic de novo formation, congenital, syndromic associations (e.g., neurofibrosis (NF)-1), and traumatic etiologies have all been reported (**Table 23.1**).
- Extradural-intradural AVM
  - High-flow AVM, irrespective of tissue boundaries. Commonly involves multiple or entire spinal segments. May interdigitate with functional cord tissue. Commonly fed by ASA and posterior spinal artery (PSA). Rare.
- Intramedullary AVM
  - High-flow AVM with diffuse and compact forms. High-risk features, including varix formation and associated aneurysms, are common.
  - Typically symptomatic early in life (10 to 30 years), with predilection for the cervical spine depending on report; represents 15 to 20% of all spinal vascular lesions
- Conus AVM: high-flow, complex shunting pattern found at conus. Multiple shunts and nidi may be pial or intramedullary. Rare (**Table 23.2**).[1]

– Signs, symptoms, and physical examination
  - Intradural-dorsal AVF: protean history of progressive myelopathy, dominated by gait and sphincter dysfunction. Pathophysiology relates to venous vascular congestion.
  - Intradural ventral: similarly protean, progressive, and variable history dominated by myelopathic findings. Symptomatic progression due to steal, compression, and hemorrhage increases with grade and flow rate.
  - Extradural: Myeloradiculopathy is common, with symptoms due to compression, steal, and hemorrhage. Venous congestion is typically rare.
  - Extradural-intradural AVM: malignant natural history characterized by progressive myelopathy. Radicular pain referable to the involved segment is typical. Pathophysiology involves mass effect, steal, hemorrhage, and compression.

Table 23.1 Spetzler et al AVF Classification[1]

Type	Shunt location	Pathophysiology	Symptoms	Imaging	Treatment
Intradural dorsal A (single-level feeder) B (multiple feeders)	Intradural entry of radiculomedullary artery at root sleeve	Vascular congestion due to venous outflow obstruction	Progressive myelopathy	MRI shows dorsal flow voids and T2 cord change DSA gold standard	Surgery vs endovascular
Intradural ventral* A B C	Direct fistula to anterior spinal artery	Mass effect, steal, or hemorrhage progressive with grade	Progressive myelopathy	MRI shows ventral flow voids DSA gold standard	Surgery. Endovascular may be more appropriate alternative with progressive grade
Extradural	Epidural artery and vein	Primarily compression and steal over congestion May hemorrhage	Progressive myelopathy and/or radiculopathy	MRI shows epidural engorgement DSA gold standard	Primarily endovascular, except when decline due to hemorrhage

*Types are characterized by increasing flow rate, varix formation, and venous dilation.
Abbreviations: AVF, arteriovenous fistula; DSA, digital subtraction angiogram; MRI, magnetic resonance imaging.

Table 23.2 Spetzler et al AVM Classification[1]

Type	Distinguishing features	Pathophysiology	Symptoms	Treatment
Extradural-intradural	Irrespective of normal tissue planes. May involve entire metamere	Steal, compression, hemorrhage	Progressive myelopathy, often with radicular-type pain	Multimodality, typically palliative
Intramedullary Compact nidus Diffuse nidus	Typically with at least one ASA feeder. PSA feeders also common. High flow–associated aneurysms and varices	Hemorrhage, steal, compression	Acute or stepwise progression of radicular pain and long-tract signs (e.g., myelopathy)	Primarily surgical. Preoperative embolization typically useful
Conus	Complex shunting and nidal patterns typically involve ASA and PSA	Steal, hemorrhage, venous congestion	Progressive myelopathy and/or radiculopathy. Symptoms referable to conus location	Multimodality (endovascular + surgery)

Abbreviations: ASA, anterior spinal artery; AVM, arteriovenous malformation; PSA, posterior spinal artery.

- Intramedullary AVM: malignant natural history characterized by progressive myeloradiculopathy. Stepwise deterioration or acute decline attributable to repeated hemorrhage, steal, and compression.
- Conus AVM: progressive myeloradiculopathy, symptoms referable to conus[1]
  - Workup
    - Spinal MRI/magnetic resonance angiography (MRA) has proven especially useful for intradural dorsal lesions. MRA may be sufficiently sensitive to identify the fistula type, to pinpoint the level(s) of the shunt, and to confirm treatment at follow-up.
    - Spinal angiography, however, remains the gold standard imaging modality (for all spinal AVFs and AVMs) and may be directed more precisely after careful inspection of prior MRA.
  - Neuroimaging
    - AVMs
      - MRI is most useful to delineate the size and configuration of the nidus (compact vs diffuse), to evaluate for hemorrhage, and to assess the angioarchitecture.
    - Intradural dorsal AVF
      - MRI: In the appropriate clinical setting, extensive intramedullary T2 hyperintensity along with intradural flow voids along the dorsal pial surface is nearly pathognomonic. Enhancement may be variable.
      - Angiography: Venous outflow is sluggish, and long venous phase may be necessary. Suspected but occult intradural-dorsal fistulas require surgical exploration.
    - Intradural ventral
      - MRI: reveals variable T2 hyperintensity and/or enhancement with dilated flow voids along the ventral surface of the spinal cord. Identifies varix formation.
      - Angiography: reveals a direct fistula between the radiculomedullary artery and ASA. The ASA is identified by the classic hairpin loop and may be displaced from midline. The ventral arterialized vein often harbors a prominent venous varix.
    - Extradural: MRI/MRA: prominent epidural flow voids and enhancement, typically with significant mass effect. Variable T2 intramedullary signal change.[3]
  - Treatment
    - Intradural-dorsal AVF: Microsurgical clip occlusion at intradural fistulous point remains the gold standard. Embolization with liquid agent now acceptable first-line treatment, but associated with greater risk of recurrence.[5]

- Intradural-ventral AVF: Microsurgical fistula obliteration remains treatment of choice, but embolic strategies often used as well. Vessel caliber (particularly type A and B) and proximity to ASA present challenges to endovascular management.
- Extradural AVF: Large-caliber feeding vessels favor coil embolization.
- Extradural-intradural AVM: Curative resection is atypical. Multimodal palliation strategies ameliorate symptoms due to steal, compression, and/or hemorrhage.
- Intramedullary AVM: Surgical resection, typically via a posterior or posterolateral approach, remains the gold standard and is typically preceded by attempts at embolization in appropriately selected patients.[6]
- Conus AVM: Multimodal strategies include aggressive embolization and resection.[1]

– Surgical pearls
- Indocyanine green angiography (ICG) is ideal for intraoperative confirmation of location and essential for the identification of angiographically occult lesions.
- Intramedullary AVMs are commonly fed by at least one branch of the ASA. Steal phenomena may obscure ASA involvement on preoperative angiography, but serial runs mid-resection may reveal the ASA as shunting is progressively eliminated.
- Arterial supply is circumferentially addressed first for intramedullary AVMs. Venous outflow is spared until the lesion is sufficiently devascularized.

Common Clinical Questions

1. The Spetzler et al nomenclature divides arteriovenous lesions solely on the basis of what characteristic?
2. What imaging modality is the gold standard and is mandatory for all spinal arteriovenous lesions?
3. Describe the typical imaging findings of an intradural-dorsal fistula on MRI.

References

1. Spetzler RF, Detwiler PW, Riina HA, Porter RW. Modified classification of spinal cord vascular lesions. J Neurosurg 2002;96(2, Suppl):145–156
2. Perrini P, Uygur E, Spetzler RF, Lanzino G. Cavernous malformations of the spinal cord. In Lanzino G, Spetzler RF, eds. Cavernous Malformations of the Brain and Spinal Cord. New York: Thieme Medical Publishers; 2008:88–93
3. Jackson J, Partovi S. Imaging of spinal cord vascular malformations. Operative Techniques in Neurosurgery. 2003;6(3):125–140
4. Vishteh AG, Sankhla S, Anson JA, Zabramski JM, Spetzler RF. Surgical resection of intramedullary spinal cord cavernous malformations: delayed complications, long-term outcomes, and association with cryptic venous malformations. Neurosurgery 1997;41(5):1094–1100, discussion 1100–1101
5. Steinmetz MP, Chow MM, Krishnaney AA, et al. Outcome after the treatment of spinal dural arteriovenous fistulae: a contemporary single-institution series and meta-analysis. Neurosurgery 2004;55(1):77–87, discussion 87–88
6. Connolly ES Jr, Zubay GP, McCormick PC, Stein BM. The posterior approach to a series of glomus (Type II) intramedullary spinal cord arteriovenous malformations. Neurosurgery 1998;42(4):774–785, discussion 785–786

Answers to Common Clinical Questions

1. Anatomic location; all other characteristics follow suit
2. Angiography
3. Dorsal flow voids, extensive T2 signal change, variable and patchy enhancement

24 Spondyloarthropathies

Amir Ahmadian and Fernando L. Vale

I. Key Points

- Spondyloarthropathies are subdivided into seronegative and seropositive arthropathies (positive vs. negative antinuclear antibody [ANA] or rheumatoid factor [RF]).
- A family of described disorders/syndromes with overlapping symptomology with varying human leukocyte antigen (HLA) associations, including ankylosing spondylitis (AS), psoriatic arthritis, enteropathic arthritis, Reiter syndrome, ossification of the posterior longitudinal ligament (OPLL), and rheumatoid arthritis (RA)
- RA with high incidence of C-spine involvement (>85%)[1]
- In RA, atlantoaxial subluxation (AAS) classified by anterior atlantodental interval (ADI) ≤3 mm (stable) and posterior atlantodental interval (PADI) ≤14 mm (increased risk of injury)
- OPLL: Asians, mostly asymptomatic, surgical approach controversial. Computed tomography (CT) for evaluation of posterior longitudinal ligament (PLL) calcification/ossification.
- Diffuse idiopathic skeletal hyperostosis (DISH): sacroiliac sparing, osteophytic change, associated with globus and dysphagia

II. Ankylosing Spondylitis Seronegative Arthropathy

- Background
  - Also called Marie-Strümpell disease.[1] Affects 0.1 to 0.2% of the population, with a male : female ratio of 3 : 1. Peak age of onset: teens to fourth decade of life.[2]
  - A chronic systemic inflammatory disease (strongest correlation with HLA-B27). CD4, CD8, and cytokine (tumor necrosis factor [TNF]-α and -β) mediated.[3–5]
  - AS specifically involves the sacroiliac joints and progresses to involve the entire spine. It may also variably involve peripheral joints, eyes, skin, and the cardiac and intestinal systems.
  - Increased risk (up to 20%) if there is a first-degree relative with HLA-B27 and AS[6]
  - Enthesitis: chronic inflammation at the insertion point of tendons that leads to ossification[5]

- Enthesopathy leads to osteoporosis of vertebral bodies and disc with sparing of nucleus pulposus (bridging osteophytes), producing the so-called bamboo spine.[1]
- Signs, symptoms, and physical exam[1,5]
  - Initial nonradiating back pain and morning stiffness (>45 minutes) that improves with exercise/activity
  - Stiffness of the gluteal and lumbosacral junction (sacroiliitis)
  - Progression of symptoms to entire spinal axis
  - Eventual decrease in range of motion (autofusion)
  - Tendon/ligament involvement (plantar fasciitis/Achilles tendonitis)
  - Differential diagnosis: rheumatoid arthritis (RF+), DISH (also called Forestier disease) (spares facet and sacroiliac [SI] joint, later age of onset than AS), psoriatic arthritis/Reiter syndrome (milder with asymmetric sacroiliitis)
  - The Patrick or FABERE (flexion, abduction, external rotation, extension) test: flex hip, flex knee, and place the lateral malleolus on contralateral knee; then press the ipsilateral knee downward (by stressing the hip joint); will cause pain in bursitis, sacroiliitis, and other hip joint pathology
  - Cauda equina syndrome: usually no obvious etiology or compression
  - Unstable rotatory subluxation (occipitoatlantal or atlantoaxial joint)
  - Myelopathy: due to bow stringing of cord
  - Significant fractures with minimal trauma
- Workup
  - Modified New York criteria (radiographic sacroiliitis and back pain >3 months, limited spine motion in sagittal/frontal planes, or limited chest expansion)
- Neuroimaging
  - Plain x-rays (crucial for diagnosis): obtain x-rays of entire spine (bamboo spine) and pelvis (SI joint) (**Fig. 24.1**)
  - Magnetic resonance imaging (MRI): for further evaluation of disc spaces and ligamentous changes
  - Bone scan: increased uptake at SI joint
- Treatment
  - Medical management with nonsteroidal antiinflammatory drugs (NSAIDs), sulfasalazine, TNF-α antagonists, and corticosteroids
  - Stable fracture: treatment with rigid brace
  - Surgical decompression for inpatients with unstable fractures and/or progressive neurologic deficit

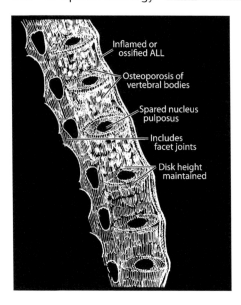

Fig. 24.1 "Bamboo spine" in ankylosing spondylitis.

- Surgical pearls[1,5]
  - Special care needed with routine neck immobilization after trauma intraoperatively in patients with AS. These patients tend to have the neck fixed in flexed position. Forced inline fixation may be deleterious, so fix neck in natural position.
  - If patient is placed in traction, special attention to degree of kyphosis is necessary. Traction must be in line with patient's natural kyphosis and not directly horizontal.
  - No consensus on treatment for cord injury in AS patients (halo vs internal fixation) without obvious compression
  - Root/cord compression: laminectomy and fusion recommended
  - Posterior approach should be strongly considered secondary to anterior bridging osteophytes and concerns with fixation of anterior plate for osteoporotic vertebral body.
  - Consider posterior osteotomy and fusion for correction of severe kyphotic deformity

III. Rheumatoid Arthritis

- Background
  - Very high incidence of C-spine involvement (atlantoaxial subluxation [anterior > posterior], basilar impression, pannus granulation of odontoid)[5,7]

- 2 : 1 female : male ratio; peak incidence in fourth to fifth decade of life
- Serum RF+: 1 to 2% prevalence
- AAS: erosion at C1-C2 joint and at transverse ligament insertion
– Signs, symptoms, and physical exam
  - Morning stiffness, symmetric multi-joint arthritis (particularly the proximal interphalangeal [PIP], metacarpophalangeal [MCP], and metatarsophalangeal [MTP]), rheumatoid nodule (extensor surface)
  - Radiographic decalcification at joints (x-ray hand)
  - Neck pain with possible C2 radiculopathy
  - Headache, paresthesias, difficulty with ambulation, and signs of cervicomedullary junction compression (basilar impression)
– Workup
  - ADI: ≤3 mm for evaluation of integrity of the transverse ligament; does *not* correlate with risk of injury[8]
  - PADI: essentially the amount of space for the cord at C1-C2; *does* correlate with risk of injury if ≤14 mm[5,8]
  - Look for basilar impression and cervicomedullary junction compression
– Neuroimaging
  - Lateral C-spine x-ray: ADI (anterior aspect of odontoid to arch of C1) / PADI (posterior aspect of vertebral body to spinolaminar line)
  - MRI for evaluation of degree of stenosis (pannus)
– Treatment
  - Surgical treatment of asymptomatic AAS can be considered when ADI >6 to 10 mm.[9]
  - AAS in RA will progress with time; therefore, treatment is recommended, especially if myelopathy exists.
  - Rigid collar does not support C1-C2 and is therefore a poor option.
  - Immobilization of the C1-C2 joint via halo or posterior fusion alone may reduce the size of pannus over time.
  - May use halo traction to align the odontoid and return it to its neutral position (start with 5 lb).
– Surgical pearls[5]
  - Anterior, posterior, or vertical subluxation: most cases will require 360 degrees of fusion.
  - Rotational or lateral subluxation: posterior-only approach is adequate.

- Posterior fusion with or without laminectomy (C1): C1-C2 fusion, C2-occiput
- Anterior approach: odontoidectomy. For transoral approach the patient's mouth must be able to open at least 25 mm.[1] Patient is to remain in halo traction until fusion.
- RA with concomicant basilar impression should first be reduced and then fused.
- Transoral approach is associated with higher morbidity and usually reserved as a second option to posterior fusion.

IV. Diffuse Idiopathic Skeletal Hyperostosis

- Background
  - Significant osteophyte formation in absence of significant degeneration. Distinct from degenerative disease, OPLL, and AS (**Fig. 24.2**).[10]
  - Males in seventh decade of life
  - SI joint spared[11]
  - Osteophytes do not stabilize, and unfused they are unstable. Minor trauma can lead to significant injury.
- Signs, symptoms, and physical exam
  - Morning stiffness (milder than with AS)
  - Globus: sensation of lump in the throat, secondary to large anterior vertebral body osteophyte adjacent to esophagus
  - Dysphagia with or without weight loss[1]

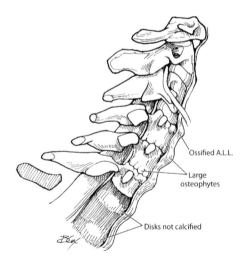

Fig. 24.2 Diffuse idiopathic skeletal hyperostosis in the cervical spine. Note the continuous osteophyte formation along the anterior border of the cervical spine.

- Neuroimaging/workup/treatment
    - Dysphagia: speech therapy consult to rule out primary esophageal pathology, diet modification, barium swallow (to localize obstruction). Progressive dysphagia with weight loss may benefit from surgical debulking.[5]
    - CT scan superior to x-ray for evaluation of osteophytic structures
    - Conservative treatment unless mass effect on esophagus or surrounding structures causes significant health risk (i.e., weight loss from dysphagia, pneumonia, and respiratory difficulty)
    - Initially a change in diet to soft mechanical may be beneficial.
- Surgical pearls
    - Anterior approach, drill down osteophyte. Special attention needed for protection of surrounding structures.
    - No instrumentation needed. Debulking only. Do not violate disc space.[7]
    - Initially, postop patients may have increased dysphagia. Risk of gastrostomy tube requirement.[1]

V. Ossification of the Posterior Longitudinal Ligament

- Background
    - Calcification with subsequent ossification of PLL. Can occur in any part of the spinal column and can extend into dura. Most commonly cervical (C3-C6).
    - Classified as segmental when ossification skips area behind disc space and is present only behind each vertebral body. (Mixed type and focal form exist.)
    - Increased incidence in Asian (Japanese) population (prevalence around 2%).[5,12] Prevalence increases with age (average age at time of diagnosis is mid-50s).
- Signs, symptoms, and physical exam
    - Most are asymptomatic but can progress to myelopathy over time.[13]
    - Symptoms can range from subjective neck pain to severe myelopathy.
- Neuroimaging/workup
    - Plain x-rays will miss the ossification. Therefore, CT is suggested when OPLL is suspected.
    - MRI or CT with intrathecal contrast for evaluation of degree of stenosis
    - MRI: ossified PLL is dark on T1 and T2.

- Consider glucose level check given the higher frequency of OPLL patients with diabetes mellitus (DM)
- Treatment
  - Surgical treatment required to decompress the spinal cord. Patients with myelopathy can benefit from early decompression.
  - Patients with mild subjective complaints can be treated conservatively.
- Surgical pearls
  - Nasotracheal/fiberoptic intubation should be strongly considered to prevent hyperextension.
  - Surgeon's prerogative as to whether or not to leave a thin rim of ossified PLL attached to the dura during decompression. Note that the ossification usually extends into the dura and is inseparable.[1]
  - Anterior approach (corpectomy) as opposed to posterior (laminectomy/laminotomy) decompression is controversial because of the significant risk associated with resecting all of the OPLL.[14] Leaving a thin layer of bone that is adherent to the dura is recommended. Nerve root decompression is required.[7]
  - Somatosensory evoked potential (SSEP) monitoring highly recommended.

24 Spondyloarthropathies

Common Clinical Questions

1. A 65-year-old male comes to the hospital after a motor vehicle accident complaining of neck and back pain. Further questioning reveals that the patient has had a history of chronic neck ache with morning "back stiffness." He also admits to having mild dysphagia with the sensation of a lump in his throat. Initial x-rays show significant vertebral osteophyte formation but are otherwise negative. Hip x-rays show normal hip and pelvic joints with no fractures. What is the patient's most likely diagnosis?
   A. OPLL
   B. DISH
   C. Ankylosing spondylitis
   D. Acute cervical fracture

2. A 65-year-old Japanese male comes to your office complaining of not being able to keep objects in his hands and "dropping things." Your exam is positive for bilateral Hoffman 3+ reflexes and 4/5 weakness of intrinsic hand muscles. Cervical spine MRI with central canal stenosis and cervical dynamic x-rays are normal. Careful analysis of MRI indicates a hypointense signal on T1 and T2 lining the posterior side of the vertebral body at C3-C5 with sparing of disc space. What is the most likely diagnosis?
   A. Primary bone tumor
   B. Metastatic disease
   C. DISH
   D. Segmental OPLL

3. True or false: An ADI >3 mm correlates with increased risk of cervical injury.

4. Dynamic imaging indicates C1-C2 instability. Which of the following is *not* a recommended treatment?
   A. Cervical fusion secondary to ADI >10 mm
   B. Rigid cervical collar with close follow-up
   C. Halo fixation with subsequent close follow-up imaging in an effort to decrease pannus size
   D. Cervical fusion and decompression secondary to symptoms of myelopathy

5. True or false: Enthesitis is a chronic inflammation at the insertion point of the tendons into the spine that can become ossified.

References

1. Greenberg MS. Handbook of Neurosurgery. 7th ed. New York: Thieme Medical Publishers; 2010
2. Braun J, Sieper J. Ankylosing spondylitis. Lancet 2007;369(9570):1379–1390
3. Reveille JD, Ball EJ, Khan MA. HLA-B27 and genetic predisposing factors in spondyloarthropathies. Curr Opin Rheumatol 2001;13(4):265–272
4. Reveille JD, Arnett FC. Spondyloarthritis: update on pathogenesis and management. Am J Med 2005;118(6):592–603
5. Schmidek HH, Roberts DW. Schmidek & Sweet Operative Neurosurgical Techniques: Indications, Methods, and Results. 5th ed. Philadelphia, PA: Saunders Elsevier; 2006
6. Khan MA. Update on spondyloarthropathies. Ann Intern Med 2002;136(12):896–907
7. Burkus JK. Esophageal obstruction secondary to diffuse idiopathic skeletal hyperostosis. Orthopedics 1988;11(5):717–720
8. Boden SD, Dodge LD, Bohlman HH, Rechtine GR. Rheumatoid arthritis of the cervical spine. A long-term analysis with predictors of paralysis and recovery. J Bone Joint Surg Am 1993;75(9):1282–1297
9. Papadopoulos SM, Dickman CA, Sonntag VKH. Atlantoaxial stabilization in rheumatoid arthritis. J Neurosurg 1991;74(1):1–7
10. Resnick D, Guerra J Jr, Robinson CA, Vint VC. Association of diffuse idiopathic skeletal hyperostosis (DISH) and calcification and ossification of the posterior longitudinal ligament. AJR Am J Roentgenol 1978;131(6):1049–1053
11. Olivieri I, D'Angelo S, Palazzi C, Padula A, Mader R, Khan MA. Diffuse idiopathic skeletal hyperostosis: differentiation from ankylosing spondylitis. Curr Rheumatol Rep 2009; 11(5):321–328
12. Nakanishi T, Mannen T, Toyokura Y. Asymptomatic ossification of the posterior longitudinal ligament of the cervical spine. Incidence and roentgenographic findings. J Neurol Sci 1973;19(3):375–381
13. Matsunaga S, Sakou T, Taketomi E, Komiya S. Clinical course of patients with ossification of the posterior longitudinal ligament: a minimum 10-year cohort study. J Neurosurg 2004;100(3, Suppl Spine):245–248
14. Epstein N. Diagnosis and surgical management of cervical ossification of the posterior longitudinal ligament. Spine J 2002;2(6):436–449

Answers to Common Clinical Questions

1. B. Diffuse idiopathic hyperostosis (DISH) is the most likely diagnosis. The patient admits to morning stiffness, chronic axial spine pain, sensation of throat lump ("globus") with dysphagia. The formation of osteophytes and the sparing of the sacroiliac joints also point to DISH as the most likely diagnosis. These bridging osteophytes seen with DISH do not provide any added stability.
2. D. The patient's diagnosis is most consistent with segmental OPLL. Calcified lesions are hypointense on T1 and T2. In addition, OPLL has a high incidence in the Japanese population. Finally, because the area behind the disc was spared, the OPLL is classified at segmental.
3. False. A PADI >14 mm does, not an ADI.
4. B. A rigid collar is a poor choice here because it does not provide stability at C1-C2.
5. True. It is seen particularly in patients with ankylosing spondylitis, but it can also be seen in a variety of spondyloarthropathies.

25 Spinal Emergencies

Mohammed Eleraky and Frank D. Vrionis

I. Key Points

- Prompt and accurate diagnosis of spinal emergencies is critical because return of function is highly dependent on early intervention.
- Magnetic resonance imaging (MRI) is often the imaging modality of choice in diagnosing spinal hematomas, acute herniated nucleus pulposus, and spinal epidural abscesses.
- Trauma and tumors may also present as "spinal emergencies" and are discussed elsewhere.

II. Spinal Hematomas

- Background
  - As in the cranium, these include subdural, epidural, and subarachnoid hematomas.
  - In up to one-third of cases, no etiologic factor can be identified.
  - Anticoagulant therapy and vascular malformations represent the second and third most common causes.
  - Spinal hematomas are typically localized dorsally to the spinal cord at the cervicothoracic and thoracolumbar regions.[1,2]
  - Subarachnoid hematomas can extend along the entire length of the subarachnoid space.
  - Intramedullary hemorrhages, caused by cavernomas or arteriovenous malformations (AVMs), typically produce devastating neurologic symptoms but are often not managed with emergent surgical decompression.
- Signs, symptoms, and physical exam
  - Epidural and subdural spinal hematomas present with intense, knife-like pain at the location of the hemorrhage ("coup de poignard").
  - This may be followed by a pain-free interval of minutes to days.
  - Subarachnoid hematoma can be associated with meningitis-like symptoms, disturbances of consciousness, and epileptic seizures (often misdiagnosed as cerebral hemorrhage based on these symptoms).
  - Symptoms depend on the location and extent of hemorrhage and may include motor weakness, sensory and reflex deficits, and acute bowel/bladder dysfunction.[1]

25 Spinal Emergencies

- Workup
    - Hematology (including platelets), electrolytes, and partial thromboplastin time (PTT)/prothrombin time (PT)/International Normalized Ratio (INR)
    - Disseminated intravascular coagulation (DIC) panel and specific hematology factors may need to be assessed.
    - Appropriate neuroimaging
- Neuroimaging
    - The imaging modality of choice is MRI with or without gadolinium (**Fig. 25.1**).
    - The appearance of hematomas in MRI is highly dependent on the age of the clot.
    - Hyperacute bleeding (<24 hours): T1 isointense, T2 slightly hyperintense
    - Acute bleeding (1 to 3 days): T1 slightly hyperintense, T2 hypointense
    - Subacute bleeding (>3 days): T1 hyperintense, T2 hypointense (T2 may be hyperintense for late subacute)
- Treatment
    - The treatment of choice is correction of coagulopathy, if present, and emergent surgical decompression.[1]

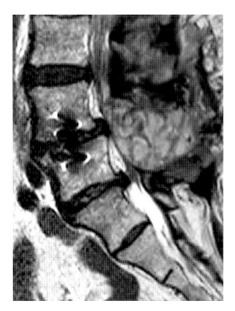

Fig. 25.1 T2-weighted MRI of the lumbar spine showing postoperative mixed signal fluid collection (consistent with epidural hematoma) in the epidural space compressing the dural sac.

- Benefit of surgical intervention is debatable if only symptom is pain.
- Surgery typically involves laminectomy without the need for fusion.
- For cervicothoracic and thoracolumbar junction multilevel laminectomies, consider instrumentation and fusion.
  - Surgical pearls
    - Subfascial drains may diminish the incidence of symptomatic epidural blood collections following multilevel laminectomy procedures.

III. Cauda Equina and Conus Syndromes

- Background
  - Cauda equina syndrome (CES) refers to the clinical condition that results from compressive, ischemic, and/or inflammatory neuropathy of multiple lumbar and sacral nerve roots in the lumbar spinal canal.[3,4]
  - Conus syndrome has features similar to those of CES but involves compression at the level of the conus medullaris (T12-L1 typically).
  - The most common cause is disc herniation in the lumbar region.
  - It may also be caused by traumatic injury, lumbar spinal stenosis, primary or metastatic tumors, epidural abscess, ankylosing spondylitis, spinal subdural or epidural hematoma, spinal manipulation, and vascular malformation.[3,4]
- Signs, symptoms, and physical exam
  - Urinary retention is the most consistent finding, occurring in 90% of patients presenting with CES.
  - Anal sphincter tone diminished in 80% of patients.
  - Saddle anesthesia is the most common sensory deficit (75% of patients).
  - Once total perineal anesthesia develops, patient will likely have permanent bladder dysfunction.
  - Low back pain and radicular symptoms
  - Conus lesions have the same features except that motor and sensory loss is typically asymmetric.
- Workup
  - Basic laboratory studies and appropriate neuroimaging
  - If imaging demonstrates pathology other than herniated nucleus pulposus (HNP), further workup is indicated (e.g., tumor or infection workup).

- Neuroimaging
    - MRI is the best initial study if CES or conus syndrome is suspected.
    - MRI assesses soft tissue compression as well as signal changes within the spinal cord.
- Treatment
    - Prompt surgical decompression (<24 hours)
    - Surgical strategy is usually focused on the underlying causes.
    - Typically involves laminectomy and discectomy (for HNP)
    - More extensive surgery (e.g., vertebrectomy, tumor removal) may be necessary for other pathologies.
    - Return of function is dependent on the extent and duration of preoperative deficits.
- Surgical pearls
    - Complete hemilaminotomy or laminectomy may be required for removal of large central disc fragment causing conus or cauda equina syndrome.

IV. Spinal Epidural Abscess

- Background
    - Spinal epidural abscess (SEA) is responsible for 0.2 to 2 cases per 10,000 hospitalizations.
    - Thoracic level is the most common site (50%), followed by lumbar (35%).
    - Often associated with vertebral osteomyelitis/discitis
    - Risk factors include diabetes mellitus, trauma, intravenous drug abuse, alcoholism, and epidural anesthesia or analgesia.
    - Skin abscesses and furuncles are the most common sources of infection.
    - Gram-positive *Staphylococcus aureus* is the most common causative agent.
- Signs, symptoms, and physical exam
    - Diagnosis is often achieved in delayed fashion due to vagueness of presenting signs and symptoms.
    - The most common presenting symptoms include excruciating pain localized over the spine, radicular pain, weakness, and sensory deficits.
    - Average time from back pain to root symptoms is 3 days, and 4.5 days from root pain to weakness.
    - Leukocytosis and fever may be absent.

- Workup
  - Hematology (complete blood count [CBC] with differential), electrolytes (comprehensive metabolic panel [CMP]), acute phase reactants (erythrocyte sedimentation rate [ESR], C-reactive protein [CRP]), blood cultures. Cardiac echo to rule out endocarditis may be indicated.
- Neuroimaging
  - MRI with gadolinium is the modality of choice in diagnosing SEA.
  - Typical finding: T1 shows hypo- or isointense epidural mass; vertebral osteomyelitis shows up as reduced signal in bone. T2 shows high-intensity epidural mass that often enhances with gadolinium but may show minimal enhancement in the acute stage when composed primarily of pus with little granulation tissue.[5]
  - Plain radiographs often helpful for suspected discitis and will show chronic, erosive changes in the end plates.
- Treatment
  - For SEAs that show clear involvement of the spinal canal and cause dural compression, surgical decompression and intravenous antibiotic therapy are the treatments of choice.
  - SEA is often seen in association with discitis/osteomyelitis. In these cases, typically only a thin film of epidural enhancement is seen. Surgical intervention not necessarily indicated in these situations.
  - Patients with severe neurologic deficit may show minimal improvement even with surgical intervention.
  - SEA is fatal in up to one-third of elderly patients, and mortality is usually due to the original focus of infection or as a complication of neurologic compromise.
- Surgical pearls
  - Most spinal instrumentation is safe, effective, and at times necessary in the treatment of epidural abscess or discitis/osteomyelitis of the spine.

Common Clinical Questions

1. Cauda equina syndrome describes the clinical condition that results from what neuropathy involving multiple lumbar and sacral nerve roots?
   A. Compressive
   B. Ischemic
   C. Inflammatory
   D. All of the above

2. Conus lesions have the same features as cauda equina except:
   A. Urinary retention
   B. Anal sphincter tone diminished in 80% of patients
   C. Saddle anesthesia
   D. Motor and sensory loss typically asymmetric

References

1. Groen RJ. Non-operative treatment of spontaneous spinal epidural hematomas: a review of the literature and a comparison with operative cases. Acta Neurochir (Wien) 2004;146(2):103–110
2. Liu WH, Hsieh CT, Chiang YH, Chen GJ. Spontaneous spinal epidural hematoma of thoracic spine: a rare case report and review of literature. Am J Emerg Med 2008;26(3):384, e1–e2
3. Ahn UM, Ahn NU, Buchowski JM, Garrett ES, Sieber AN, Kostuik JP. Cauda equina syndrome secondary to lumbar disc herniation: a meta-analysis of surgical outcomes. Spine (Phila Pa 1976) 2000;25(12):1515–1522
4. Hussain SA, Gullan RW, Chitnavis BP. Cauda equina syndrome: outcome and implications for management. Br J Neurosurg 2003;17(2):164–167
5. Karikari IO, Powers CJ, Reynolds RM, Mehta AI, Isaacs RE. Management of a spontaneous spinal epidural abscess: a single-center 10-year experience. Neurosurgery 2009;65(5):919–923, discussion 923–924

Answers to Common Clinical Questions

1. D
2. D

IV
Surgical Techniques

26 Occipitocervical Fusion

Edwin Ramos and Juan S. Uribe

I. Key Points

- Maintaining occipitocervical (OC) alignment, decompressing neural elements, and achieving a strong arthrodesis are the main goals of this procedure. This is accomplished by judicious use of fluoroscopy/image guidance and meticulous technique in decorticating and placing the graft material.
- Traction is not applied in cases of occipitocervical dislocation or significant ligamentous injury on magnetic resonance imaging (MRI).
- As part of preoperative planning, make sure to review the depth of the midline suboccipital keel, thickness of the paramedian cranium, and course of the vertebral artery.
- Prior to locking in the construct, verify that a neutral occipitocervical relationship has been achieved.

II. Indications

- Occipitocervical instability due to trauma, infections, rheumatoid arthritis, tumors, iatrogenic injury (after transoral odontoidectomy), congenital anomalies, cranial settling with brainstem or cord compression[1]

III. Technique

- For most of these patients fiberoptic intubation is performed, and then baseline somatosensory evoked potentials (SSEPs) and motor evoked potentials (MEPs) are obtained with the patient still supine.
- Maintaining cervical alignment, rotate the patient to the prone position onto chest rolls or a Jackson frame.
- The head is secured with a Mayfield cranial fixation system (Schaerer Mayfield, Randolph, MA) or in modest traction with tongs when not contraindicated (OC dislocation).
- Cervical alignment is maintained and checked with fluoroscopy to ensure a neutral OC relationship.
- The suboccipital area is shaved and cleansed. If autograft is required, the hip harvest site is incorporated in the prepped area.

- A midline incision is extended from the inion to the lowest level to be incorporated in the construct.
- Subperiosteal dissection with Bovie electrocautery (Bovie Medical Corporation, Clearwater, FL) is performed to expose the suboccipital bone. Special care is taken to leave a cuff of fascia near the inion for subsequent closure. This ensures that the occipital plate will be fully covered by muscle, reducing the chances of hardware eroding through the skin.
- Subperiosteal dissection is also used to expose the dorsal elements of the cervical spine. When exposing the arch of C1, blunt dissection with a Penfield 1 is recommended to avoid injury to the vertebral artery.
- Any decompression required (suboccipital or cervical) is now performed, with the bone saved for autograft.
- Occipital fixation can be performed using a variety of methods: occipital wiring, occipital in/out buttons, occipital screw fixation (occipital plate) (**Fig. 26.1**), or occipital condyle screw fixation. The current evidence supports the superiority of cranial screw fixation over wire and cable constructs with respect to both clinical outcomes and fusion rates.
- First place the suboccipital plate in position and use one of the plate apertures to mark the midline keel with a marking pen.

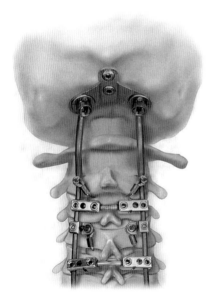

Fig. 26.1 Occipital plate and rod system. Illustration of the Summit occipital plating and rod system (DePuy Spine, Raynham, MA). Note that the occipital anchor plate is extended to the cervical spine via rods anchored by sublaminar wires that pass through custom cable connectors (reprinted with permission from DePuy Acromed; SCSCT pg. 434, Fig. 26-14).

The plate is removed and a hand-held power drill is used to make a bicortical hole. To avoid injury to the suboccipital neural structures, drill in a progressive fashion—first to a depth of 8 mm, then slowly increasing the depth in 2 mm increments until bicortical penetration is felt, usually around 10 to 14 mm. The hole is tapped (this is mandatory; the occipital keel is only cortical bone) and then the plate is repositioned over this hole and secured with an appropriate-length screw with a 4.5 mm diameter. The other midline holes can now be drilled with the plate in position.
- Some plates provide the option of paramedian holes for screw placement. Keep in mind that the paramedian bone in the suboccipital region is not as thick as the midline keel.
- The cervical instrumentation can now be placed and incorporated to the suboccipital plate using rods bent to the appropriate shape.
- The plate should be placed high in the suboccipital bone (closer to the inion than to the foramen magnum) to leave a small area of bone caudal to the plate for fusion surface.
- An alternative to plate systems is the occipital condyle screw fixation.[2] It is particularly useful in situations where a suboccipital decompression is required. With this technique a 3.5 mm × 20 to 22 effective length and 10 to 12 mm lag shank screw (30 to 34 mm) is placed in the center of the condyle, inferior to the hypoglossal canal. Although different techniques for its placement have been described, in general the screw has a medial trajectory (10 to 25 degrees) from an entry point about 5 mm lateral to the foramen magnum on the condyle itself. Image guidance and free-running electromyography (EMG) monitoring of the hypoglossal nerve are highly recommended with this technique.

IV. Complications

- In contemporary series, complication rates (minor and major) range from 12 to 30%.[3,4]
  - Wound infection, cerebrospinal fluid (CSF) leak, intracranial injury (sub-/epidural hematoma), spinal cord injury (instrumentation into spinal canal), vascular injury (hardware into vertebral artery)
  - Hardware failure (loosening, pullout, breakage)
  - Nonunion requiring re-operation
  - Fixation of patient's neck in exaggerated flexion or extension

V. Postoperative Care

- Upright x-rays with cervical collar
- Subfascial drain
- Prophylactic antibiotics for 24 hours
- Prompt mobilization with collar

VI. Outcomes

- Fusion rates of 94 to 97% with screw-rod constructs and more than 85% neurologic improvement have been achieved in patients with myelopathy.[1,4]
- Screw-rod constructs have a much lower pseudarthrosis rate compared with wiring techniques (6 vs 27%) and result in a higher rate of neurologic improvement (86 vs 40%).[5]
- Early biomechanical studies suggest that condyle screw fixation is biomechanically equivalent to suboccipital plate systems in terms of providing craniocervical stability.[2]

VII. Surgical Pearls

- Cervical traction is not applied in cases of occipitocervical dislocation.
- As part of the preoperative planning, make sure to review the depth of the midline suboccipital keel, thickness of paramedian cranium, and course of the vertebral artery.
- Prior to locking in the construct, verify that a neutral occipitocervical relationship has been achieved.

Common Clinical Questions

1. Cervical traction is contraindicated in which occipitocervical instrumentation cases?
2. Before locking the construct down, why are anteroposterior and lateral fluoroscopy views obtained?
3. Which construct has the lowest pseudarthrosis rate?

References

1. Lu DC, Roeser AC, Mummaneni VP, Mummaneni PV. Nuances of occipitocervical fixation. Neurosurgery 2010;66(3, Suppl):141–146
2. Uribe JS, Ramos E, Youssef AS, et al. Craniocervical fixation with occipital condyle screws: biomechanical analysis of a novel technique. Spine (Phila Pa 1976) 2010;35(9):931–938
3. Deutsch H, Haid RW Jr, Rodts GE Jr, Mummaneni PV. Occipitocervical fixation: long-term results. Spine (Phila Pa 1976) 2005;30(5):530–535
4. Nockels RP, Shaffrey CI, Kanter AS, Azeem S, York JF. Occipitocervical fusion with rigid internal fixation: long-term follow-up data in 69 patients. J Neurosurg Spine 2007; 7(2):117–123
5. Grob D, Crisco JJ III, Panjabi MM, Wang P, Dvorak J. Biomechanical evaluation of four different posterior atlantoaxial fixation techniques. Spine (Phila Pa 1976) 1992;17(5): 480–490

Answers to Common Clinical Questions

1. Those performed for occipitocervical dislocation or when significant ligamentous injury is suspected
2. To ensure adequate alignment and avoid exaggerated flexion or extension
3. Screw-and-rod-based constructs

27 Chiari I Decompression

Mark S. Greenberg

I. Key Points

- Consistent feature of Chiari I: disruption of normal cerebrospinal fluid (CSF) flow through the foramen magnum. Most symptomatic cases have descent of cerebellar tonsils ≥5 mm below the margins of the foramen magnum, which is best seen on magnetic resonance imaging (MRI).
- Surgical treatment for symptomatic patients consists of enlarging the foramen magnum (suboccipital decompression), usually with C1 laminectomy.
- Syringomyelia, if present, will usually respond to suboccipital decompression alone.

II. Indications

- Symptoms include
  - Pain (the most common symptom; mostly suboccipital headache that is exacerbated by neck extension), neck pain, arm pain, weakness/numbness in one or more limbs, loss of temperature sensation (dissociated sensory loss),[1] balance difficulties. Fifteen to 30% of patients meeting radiographic diagnostic criteria are asymptomatic.[2]
- Signs[3] include
  - Hyperactive lower-extremity (LE) reflexes, downbeat nystagmus, gait disturbance, hand muscle atrophy, cerebellar signs, Babinski sign

III. Technique

- Position: Patient is prone on chest rolls with the neck flexed and the head in a Mayfield head holder (Schaerer Mayfield, Randolph, MA) or on a horseshoe head rest.
- Skin incision: midline incision from the inion down to the C2 spinous process
- The fascia is opened in a Y or T, leaving a cuff of tissue attached to the occiput for use during closure.
- The occipital bone is exposed down to the foramen magnum (FM). The posterior C1 arch is exposed (taking caution regarding the vertebral arteries).

- At a minimum, the surgery consists of enlargement of the FM (suboccipital decompression) often combined with C1 laminectomy. The area of removal of occipital bone should be as wide as the FM, but should be no more than 2.5 to 3 cm above the FM (to avoid cerebellar herniation). Techniques include thinning the bone with a high-speed drill and removing the residual bone with a Kerrison rongeur (**Fig. 27.1**). Options to suboccipital decompression include
  - C2 laminectomy: reserved for cases with severe tonsillar descent below the superior margin of C2 (**Table 27.1**)
  - Duraplasty: A Y-shaped incision is made in the dura (some surgeons preserve the arachnoid[4]) and a patch graft is sewn in watertight closure with 4-0 Nurolon (Ethicon, Johnson & Johnson, Piscataway, NJ). Options for sources of graft: pericranium, fascia lata, and dural substitutes. Pericranium can be harvested through the same incision by subcutaneous dissection.[5]
  - Instead of opening the dura in all cases, some surgeons simply lyse extradural constricting bands. Then intraoperative ultrasound may be used to determine if there is adequate room for CSF circulation. If not, a duraplasty is performed.
  - An alternative to duraplasty (primarily in pediatrics): partial thickness scoring of the dura with several parallel passes of a scalpel
- Closure: A multilayered water-tight closure is performed. Skin approximation with sutures is preferred over staples. A wound drain is *not* used. A lumbar drain is occasionally used for 2 to 3 days.

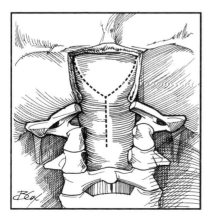

Fig. 27.1 Posterior exposure of the dura after bony removal, showing an outline of the Y-shaped dural incision. (From Vaccaro AR and Albert TJ, Spine Surgery: Tricks of the Trade, Thieme; 2009. Reprinted with permission.)

IV. Complications

- The major complication from surgery is CSF leak. This may be external (and can be initially treated by oversewing the site of leak and temporary lumbar drainage) or subcutaneous (pseudomeningocele).
- Overaggressive removal of occipital bone can lead to cerebellar ptosis (sagging of the tonsils).
- Injury to brainstem or posterior inferior cerebellar arteries (PICAs). Avoid aggressive treatment of tonsillar adhesions. Use an operating microscope if needed.
- Post-op apnea or respiratory depression: tends to occur within the first few days post-op. Monitor for apnea and increasing arterial pCO_2.

V. Outcomes

Pre-op symptoms of headache or pain respond in 82% with a 4 year follow-up.[1] Weakness is less responsive to surgery, especially if atrophy has occurred. Symptoms of greater than 2 years' duration have a worse prognosis.

Postoperative Care
- Intensive care unit (ICU) observation overnight with head computed tomography (CT) the next morning to rule out epidural hematoma.
- Mobilize and discharge typically in 24 to 48 hours postoperatively.
- Early follow-up in clinic recommended to assess wound, d/c sutures/staples, and ensure no pseudomeningocele has developed.

VI. Surgical Pearls

- Treating the Chiari malformation via suboccipital decompression corrects syringomyelia in the majority of cases without the need for any other procedure.
- Fifteen to 30% of patients with radiographic criteria of Chiari I malformation are asymptomatic.[2]

Table 27.1 Variation with Age of the Location of the Inferior Tonsillar Pole Relative to the Foramen Magnum[6]

Age (years)	Two standard deviations below the FM (mm)
0–9	6
10–29	5
30–79	4
80–89	3

Abbreviation: FM, foramen magnum.

Common Clinical Questions

1. Three weeks following a suboccipital decompression with duraplasty for a symptomatic Chiari I malformation, a patient develops a tense, very painful fluid collection under the incision and an MRI shows it has the appearance of CSF without any other significant abnormalities. The best management options are:
   A. Percutaneous tapping of the fluid after careful skin prep, and then tightly wrapping the head with bandages to prevent reaccumulation
   B. Placement of a lumbar drain and having the patient lie flat in bed for 3 days
   C. Surgical exploration of the wound in the OR with repair of dural defect, and placement of lumbar drain for 3 days with the head of bed greater than 30 degrees
   D. Placement of an external ventricular drain to divert the CSF from the wound, and conversion to a ventriculoperitoneal (VP) shunt if the patient is drain dependent after 5 days

2. A 48-year-old female elementary school teacher presents with a 20-year history of headaches that occur almost every day at the same time. They vary from the left to right side and are often associated with neck pain. No medication or change in position has provided any relief. Her primary care physician ordered a brain MRI, on which the only abnormality identified is that the inferior pole of the cerebellar tonsils is 4 mm below the foramen magnum. She is neurologically intact. You should:
   A. Order a cine flow MRI
   B. Have her see a neurologist to rule out other causes of chronic headache
   C. Order a cervical MRI
   D. All of the above

References

1. Paul KS, Lye RH, Strang FA, Dutton J. Arnold-Chiari malformation. Review of 71 cases. J Neurosurg 1983;58(2):183–187
2. Bejjani GK, Cockerham KP. Adult Chiari malformation. Contemp Neurosurg 2001; 23(26):1–7
3. Levy WJ, Mason L, Hahn JF. Chiari malformation presenting in adults: a surgical experience in 127 cases. Neurosurgery 1983;12(4):377–390
4. Sindou M, Gimbert E. Decompression for Chiari type I-malformation (with or without syringomyelia) by extreme lateral foramen magnum opening and expansile duraplasty with arachnoid preservation: comparison with other technical modalities (Literature review). Adv Tech Stand Neurosurg 2009;34:85–110
5. Stevens EA, Powers AK, Sweasey TA, Tatter SB, Ojemann RG. Simplified harvest of autologous pericranium for duraplasty in Chiari malformation Type I. Technical note. J Neurosurg Spine 2009;11(1):80–83
6. Mikulis DJ, Diaz O, Egglin TK, Sanchez R. Variance of the position of the cerebellar tonsils with age: preliminary report. Radiology 1992;183(3):725–728

Answers to Common Clinical Questions

1. C. The patient probably has a "ball-valve" effect through a dural flap. Tapping the fluid will not prevent reaccumulation. Placing the patient flat will actually put more pressure on the incision. An external ventricular drain (EVD) and/or shunt has no role in the absence of hydrocephalus.

2. D. The headaches sound atypical for Chiari malformation, and she is borderline for the tonsillar descent (which is at two standard deviations below normal for her age; see **Table 27.1**). The cine MRI may give additional helpful data, but before recommending surgery it is critical to rule out other explanations for her headache. A cervical MRI will rule out cervical spondylosis, which may cause neck pain and headache, and it is also necessary to rule out a syrinx associated with the tonsillar descent. Since she is neurologically intact, there should be little risk in proceeding cautiously.

28 Transoral Odontoidectomy

Frank M. Phillips and Colin B. Harris

I. Key Points

- The transoral approach allows the surgeon ventral midline access from the top of the arch of the atlas to the C2-C3 disc space.[1]
- A thorough preoperative assessment is necessary to ensure that the patient is free from any oral or dental pathology, which are contraindications to this approach.
- A minimum of 2.5 to 3 cm of dental clearance should be present to allow adequate exposure for odontoid resection.[2]

II. Indications

- Ventral spinal cord compression from rheumatoid pannus not amenable to posterior decompression and fusion
- Midline ventral cord compression from intradural or extradural spinal tumors
- Irreducible atlantoaxial subluxation with myelopathy and cord compression[1]

III. Technique

- The patient is positioned supine on the operating room table with a Mayfield headrest (Schaerer Mayfield, Randolph, MA), or in Mayfield tongs for greater control if there is instability of the occipitocervical junction.
  - Prophylactic antibiotics consist of intravenous cephalosporin and metronidazole preoperatively and for 72 hours postoperatively.
  - Nasotracheal intubation is preferred to avoid manipulation of the occipitocervical junction, and a nasogastric tube should be placed to prevent postoperative wound contamination.
- A transoral tongue retractor is inserted to visualize the oropharynx.
- A lateral fluoroscopic image is taken to localize the odontoid process and anterior arch of the atlas, followed by infiltration of 1% lidocaine with epinephrine into the planned incision site.
- A 2 cm full-thickness vertical incision is made in the midline, dividing the mucosa and pharyngeal constrictor musculature.

- A pharyngeal retractor is placed in a horizontal fashion, exposing the anterior tubercle of the atlas, origin of the longus colli, and anterior longitudinal ligament (**Fig. 28.1**).
- Cautery is used to skeletonize the ventral aspect of the arch of the atlas and the odontoid.
- The central 10 to 15 mm of the arch of the atlas is removed using a high-speed burr to expose the odontoid process in its entirety.[1]
- The odontoid is then resected using a high-speed burr for the anterior cortex and cancellous portion.
- Angled curettes are used to detach the apical and alar ligaments to allow the tip of the dens to be removed.
- Kerrison rongeurs (1 and 2 mm) and microcurettes are then used to complete the resection of the posterior dens cortical shell until the posterior longitudinal ligament and dura are identified.
- In patients with rheumatoid arthritis, the retrodental soft-tissue pannus is exposed following odontoid resection. Only loose

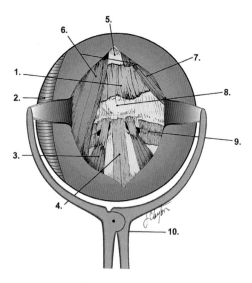

Fig. 28.1 Retropharyngeal anatomy and retractor. 1, anterior atlanto-occipital membrane; 2, armored nasotracheal tube; 3, longus colli muscle; 4, anterior longitudinal ligament; 5, clivus; 6, longus capitis muscle; 7, rectus capitis anterior muscle; 8, anterior tubercle of C1; 9, lateral atlantoaxial joint capsule; 10, retropharyngeal soft-tissue retractor. (From Haher T, Merola A, Surgical Technique for the Spine, Thieme; pg. 5, Fig. 1-5. Reprinted with permission.)

fragments should be debulked, as complete pannus removal is usually unnecessary and risks a cerebrospinal fluid (CSF) leak.[2]
- The incision is irrigated with antibiotic solution, followed by closure of the muscle and mucosa in two layers with absorbable 3-0 suture.
- The retractors are removed, and 1% cortisone cream may be applied to the lips and tongue to decrease postoperative edema.
- The patient may be repositioned prone with the Mayfield tongs if a posterior stabilization and fusion procedure is planned.

IV. Complications

- Neurologic injury
  - Awake nasotracheal intubation avoids manipulation of the craniocervical junction.
  - Somatosensory evoked potentials (SSEP) and motor evoked potentials (MEP) can provide intraoperative warning of spinal cord compromise.
  - Keep mean arterial pressure (MAP) high to prevent ischemic spinal cord injury.
- CSF leak
  - Direct dural repair (if possible), followed by fascial or fat graft
  - Placement of subarachnoid lumbar drain postoperatively can be helpful.
- Airway obstruction
  - Avoid premature extubation as reintubation can be very difficult and require emergency tracheostomy. Prior to extubation, evaluate for:
    - Resolution of retropharyngeal swelling on lateral radiograph (usually 24 to 48 hours postoperatively)[1]
    - Ability to breathe around orotracheal airway[2]
- Infection
  - Can be minimized with meticulous wound closure and 72 hours of intravenous antibiotics
  - Delay removal of nasogastric tube and oral fluid administration for 4 to 5 days postoperatively to allow for mucosal healing.
- Vertebral artery injury
  - Preoperative CT or MRI scans should be reviewed to determine if there is an aberrant medial course of the vertebral

artery, which is more common in patients with atlantoaxial rotatory subluxation.
- Dissection of the atlas should stay within 2 cm of the midline, and dissection at the level of the C2-C3 disc should stay within 1 cm of the midline.[1]

V. Postoperative Care

- The patient should be kept intubated for 2 to 3 days postoperatively to allow airway edema to subside.[2]
- Temporary use of an endotracheal cuff leak and tube changer can help anesthetist to guard against a difficult reintubation.[2]
- Once extubated, patient can be mobilized out of bed to chair in a cervical collar or orthosis depending on stability.

VI. Outcomes

- No level I studies have been performed to evaluate outcomes following transoral odontoid resection.
- Based on a review of smaller case series, improvement of preoperative neurologic deficits can be expected but is dependent on chronicity of spinal cord compression.
- In one 10-year review of 72 cases, there were two postoperative deaths and one pharyngeal infection requiring a repeat operation, with improvement seen in all patients' neurologic function.[3]

VII. Surgical Pearls

- Care should be taken to avoid entrapment of the tongue against the teeth with the retractor system.
- As an alternative to palatal retractors, a red rubber catheter can be passed through the nares and sutured to the soft palate; it can then be used as a retractor.[2]
- The soft palate and mandible can be split to provide extensile exposure in the proximal and distal directions, respectively, although the increased morbidity should be considered.

Common Clinical Questions

1. Which of the following is the minimum clearance between the upper and lower teeth needed for performing transoral odontoid resection?
   A. 1 cm
   B. 2 cm
   C. 3 cm
   D. 4 cm

2. Which of the following is *not* an indication for transoral (anterior) odontoid resection?
   A. Irreducible atlantoaxial subluxation with spinal cord compression
   B. Spinal cord tumors at the C1 level causing ventral spinal cord compression
   C. Rheumatoid pannus not amenable to posterior decompression and fusion
   D. Atlantooccipital instability with myelopathy

3. Which of the following is the minimum average distance to the vertebral artery from the midline (in the medial to lateral direction) in the transoral approach to the odontoid?
   A. 1 cm at the atlas
   B. 2 cm at the C2-C3 disc
   C. 2 cm at the atlas
   D. 3 cm at the C2-C3 disc

References

1. Mendoza N, Crockard A. Anterior transoral procedures. In An HS, Riley LH III. An Atlas of Surgery of the Spine. London: Martin Dunitz Ltd; 1998:55–69
2. Mummaneni PV, Haid RW. Transoral odontoidectomy. Neurosurgery 2005; 56(5):1045–1050
3. Menezes AH, VanGilder JC. Transoral-transpharyngeal approach to the anterior craniocervical junction. Ten-year experience with 72 patients. J Neurosurg 1988;69(6):895–903

Answers to Common Clinical Questions

1. C. A minimum of 2.5 to 3 cm of clearance is necessary for odontoid resection. If less space is present, either splitting of the soft palate (for more cephalad extension) or mandible (for caudal extension) may be necessary if this approach is chosen.

2. D. Cases presenting with instability should be treated with a posterior decompression and fusion, as anterior decompression alone would not address the instability.

3. C. The vertebral artery sits about 2 cm from the midline at the level of the atlas, and lies more medial (1 cm from the midline) in the transverse foramen at the level of the C2-C3 disc.

29 C1-C2 Techniques

Jau-Ching Wu and Praveen V. Mummaneni

I. Key Points

- Fixation choices are (1) C1 lateral mass screws in combination with C2 pars screws, pedicle screws, or translaminar screws; (2) C1-C2 transarticular screw (Magerl's technique); or (3) wiring techniques.
- Posterior C1-C2 fusion techniques are technically demanding and caution should be used to avoid vascular (vertebral and carotid arteries) injury during screw placement.
- Preoperative computed tomography (CT) scan (with or without CT angiography) is helpful to assess the position of the foramen transversarium of C1 and C2.

II. Indications

- Most C1-C2 ligamentous instabilities (>3 mm atlantodental interval [ADI] on flexion-extension x-rays in an adult without rheumatoid arthritis)
- Traumatic fractures are among the most frequent indications for posterior C1-C2 fixation.
- Certain subsets of type 2 and type 3 odontoid fractures are amenable to posterior C1-C2 fixation.
  - Type 2 odontoid fracture associated with
    - Fracture of the atlantoaxial joint
    - Anterior-inferior oblique fracture in the coronal plane
    - Oblique fracture in the frontal plane
    - Jefferson fracture
    - Ruptured transverse ligament
    - Old, unhealed type 2 odontoid fracture
  - Type 3 odontoid fracture associated with
    - Fracture of the atlantoaxial joint
    - Jefferson fracture
    - Chronic unhealed odontoid fracture after immobilization; rotatory subluxation of C1-C2
- Congenital malformations of C2 (e.g., os odontoideum and odontoid agenesis with C1-C2 dynamic instability)
- Inflammatory diseases (e.g., rheumatoid arthritis with >7 mm ADI)
- Degenerative diseases (with instability and abnormal ADI)

- Infections (with instability and abnormal ADI)
- Neoplasms (with instability and abnormal ADI)

III. Techniques

The procedure is technically demanding, and an exact three-dimensional (3D) understanding of the anatomy of the region and of the vertebral artery is mandatory.

The patient is positioned prone with head fixed by a Mayfield head holder (Schaerer Mayfield, Randolph, MA). The neck should be in the neutral position and the head kept in the military chin tuck position. A midline posterior neck incision is then made from the suboccipital area to the spinous process of C3, allowing exposure of C2-C3 facet joints and the posterior C1 arch.

C1 Lateral Mass Screw with C2 Pars, Pedicle, or Translaminar Screws[1,2]
- C1 lateral mass screw[5,6]
  - Control of hemorrhage from the venous plexus between C1 and C2 must be achieved by bipolar coagulation or hemostatic agents. It is not necessary to expose the vertebral artery on the superior aspect of the C1 arch (sulcus arteriosus). Usually the C2 nerve root is mobilized caudally for exposure of the C1 lateral mass inferior to the C1 arch. The medial border of the C1 lateral mass is palpated. A pilot hole can be made with a 3 mm drill bit at the center of C1 lateral mass. The screw trajectory is 10 degrees medial angulation in the axial plane. On lateral fluoroscopic imaging the drill is aimed toward the anterior tubercle of C1. Stop the drill at the "back side" of the anterior C1 tubercle to prevent plunging the bit into the retropharynx. After tapping of the hole, the C1 lateral mass screw is placed (usually 34 to 36 mm in length).
- C2 pars screws (**Fig. 29.1**)[5,6]
  - The C2 pars is defined as the portion of C2 vertebra connecting the superior and inferior articular surfaces. A C2 pars screw is placed in a trajectory similar to that of a C1-C2 transarticular screw, except that it is shorter. Its entry point is about 3 mm rostral and 3 mm lateral to the inferior medial aspect of the inferior articular surface of C2. The screw should follow a steep trajectory, 45 to 60 degrees, with 10 to 15 degrees of medial angulation. Typical screw length is 16 mm, but the screw must stop short of the transverse foramen (check with preoperative CT scan). The risk of vertebral artery injury for C2 pars screws is lower than that for C1-C2 transarticular screws.

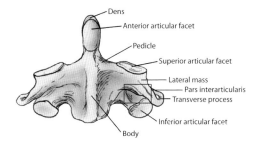

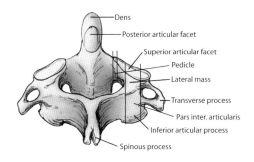

Fig. 29.1 Anatomy of the axis (C2). (From Fessler/Sekhar, Atlas of Surgical Techniques, Thieme, pg. 138, Fig. 16.3A,B. Reprinted with permission.)

- C2 pedicle screws
  - The C2 pedicle is the portion of the C2 vertebra that connects its posterior elements to the vertebral body. The entry point of the C2 pedicle screw is in the pars of C2, lateral to the superior margin of the C2 lamina. This is usually 2 mm lateral and 2 mm superior to the C2 pars screw entry point described above. The pedicle screw requires a medial angulation of 15 to 25 degrees with 20 degrees upward trajectory. For those with very narrow C2 pedicles, risk of breach into the neural canal or transverse foramen is high (check with preoperative CT scans).
- C2 translaminar screws
  - Translaminar screws serve as a salvage technique for C2 pars screws or pedicle screws in cases of the anomalous high-riding vertebral artery or very thin pedicle. The entry point is at the junction of the spinous process and lamina. The trajectory has to meet the slope of the lamina while aiming mildly dorsally to avoid canal breach. If bilateral translaminar screws are used, offset the entry points craniocaudal to keep the two screw paths from intersecting.
  - Using polyaxial screws, the C1 lateral mass screws can be easily connected with either of the three kinds of C2 screws described above.

- C1-C2 transarticular screws
  - The advantage of the C1-C2 transarticular screw technique is the complete obliteration of the rotational motion of the atlantoaxial joint. The drawbacks of this procedure are the need for anatomical reduction of C1-C2 and the potential for vertebral artery injury. If placement of the first screw likely caused vertebral artery injury, then screw insertion into the contralateral side should not be attempted, because bilateral vertebral artery laceration could result in brain stem infarction and death. The preoperative CT scan must be carefully examined to exclude a high-riding vertebral artery or destruction of bone at the site of intended screw placement.
  - The screw entry point is approximately 3 to 4 mm rostral and 3 to 4 mm lateral to the inferior medial portion of the C2-C3 facet joint. The K-wire trajectory is typically 15 degrees medial with the superior angle visualized by fluoroscopy aiming at the C1 anterior tubercle (often 60 degrees). While the K-wire is drilling, subtle changes in resistance may be perceived as the K-wire traverses the four cortical surfaces along the path into the C1 lateral mass: (1) the posterior C2 entry point, (2) the superior articular surface of C2, (3) the inferior articular surface of C1, and (4) the anterior cortex of the C1 ring. After the K-wire is placed, a cannulated drill bit, tap, and screw can be placed. Typical screw length is 36 to 46 mm.
- Wiring techniques
  - Posterior wiring techniques require an intact posterior arch in each of C1 and C2. Therefore, in cases of Jefferson fracture or hangman's fracture the K-wire is of no use. Double-braided titanium cables are preferred (over steel wires) because they are more flexible and have less chance of causing cord or dural injury during the sublaminar passage. Several techniques of sublaminar wiring and bone graft placement have been reported, including the Sonntag wiring, the Brooks wiring, and the Gallie wiring.

IV. Complications

- Vertebral artery laceration (unilateral vertebral artery occlusion could be asymptomatic, but bilateral vertebral artery injury could result in a large posterior circulation infarction and death). If there is a unilateral vertebral artery injury, consider placing the screw into the bone to tampanade the bleeding. Consider not placing the contralateral screw. Consider taking the patient for a postoperative angiogram to ensure there is no artery dissection.
- Dural injury or cord injury

V. Postoperative Care

- No need for external orthosis if rigid screw fixation is achieved.

VI. Outcomes

- Transarticular screws together with the Sonntag wiring technique and bone graft essentially create a three-point fixation that completely obliterates the rotational and flexion-extension motion of the C1-C2 joint. Apfelbaum reports that fusion was achieved in 99% of 198 patients undergoing transarticular screw fixation. However, Apfelbaum also reported a 16.7% complication rate, including 5 patients with vertebral artery injuries, one of which was bilateral and fatal.[3]
- C1 lateral mass screws connected to C2 pars/pedicle, or translaminar screws, provide biomechanical strength and actually facilitate anatomic reduction with a fusion rate higher than 95%.[4]
- Biomechanical analysis in cadaveric specimens showed crossed translaminar fixation to be superior to pars screws in strength.

VII. Surgical Pearls

- Preoperative planning is crucial. The CT scan must be evaluated to rule out an anomalous vertebral artery path and to assess the bony anatomy.
- A thorough understanding of the 3D anatomy of the axis and atlas is mandatory.
- Be aware of the robust venous plexuses around the C1-C2 region and use a hemostatic agent to diminish bleeding in this area.

Common Clinical Questions

1. Where is the entry point for the C2 pars screw?
2. Where is the entry point for the C1-C2 transarticular screw?
3. Should you place a contralateral C2 pars screw if you have an ipsilateral vertebral artery laceration during insertion of the first C2 pars/pedicle or transarticular screw?

References

1. Mummaneni PV, Haid RW. Atlantoaxial fixation: overview of all techniques. Neurol India 2005;53(4):408–415
2. Yanni DS, Perin NI. Fixation of the axis. Neurosurgery 2010;66(3, Suppl): 147–152
3. Finn MA, Apfelbaum RI. Atlantoaxial transarticular screw fixation: update on technique and outcomes in 269 patients. Neurosurgery 2010;66(3, Suppl):184–192
4. Mummaneni PV, Lu DC, Dhall SS, Mummaneni VP, Chou D. C1 lateral mass fixation: a comparison of constructs. Neurosurgery 2010;66(3, Suppl):153–160
5. Goel A, Kulkarni AG, Sharma P. Reduction of fixed atlantoaxial dislocation in 24 cases: technical note. J Neurosurg Spine 2005;2(4):505–509
6. Harms J, Melcher RP. Posterior C1–C2 fusion with polyaxial screw and rod fixation. Spine 2001;26(22):2467–2471

Answers to Common Clinical Questions

1. The C2 pars screw entry point is approximately 3 mm rostral and 3 mm lateral to the inferior medial aspect of the inferior articular surface of C2.
2. The same as for the C2 pars screw
3. No. Patients may tolerate a one-sided vertebral artery injury, but a bilateral vertebral injury could be fatal.

30 Direct Fixation of Odontoid Fractures

Andrew T. Dailey and Jose Carlos Sauri-Barraza

I. Key Points

- Odontoid screw fixation is suitable for acute type II odontoid fractures, which represent 60% of all dens fractures.[1]
- Rigid immobilization alone has been associated with nonunion in over 50% of cases in many series. Risk factors for nonunion include age greater than 50, displacement more than 6 mm, angulation, and smoking history.[1]
- Odontoid screws allow for direct fixation of the fracture fragments and have been reported to result in successful stabilization in 80 to 90% of cases.[2]

II. Indications

- Type II or shallow type III fractures that are acute or subacute
- Contraindications include pathologic fracture, injuries with associated rupture of the transverse atlantal ligament, chronic nonunion of odontoid (fractures present for more than 3 to 6 months), and comminuted fractures.
- Contraindications include severe osteoporosis, irreducible fractures, barrel chest, and thoracic kyphosis where the trajectory for a screw is not possible.

III. Technique

- Intraoperative fluoroscopy is essential to these procedures and should be performed in the anteroposterior (AP) and lateral planes (i.e., use two C-arms, **Fig. 30.1**).
- Place patient supine in halter traction or Gardner-Wells tongs.
- A bite block (cork) is useful for obtaining the AP image.
- Proper patient positioning with fracture reduction and extension of the neck to allow for proper screw trajectory is the most important aspect of the procedure.
- A transverse incision at C5-C6 provides the proper trajectory.
- Dissection is carried down to precervical fascia exactly as in approach for anterior cervical decompression.
- Medial-lateral retractors are placed under longus at C5 and blunt dissection is carried up to C2-C3 disc space.

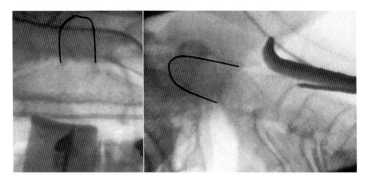

Fig. 30.1 Simultaneous AP and lateral fluoroscopy with retractors in place and K-wire pointing to the entry point for the screw. (Reproduced with permission of Springer from Dailey et al 2010.)[1]

- A cephalad retractor is used to protect the esophagus.
- Two general techniques may be used to place the screw: a cannulated screw system that allows the screw to be placed over a K-wire, or a non-cannulated screw that is placed directly down the path of the drill.
- The author prefers to use a non-cannulated system with specialized retractors and drill guides that allow for optimal position of the screw in the dens (**Fig. 30.1**).
- The trajectory is chosen so that the screw enters the C2 body in the anterior portion of the C2-C3 disc and not along the anterior border of the body of C2.
- Once the entry point is chosen, three steps remain: drill, tap, screw.
- Drilling is performed with fluoroscopic imaging to ensure that the path of the screw is acceptable and that the distal fracture fragment is not displaced cephalad during the drilling.
- The drill should engage the cortex at the distal tip of the dens to allow the screw to penetrate and lag the two fragments of the dens together (**Fig. 30.2**). It is this distal cortex that provides the strength for the fixation. If not engaged, the screw can back out and fixation will fail.
- The entire length of the screw trajectory is tapped, including the distal cortex.
- Either one or two screws can be used. The first screw should be a partially threaded or lag screw that will draw the fragments

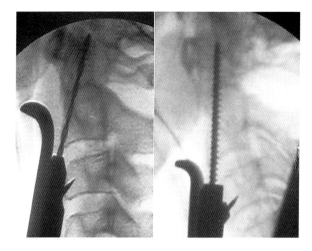

Fig. 30.2 Lateral fluoroscopy showing the correct position of the tip of the drill (left) and tap (right) so that the screw will engage the distal cortex of the dens. (Reproduced with permission of Springer from Dailey et al 2010.)[1]

together once the distal cortex is engaged. The second screw is fully threaded.
- Once the screws are placed, the retractors are carefully removed, the wound irrigated, and the incision closed like that for an anterior cervical decompression and fusion. Meticulous hemostasis is performed prior to closure to prevent a retropharyngeal hematoma.

IV. Complications

- Nonunion. This can be treated with a posterior C1-C2 arthrodesis.
- Screw back-out
- Screw breakage. Rare with non-cannulated 3.5 mm screws.
- Dysphagia and hoarseness. In the elderly population, patients may temporarily need a feeding tube due to dysphagia up to 25% of the time.[3]
- Aspiration pneumonia
- Retropharyngeal hematoma

V. Postoperative Care

- Mobilize patients immediately, particularly elderly patients.

- Observe for signs of dysphagia and aspiration, particularly in older patients. Advance diet with caution.
- A collar may provide some additional support, particularly in osteopenic patients. Biomechanical studies show that the odontoid is restored to half its intact strength with fixation using either one or two screws.
- Patients should be followed with serial x-rays for at least one year, including flexion and extension films at 3, 6, and 12 months.

VI. Outcomes

- The largest series in the literature report fusion rates of around 90% in all patients regardless of age (**Fig. 30.3**).[2] Other studies have reported similar rates of fusion.[4]
- There has generally been no reported difference in fusion rates if one versus two screws are used.[1,2]
- Two screws may lead to a better stabilization rate in patients over 70, as a recent series reports a 96% stability rate with two screws, but only a 56% rate with the use of one screw.[3]

VII. Surgical Pearls

- Preoperative planning and careful patient selection are key to obtaining success with an odontoid screw.
- Proper positioning is crucial to successful screw placement.
- Always make sure that the screw tip engages the distal cortex of the dens.
- Counsel patients and their families that if the procedure cannot be completed, a posterior C1-C2 fusion will provide a suitable alternative or "salvage" procedure.
- So-called anterior oblique dens fractures where the fracture line runs posterior-superior to anterior-inferior are difficult to realign with an odontoid screw, and higher failure rates have been reported with this procedure.

30 Direct Fixation of Odontoid Fractures

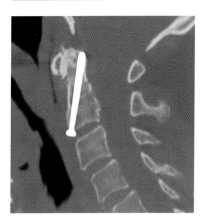

Fig. 30.3 Sagittal computed tomography with odontoid screw in position, demonstrating healing of fracture at 1 year after surgery. (Reproduced with permission of Springer from Dailey et al 2010.)[1]

Common Clinical Questions

1. Contraindications to odontoid screw placement include all of the following except:
   A. Pathologic fracture
   B. Chronic nonunion
   C. Type II fracture with associated stable C1 fracture
   D. Type I fracture with associated atlantooccipital dislocation

2. The most common cervical spine fracture in the population over age 65 is:
   A. Hangman's fracture
   B. Type II odontoid fracture
   C. Type III odontoid fracture
   D. Type I odontoid fracture

3. What is the most common immediate postoperative complication following odontoid screw fixation in patients over age 65?

References

1. Dailey AT, McCall TD, Apfelbaum RI. Direct anterior screw fixation of odontoid fractures. In Patel VV, Burger E, Brown C, eds. Spine Trauma Surgical Techniques. Berlin: Springer; 2010:Chapter 3
2. Apfelbaum RI, Lonser RR, Veres R, Casey A. Direct anterior screw fixation for recent and remote odontoid fractures. J Neurosurg 2000;93(2, Suppl):227–236
3. Dailey AT, Hart D, Finn MA, Schmidt MH, Apfelbaum RI. Anterior fixation of odontoid fractures in an elderly population. J Neurosurg Spine 2010;12(1):1–8
4. Platzer P, Thalhammer G, Ostermann R, Wieland T, Vécsei V, Gaebler C. Anterior screw fixation of odontoid fractures comparing younger and elderly patients. Spine (Phila Pa 1976) 2007;32(16):1714–1720

Answers to Common Clinical Questions

1. C. If there is no associated injury to the transverse atlantal ligament and a C1 fracture could be treated using a collar, an odontoid screw can treat the dens fracture and a collar placed for the associated C1 fracture.

2. B. The other fractures are much more common in the younger trauma population and are associated with higher-energy mechanisms of injury.

3. Any anterior cervical procedure in older patients is associated with difficulty with swallowing, and patients should be counseled about this potential development preoperatively.

31 Cervical Arthroplasty

Jau-Ching Wu, Ali A. Baaj, and Praveen V. Mummaneni

I. Key Points

- Anterior cervical discectomy and fusion (ACDF) remains the gold standard in the surgical management of symptomatic cervical spondylosis and central disc herniation.
- The emerging option of cervical arthroplasty is aimed at preservation of segmental motion with maintenance of adequate stability.[1]
- Key elements to achieving a good result and avoiding complications with cervical arthroplasty:
    - Appropriate patient selection (competent posterior elements, without spondylolisthesis)
    - Correct neck positioning during surgery (neutral to slightly lordotic cervical curvature)
    - Generous decompression with resection of the bilateral uncovertebral joints and posterior longitudinal ligament
    - Precise end plate preparation (parallel or domed according to device, with preservation of cortical end plates)
    - Accurate midline acquisition
    - Proper implant sizing (footprint coverage of disc space and avoidance of overdistraction)

II. Indications

- The current indications for cervical arthroplasty in the United States include symptomatic one-level cervical radiculopathy or myelopathy in patients who have failed nonsurgical management.
- Relative contraindications include (1) cervical kyphosis, (2) cervical spondylosis with incompetent or significantly degenerated facets (>2 to 3 mm subluxation on flexion-extension x-rays), (3) cervical ankylosis, (4) osteoporosis, and (5) cervical trauma with ligamentous or facet injury.

III. Technique

- Prophylactic antibiotics should be given; perioperative dexamethasone and intraoperative neuromonitoring are optional.

- The patient is positioned supine with the neck in neutral or slight extension, with shoulder retraction to allow adequate fluoroscopic visualization of the target level.
- Create a transverse skin incision along preexisting skin crease near the index level.
- Perform dissection between the carotid sheath and strap muscles (anterior-medial to sternocleidomastoid muscle) to expose the retropharyngeal space.
- The trachea and esophagus are retracted and protected medially by self-retaining retractors placed under the elevated longus colli muscles for exposure of the anterior cervical spine.
- After confirmation of the index level by lateral fluoroscopic x-ray, anterior cervical discectomy is performed with curettes, rongeurs, or drill.
- Full bilateral nerve canal decompression must be achieved, including removal of the uncovertebral joints.
- End plate preparation is crucial in cervical arthroplasty and may differ between prostheses. Caution must be taken not to violate the cortical surface, which would increase the risk of implant subsidence or migration.
- Midline acquisition, implant sizing (including footprint size and disc height), and insertion trajectory should be controlled to allow physiological range of motion in the cervical spine after implantation of the prosthesis.
- There are several cervical artificial discs currently on the market, and each has its unique design and fixation system (**Fig. 31.1**). Therefore, there are differences in the technique of final implantation. But they all have the common feature of absolutely requiring adequate decompression of the index level. Some differences in material and biomechanics may provide advantages in certain scenarios. In choosing one, the surgeon must have a thorough understanding of the prosthesis's biomechanical design and familiarity with its implantation (**Table 31.1**).

IV. Complications

Complications are similar to those for ACDF; however, there are four primary reasons to consider revision of cervical arthroplasty:
- Radiculopathy (or other new-onset neurologic deficit) after cervical arthroplasty
- Subsidence
- Implant migration
- Ankylosed joint (formation of significant heterotopic bone around the implant)

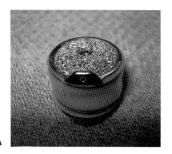
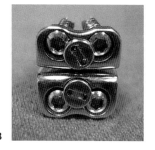
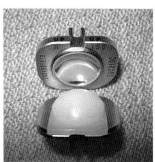

Fig. 31.1 (A–C) Photographs of the three arthroplasty devices currently approved by the U.S. Food and Drug Administration. (A) Bryan Device. (B) Prestige Device. (C) Pro-Disc C Device. (From Baaj et al, History of Cervical Arthroplasty. Neurosurgical Focus. September 2009, Figs. 2–4.)

V. Postoperative Care

Same as for ACDF, except for the following:
 – Mummaneni et al suggested that perioperative oral nonsteroidal antiinflammatory drugs (NSAIDs) for 2 weeks[2] might reduce the incidence of heterotopic bone formation.
 – Avoid neck collar (encourage normal motion).

Table 31.1 FDA-Approved Cervical Arthroplasty Devices in the United States

Device	Manufacturer	Classification	Biomaterials
ProDisc-C	Synthes Spine, West Chester, PA	Semiconstrained	CCM end plate with UHMWPE inlay
BRYAN	Medtronic Ltd., Memphis, TN	Unconstrained	Titanium alloy shells with polyurethane nucleus
PRESTIGE ST	Medtronic Ltd., Memphis, TN	Unconstrained	Metal on metal

Abbreviations: CCM, cobalt-chromium-molybdenum; FDA, Food and Drug Administration; ST, stainless steel; UHMWPE, ultra-high molecular weight polyethylene.

VI. Outcomes

To date, there have been three prospective randomized multicenter U.S. studies comparing cervical artificial disc implantation with ACDF in patients treated for single-level cervical disc disease with radiculopathy or myelopathy.

- The largest of these studies compared the PRESTIGE ST Cervical Disc System (Medtronic, Memphis, TN) with ACDF in a total of 541 patients. At 24 months' follow-up, the arthroplasty group demonstrated maintenance of physiologic segmental motion in association with improved neurologic success, improved clinical outcomes, and a reduced rate of secondary surgeries compared with conventional ACDF.[2]
- Heller et al compared the BRYAN Cervical Disc (Medtronic, Memphis, TN) with ACDF in 463 patients. At 24 months after surgery, the arthroplasty group showed a statistically greater improvement in the primary outcome variables: neck disability index score and overall success. No statistical difference was found between the arthroplasty and ACDF groups with regard to secondary surgical procedures or implant-related adverse events. The arthroplasty patients returned to work nearly 2 weeks earlier than the ACDF patients.[3]
- Murrey et al compared single-level ProDisc-C (Synthes Spine, L.P., West Chester, PA) arthroplasty with ACDF in 209 patients. At 24 months after surgery, visual analog scale (VAS), neck disability index (NDI), and neurologic success rate demonstrated no statistical difference between the arthroplasty and ACDF groups. Statistically fewer reoperations and less pain medication usage were noted in the ProDisc-C cohort.[4]

VII. Surgical Pearls

- Generous decompression of the neuroforamen bilaterally (including asymptomatic side)
- Proper end plate preparation
- Correct implant selection (footprint size, height)

Common Clinical Questions

1. How many degrees of neck range of motion loss could result from a single-level ACDF?
2. What is the incidence of development of symptomatic adjacent-level disease after single-level ACDF?
3. Why should patients take oral NSAIDs and avoid neck collar use after cervical arthroplasty?

References

1. Mummaneni PV, Haid RW. The future in the care of the cervical spine: interbody fusion and arthroplasty. Invited submission from the Joint Section Meeting on Disorders of the Spine and Peripheral Nerves, March 2004. J Neurosurg Spine 2004;1(2):155–159
2. Mummaneni PV, Burkus JK, Haid RW, Traynelis VC, Zdeblick TA. Clinical and radiographic analysis of cervical disc arthroplasty compared with allograft fusion: a randomized controlled clinical trial. J Neurosurg Spine 2007;6(3):198–209
3. Heller JG, Sasso RC, Papadopoulos SM, et al. Comparison of BRYAN cervical disc arthroplasty with anterior cervical decompression and fusion: clinical and radiographic results of a randomized, controlled, clinical trial. Spine (Phila Pa 1976) 2009;34(2):101–107
4. Murrey D, Janssen M, Delamarter R, et al. Results of the prospective, randomized, controlled multicenter Food and Drug Administration investigational device exemption study of the ProDisc-C total disc replacement versus anterior discectomy and fusion for the treatment of 1-level symptomatic cervical disc disease. Spine J 2009;9(4):275–286
5. Hilibrand AS, Carlson GD, Palumbo MA, Jones PK, Bohlman HH. Radiculopathy and myelopathy at segments adjacent to the site of a previous anterior cervical arthrodesis. J Bone Joint Surg Am 1999;81(4):519–528
6. Tu TH, Wu JC, Huang WC, Guo WY, Wu CL, Shih YH, Cheng H. Heteroptic ossification after cervical total disc replacement determination by CT and effects on clinical outcomes. J Neurosurg Spine 2011;14(4):457–465

Answers to Common Clinical Questions

1. A fusion of one level of the cervical spine typically results in the loss of 7 degrees of flexion and extension motion and 6 degrees of rotational motion.[2]
2. Symptomatic adjacent-segment disease occurs at a rate of 2.9% per year during the 10-year period after the operation (Hilibrand et al, 2008).[5]
3. NSAIDs and motion may reduce the occurrence of heterotopic bone formation around the artificial disc.[6]

32 Anterior Cervical Corpectomy

Mohammad Said Shukairy and Frank M. Phillips

I. Key Points
- Anterior cervical corpectomy is a safe and effective technique for decompression of the ventral cervical spinal cord.
- The surgical approach and exposure for corpectomy are similar to the case for the more common anterior cervical discectomy (see Chapter 33).[1]

II. Indications
- Generally corpectomy is indicated when there is ventral spinal cord compression and discectomy is inadequate for decompression.
  - Degenerative conditions, such as spondylotic myelopathy in which ventral spinal cord compression is not restricted to the disc level and/or is complicated by cervical kyphosis
  - Tumor infiltration of the vertebral body causing vertebral body collapse and spinal cord compression
  - Traumatic cervical spine injury, such as a teardrop fracture with associated spinal cord compression from retropulsion of vertebral body fragments and spinal instability
  - Osteomyelitis with epidural abscess and concomitant ventral spinal cord compression
  - Ossification of the posterior longitudinal ligament

III. Technique
- Intubation via fiberoptic technique, whether awake or asleep, is safer in cases with significant cervical spinal cord compression, myelopathic signs, myelomalacia, and/or cervical instability.
- Awake fiberoptic intubation allows for neurologic assessment immediately following intubation to assess for changes in neurologic function.
- Tape the endotracheal tube away from the side of surgical incision.
- Steroid administration preoperatively or intraoperatively lacks scientific support.
- Neurologic monitoring is prudent during operations on myelopathic patients.

- Some authors routinely use 8 to 10 lb of traction with Gardner-Wells tongs or chin strap craniocervical traction to increase disc space distraction.
- Place patient supine on the operating table.
  - Pressure points should be padded, especially the ulnar nerve.
  - A roll between the scapulae may improve lordosis and access to the level of interest. In patients with myelopathy, neck extension must be avoided.
  - Shoulders should be taped down to allow for fluoroscopic visualization of the level of interest; however, excessive traction can injure the brachial plexus.
- Localize, with fluoroscopy or using external landmarks, the approximate level of incision along the neck.
- The surgeon may approach the anterior cervical spine from the right or left side; the left-sided approach theoretically involves less risk to the recurrent laryngeal nerve.[2]
- The incision may be made transversely or longitudinally depending on the number of levels involved and surgeon preference.
- After incision, identify the platysma beneath the subcutaneous layer, and divide it sharply in a transverse or longitudinal fashion.
  - Dissecting under the platysma superiorly and inferiorly allows for better mobilization of the tissues.
- Identify the medial border of the sternocleidomastoid (SCM).
- Using Metzenbaum scissors, dissect in the areolar plane between the SCM and the medial structures.
  - The carotid artery should be palpated to ensure that the trajectory of dissection is correct.
- Using a hand-held retractor, retract the medial structures from the SCM to expose the prevertebral fascia.
- Incise the fascia to expose the cervical spine; use Kittners to sweep the prevertebral fascia superiorly and inferiorly.
- Use a spinal marker in the vertebral body (and not the disc) to confirm the level with x-ray or fluoroscopy image.
- With electrocautery or periosteal elevator, dissect the longus colli laterally from their midline attachments.
- Place self-retaining retractors and deflate the cuff of the endotracheal tube to minimize esophageal/tracheal edema.
- Caspar pins may be placed into the vertebral bodies above and below the level of interest, with distraction then applied.
- The discs above and below the level of interest should be incised and removed with curettes and pituitary rongeurs.

- When necessary, anterior osteophytes can be removed with a rongeur.
- A burr can be used to thin the vertebral body to the posterior longitudinal ligament (PLL).
- The PLL is carefully pierced with a small hook or curette.
- A small Kerrison rongeur (1 or 2 mm) can then be used to lift the PLL away from the dura and complete the decompression.
- Lateral decompression (foraminotomy) is generally completed at the level of the uncovertebral joint. The uncus can be thinned with a burr and then removal is completed with a microcurette or Kerrison rongeur (**Fig. 32.1**).
- A strut graft or cage with autograft, allograft, or bone graft substitute material is placed into the defect after contouring of the vertebral body end plates.
- An anterior plate can be used to enhance fusion and prevent graft migration. If possible, multiple points of screw fixation should be established. Posterior instrumentation does, however, provide greater stability and may be required.
- Some authors recommend rigid anterior fixation to enhance rigidity and reduce graft subsidence; others argue that variable

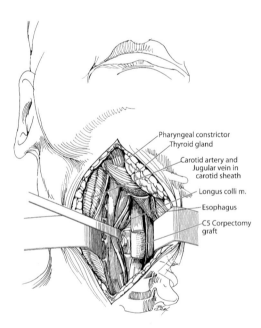

Fig. 32.1 Anterior view of the surgical field after single-level corpectomy in the cervical spine.

plates and screws may enhance fusion by dynamically loading the graft (Wolf's law). Data in support of either approach are limited to theoretical considerations and retrospective studies.[3,4]

IV. Complications

- Wound infection
- Transient hoarseness
    - Reduce risk by reducing endotracheal cuff pressure.
    - Avoid dissection into the carotid sheath.
    - Some surgeons advocate a left-sided approach to avoid risk of recurrent laryngeal nerve injury.
- Permanent hoarseness
- Transient or permanent dysphagia
- Nerve root or spinal cord injury[5]
- Acute airway obstruction from swelling or hematoma
    - Immediately stabilize the airway and intubate.
    - Open the wound at the bedside to allow for decompression of the hematoma and thereby ease intubation in an emergent setting.
- Cerebrospinal fluid (CSF) leak
    - Extremely difficult to close primarily
    - Cover with fibrin glue or dural sealant.
    - Place lumbar drain to divert CSF if there is concern about the risk of persistent drainage.
- Vascular injury
    - Vertebral artery
        - The vertebral artery lies lateral to the uncovertebral complex and is often surrounded by a collection of veins.
        - Inadvertent injury can lead to massive bleeding.
        - In the event of injury, the surgeon must immediately administer tamponade to the bleeding, usually with the aid of Gelfoam (Pfizer, New York) or another hemostatic agent. The vessel can be repaired primarily if visualized, or ligated surgically with low risk of neurologic sequelae.[6,7]
        - An emergent angiogram should be considered to rule out vertebral artery dissection and may require vertebral artery embolization.
        - The artery can be sacrificed with little consequence if it is nondominant; sacrifice of the dominant vertebral artery has a higher incidence of ischemic injury to the brain stem.[6]
- Graft dislodgment/instrumentation failure
    - Graft dislodgment may indicate pseudarthrosis, hardware failure, infection, or a combination of factors.

- Of primary importance is airway stablization; if there is significant tracheal compression, emergent intubation and reoperation may be required.
- Revision of the graft may include the use of autograft, such as iliac crest, and posterior cervical instrumentation and fusion to supplement the anterior construct.

V. Postoperative Care

- After a prolonged procedure involving concern for anterior soft-tissue swelling, consider keeping the patient intubated for 24 to 48 hours (until able to breathe around deflated airway cuff).
- Consider external immobilization of the cervical spine.
- Patients with myelopathy and gait unsteadiness may benefit from physical and occupational therapy evaluations.
- Ensure that the patient is tolerating oral intake and swallowing normally prior to discharge.

VI. Outcomes

- The goals of decompressive corpectomy are neurologic preservation, cervical spine stabilization, and/or reduction of deformity.
- Available outcomes studies are limited in their retrospective nature, but indicate excellent technical results (greater than 98% fusion rate) and improvement in radicular and myelopathic symptoms in 86%.[8]
- Even in patients with severe myelopathy resulting in a bedridden or wheelchair-bound condition, clinical outcomes showed improvement in over 60% of patients who underwent surgery.[9]

VII. Surgical Pearls

- Identify the location of vertebral artery on preoperative imaging studies.
- Avoid extension of the cervical spine during positioning.
- Generous dissection of the longus colli muscle allows better identification of midline, proper placement of retractor blades underneath the muscle fibers, and decreased pressure on vascular structures laterally or esophagus and trachea medially.
- Begin decompression with discectomy cranial and caudal to the intended corpectomy. This will assist in identification of the appropriate depth and width (uncus to uncus) of corpectomy.

– When the PLL is severely adherent, dissociation of the PLL from the adjacent structures, thus eliminating its constrictive effect on the spinal cord and preventing thecal sac manipulation, is the primary goal. Removing the PLL entirely becomes a secondary goal if it can be safely achieved.[10]

Common Clinical Questions

1. True or false: The fusion rate after anterior cervical corpectomy increases with augmented posterior fixation, especially after two- and three-level corpectomies.

References

1. Aronson N, Filtzer DL, Bagan M. Anterior cervical fusion by the Smith-Robinson approach. J Neurosurg 1968;29(4):396–404
2. Bauer R, Kerschbaumer F, Poisel S, et al. Anterior approaches. In Atlas of Spinal Operations. New York: Thieme Medical Publishers; 1993:4–12
3. Vaccaro A, Singh K. The role of anterior column reconstruction. In Anterior Spinal Column Surgery. Philadelphia, PA: Hanley & Belfus; 1998:589–590
4. Ulrich C, Woersdoerfer O, Kalff R, Claes L, Wilke HJ. Biomechanics of fixation systems to the cervical spine. Spine (Phila Pa 1976) 1991;16(3, Suppl):S4–S9
5. Flynn TB. Neurologic complications of anterior cervical interbody fusion. Spine (Phila Pa 1976) 1982;7(6):536–539
6. Rao R, David K. Anterior cervical surgery. In Complications in Orthopaedics: Spine Surgery. Rosemont, IL: American Academy of Orthopaedic Surgeons; 2006:4–16
7. Daentzer D, Deinsberger W, Böker DK. Vertebral artery complications in anterior approaches to the cervical spine: report of two cases and review of literature. Surg Neurol 2003;59(4):300–309, discussion 309
8. Eleraky MA, Llanos C, Sonntag VK. Cervical corpectomy: report of 185 cases and review of the literature. J Neurosurg 1999;90(1, Suppl):35–41
9. Scardino FB, Rocha LP, Barcelos AC, et al. Is there a benefit to operating on patients (bedridden or in wheelchairs) with advanced stage cervical spondylotic myelopathy? J Euro Spine, 2010
10. Sandhu H. Anterior cervical corpectomy. In Spine Surgery: Tricks of the Trade. New York: Thieme Medical Publishers; 2003:44–45

Answers to Common Clinical Questions

1. True.

33 Anterior Cervical Discectomy

Daniel C. Lu, Kevin T. Foley, and Praveen V. Mummaneni

I. Key Points
- Appreciation of the surgical anatomy of vital structures (carotid, esophagus, recurrent laryngeal nerve) during approach is essential.
- To decrease incidence and severity of dysphagia, endotracheal cuff pressure can be decreased during the retraction phase of the surgery. Additionally, intermittent relaxation of the retraction can be utilized.

II. Indications
- Symptomatic herniated nucleus pulposus
  - Radiculopathy (after failed conservative therapy)
  - Myelopathy
- Cervical spondylosis with radiculopathy or myelopathy
- Ossification of the posterior longitudinal ligament with myelopathy
- Cervical fracture with instability

III. Technique
- Place patient in supine position, arms tucked at sides.
  - May use horseshoe headrest with weight strap (7 to 10 lb)
  - May use foam doughnut head holder with shoulder retraction using thick tape
  - Intravenous (IV) bag placed longitudinally between shoulder blades to provide mild head extension
- Localize with fluoroscopy or utilize landmarks (cricoid cartilage approximates C5-C6).
  - If fluoroscopy is used, the incision is marked parallel to the disc space.
  - If multilevel procedure is performed, favor the incision placement at the rostral disc space.
  - A transverse incision 3 cm in length is adequate for single-level procedure; a longitudinal incision along the anterior border of the sternocleidomastoid is preferable for a procedure with three or more levels.
- Incision is made and the platysma undermined; the plane medial to the sternocleidomastoid muscle is identified and bluntly

33 Anterior Cervical Discectomy

dissected with a finger or blunt instrument in a rostral-to-caudal direction (**Fig. 33.1**). The omohyoid muscle overlies the C6 level and can be divided.[1]
- The carotid is then palpated and the plane medial to the carotid and lateral to the trachea and esophagus is developed by blunt dissection in the rostral-to-caudal direction.
- The spine is then palpated, the prevertebral fascia is entered, and the disc level is confirmed by x-ray or fluoroscopy.
- Hand-held Cloward retractors are used to retract and provide protection medially (the trachea and esphogaus) and laterally (the carotid sheath), while the longus colli muscles are mobilized with Bovie electrocautery (Bovie Medical Corp., Clearwater, FL). The midline is marked on the vertebral body to facilitate alignment of the cervical plate.
- Self-retaining retractor (Trimline [Medtronic, Memphis, TN] or equivalent) is placed underneath the longus colli. The endotracheal tube cuff may be mildly depressurized at this point.
- Disc annulectomy is performed with a number 15 blade scalpel; additional disc removal is performed with a pituitary ron-

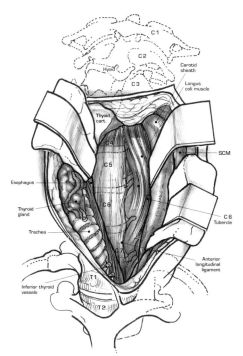

Fig. 33.1 Anterior exposure to cervical spine. (From Haher R, Merola A, Surgial Technique for the Spine, Thieme; pg. 73, Fig. 15-1B.)

geur. The cartilaginous end plate is removed from the bony end plate with curettes. Carefully remove the lateral disc demarcated by the uncovertebral joint.
- Osteophytes/calcified disc fragments are drilled down to the posterior longitudinal ligament (PLL), the angle of drilling follows the angle of the disc space as seen with intraoperative radiographs or fluoroscopy. Take care not to drill away the bony end plate.
- The PLL is defined and first entered with a fine-angle nerve hook; it is identified by round longitudinal fibers. It is resected further with fine Kerrison punches. The dural plane is now evident.
- Allograft, autograft, or polyetheretherketone (PEEK)/carbon fiber cages filled with bone may be sized and placed into the disc space.[2] Temporary sizers are introduced into the intervertebral space with head traction to assess the correct interbody spacer size.
- An anterior cervical plate is placed aligning the midline with previous mark.
- The wound is irrigated with saline (for non–bone morphogenic protein [BMP] cases).
- A small subfascial drain may be placed.
- Closure of platysma is done with interrupted 2.0 Vicryl (Ethicon, a Johnson & Johnson company, New York) and the subcutaneous layer with interrupted 3.0 Vicryl. Skin is closed with a subcuticular running 4.0 monocryl suture.
- Steri-strips (3M, St. Paul, MN) may be used for skin.

IV. Complications

- Nerve root injury (C5 nerve root palsy in up to 5%)[3]
- Spinal cord injury (especially in myelopathic patients; avoid hyperextension)
- Wound hematoma (higher in multilevel cases; may be mitigated by drain placement)
- Hoarseness
- Dysphagia (due to edema or recurrent laryngeal nerve palsy)
- Esophageal perforation
- Carotid or vertebral artery injury (0.3%)
- Pseudarthrosis (2 to 20%)
- Wound infection (<1%)

V. Postoperative Care

- Decadron may be given for 24 hours to decrease soft-tissue edema.
- Use soft cervical collar for comfort (single level) and hard collar for immobilization (multilevel cases).
- Postoperative antibiotics for 24 hours
- May be discharged the same day with 6-hour observation in recovery unit

VI. Outcomes[4]

- Anterior cervical discectomy and fusion (ACDF) is a successful procedure when performed given the right indications.
- Adjacent-level disease occurs at a rate of around 2% per year in patients undergoing one-level ACDF.

VII. Surgical Pearls

- For patient counseling, ACDF is not fully effective in patients with predominant neck pain.
- The surgeon must know the course of the recurrent laryngeal nerve (RLN) to avoid injury during surgery. On the right, the RLN loops around the right subclavian artery, and the left RLN loops around the arch of the aorta. It runs within the tracheoesophageal groove, where sharp dissection in the paratracheal muscles or prolonged retraction against an inflated endotracheal tube may cause injury. Injury causes hoarseness, cough, aspiration, mass sensation, dysphagia, and vocal cord fatigue. Studies have not demonstrated a difference in RLN injury when comparing right and left anterior cervical exposure.
- Indirect decompression by removal of central disc material and restoration of disc space height by an interbody graft may be used for a laterally herniated disc; however, the definitive procedure is to remove all lateral disc demarcated by the uncovertebral joint. It is important to achieve a direct decompression of a laterally herniated disc.

Common Clinical Questions

1. What is the course of the recurrent laryngeal nerve, and what symptoms would be manifested by a recurrent laryngeal nerve injury?
2. What measures can be undertaken to minimize the risk of dysphagia in ACDF?
3. Destruction of vertebral body end plates during discectomy may cause:
   A. Subsidence of interbody
   B. Cervical kyphosis
   C. Plate failure
   D. Successful fusion
   E. All of the above

References

1. Greenberg MS. Handbook of Neurosurgery. 6th ed. New York: Thieme Medical Publishers, 2006:304–306
2. Tumialán LM, Pan J, Rodts GE, Mummaneni PV. The safety and efficacy of anterior cervical discectomy and fusion with polyetheretherketone spacer and recombinant human bone morphogenetic protein-2: a review of 200 patients. J Neurosurg Spine 2008; 8(6):529–535
3. Fountas KN, Kapsalaki EZ, Nikolakakos LG, et al. Anterior cervical discectomy and fusion associated complications. Spine (Phila Pa 1976) 2007;32(21):2310–2317
4. Holly LT, Matz PG, Anderson PA, Groff MW, Heary RF, Kaiser MG, Mummaneni PV, Ryken TC, Choudhri TF, Vresilovic EJ, Resnick DK. Joint Section on Disorders of the Spine and Peripheral Nerves of the American Association of Neurological Surgeons and Congress of Neurological Surgeons. J Neurosurg Spine. 2009;11(2):238–244

Answers to Common Clinical Questions

1. The recurrent laryngeal nerve runs within the tracheoesophageal groove after looping around the aortic arch (left) or the subclavian artery (right). Injury would cause hoarseness, cough, aspiration, mass sensation, dysphagia, and vocal cord fatigue.
2. Decreased cuff pressure after placement of self-retaining retractors, intermittent release of retraction during surgery, and intraoperative use of Decadron
3. A

34 Anterior Cervical Foraminotomy

Matthew J. Tormenti and Adam S. Kanter

I. Key Points

- Spares disruption of the annulus fibrosus and avoids the need for interbody fusion
- Contraindicated in treating posterior pathology and centrally located anterior pathology
- Contraindicated in patients with evidence of instability

II. Indications

- Patients with cervical radiculopathy, myelopathy, or myeloradiculopathy
- Anterolateral pathology such as disc herniations or anterior osteophytes
- Lesions of the vertebral artery or foramen transversarium
- Progressive neurologic decline or failure of at least 3 months of conservative management

III. Technique

Operating Room Setup

- The operating room is set up in the same manner as for other anterior cervical approaches (e.g., anterior cervical discectomy and fusion [ACDF]).
- General endotracheal anesthesia is induced.
- The patient is placed supine with a shoulder roll to enhance cervical lordosis and access to the disc space. The patient's arms are tucked at the sides and secured with appropriate padding to avoid ulnar nerve entrapment.

Exposure

- A transverse incision is made along a natural skin crease to avoid an aesthetically unacceptable scar.
- The subcutaneous tissues and platysma are carefully dissected until the strap muscles and carotid sheath are identified.
- The carotid sheath is retracted laterally and the esophagus and trachea retracted medially with Meyerding retractors.
- Fascial dissection is performed bluntly with a cotton-tipped probe.

- Prevertebral fascia is opened using either sharp dissection or monopolar cautery.
- Radiographic localization is performed to ensure exposure of the correct level.
- Meticulous hemostasis is maintained throughout the exposure.
- Self-retaining retractors are placed in the wound.
- An operating microscope is brought to the field.

Decompression
- The ipsilateral longus colli muscle is detached from vertebral body.
- The medial borders of the transverse processes of the superior and inferior vertebral body are exposed (**Fig. 34.1**).
- Uncovertebral joints are identified (**Fig. 34.2**).
- The inferior portion of the superior vertebral body constituting the uncovertebral joint is removed.
- Approximately 4 to 5 mm of the inferior vertebral body is removed.

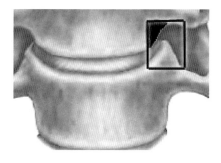

Fig. 34.1 The area of interest between the superior and inferior vertebral body is outlined. Bony removal of the inferior border of the superior vertebral body is undertaken to reach the foramen.

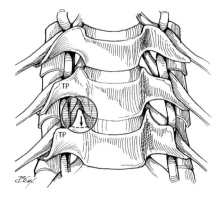

Fig. 34.2 Anterior exposure and approach for a patient with right C4-C5 foraminal stenosis. Arrow indicates the site of uncinate process takedown with 2 mm cutting burr (indicated by solid arrow within shaded circle). TP = transverse process. (From Vaccaro AR, Albert TJ, Spine Surgery: Tricks of the Trade 2nd ed, Thieme; pg. 55, Fig. 15.1.)

- Bony removal continues until the posterior longitudinal ligament (PLL) is visible.
- Osteophytectomy or fragmentectomy is performed for full decompression of the impinged nerve root.
- A nerve hook may be used to ensure decompression.

IV. Complications

- With the procedure in experienced hands, the complication rate has been reported at <5%.[1–3]
- Nerve root injury
- Spinal cord injury
- Cerebrospinal fluid (CSF) leak
- Recurrent laryngeal nerve injury
- Tracheal or esophageal injury
- Vascular injury (carotid artery, jugular vein, vertebral artery) (**Fig. 34.3**)
- Horner syndrome (sympathetic trunk injury)

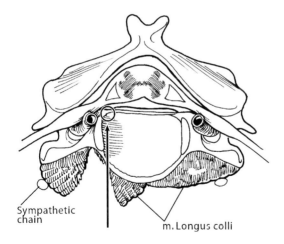

Fig. 34.3 Axial view of a vertebral body demonstrating approach for anterior foraminotomy. Operative approach includes drilling down through uncinate process to start point of foraminotomy. Special attention must always be paid to the nearby vertebral artery. (From Vaccaro AR, Albert TJ, Spine Surgery: Tricks of the Trade 2nd ed, Thieme; pg. 55, Fig. 15.2.)

V. Postoperative Care

- May be outpatient procedure or involve overnight observation
- A soft collar may be employed for comfort measures immediately after surgery, but patient should be weaned off and discontinue use shortly thereafter.
- Throat lozenges can be used to treat postoperative swallowing discomfort from esophageal irritation.

VI. Outcomes

- Jho and colleagues reported 79.8% resolution of symptoms in patients with radiculopathy.[2]
- For myelopathy, 27.5% experienced resolution of all symptoms, 52% showed improvement, and 20% were unchanged.[1]

VII. Surgical Pearls

- Proper setup and retractor placement is crucial to maximize visualization and prevent complications.
- Knowledge of the course of the vertebral artery is essential to prevent vascular injury.
- This approach is ideal for pathology located anterolateral to the neural elements.
- Minimal destabilization avoids the need for concomitant fusion.

Common Clinical Questions

1. The anterior foraminotomy may be utilized to address what type of pathology?
2. True or false: An arthrodesis procedure is necessary following anterior foraminotomy.
3. True or false: Outcomes for this operation are better for radiculopathy than for myelopathy.

References

1. Jho HD, Kim MH, Kim WK. Anterior cervical microforaminotomy for spondylotic cervical myelopathy: part 2. Neurosurgery 2002;51(5, Suppl):S54–S59
2. Jho HD, Kim WK, Kim MH. Anterior microforaminotomy for treatment of cervical radiculopathy: part 1–disc-preserving "functional cervical disc surgery." Neurosurgery 2002; 51(5, Suppl):S46–S53
3. Saringer W, Nöbauer I, Reddy M, Tschabitscher M, Horaczek A. Microsurgical anterior cervical foraminotomy (uncoforaminotomy) for unilateral radiculopathy: clinical results of a new technique. Acta Neurochir (Wien) 2002;144(7):685–694

Answers to Common Clinical Questions

1. Disc fragments or osteophytes located anterolateral to the neural elements
2. False. The procedure is not destabilizing when performed correctly. Patients with cervical instability should undergo a decompression/fusion procedure and not an anterior foraminotomy.
3. True. Approximately 80 to 100% of radicular complaints were resolved in two early series.

35 Cervical Laminectomy with or without Fusion
Ali A. Baaj and Fernando L. Vale

I. Key Points
- Conservative therapy is the initial, primary treatment modality for neck pain and/or radiculopathy caused by degenerative cervical spine disease.
- The surgical goal should be to decompress the neural elements and, when clinically warranted, provide stabilization via instrumentation/fusion.
- Focal pathology may be better treated via anterior cervical approaches or posterior foraminotomy.

II. Indications
- Multilevel degenerative disc disease causing cervical stenosis and myelopathy
- Cervical stenosis due to diffuse ossification of the posterior longitudinal ligament (OPLL)
- Epidural abscess
- Tumor

III. Technique
- Place patient in prone position.
    - Awake, fiberoptic intubation may be necessary in cases of severe stenosis or instability.
- Mayfield head fixation or the use of skull tongs to apply 5 to 10 lb of inline cervical traction is optional.
- Localize with fluoroscopy and make appropriate-length midline incision.
- Even if localization is not needed (e.g., for long occipital-cervical incisions), it is advisable to obtain at least a lateral fluoroscope shot pre-incision with patient in the prone position to (1) appreciate alignment and (2) determine if lower cervical levels can be visualized.
- Dissecting down to the spinous processes in the midline avascular plain maintains the integrity of posterior neck muscles and minimizes bleeding.
- Perform subperiosteal dissection to expose the spinous processes, the lamina, and the lateral masses of the desired levels.

35 Cervical Laminectomy with or without Fusion

- It may be desirable to reduce the monopolar cautery level as dissection is carried laterally toward the edge of the lateral mass to avoid denervation/atrophy of neck muscles.
- Perform the posterior cervical laminectomy.
  - One technique is to use an AM-8 drill bit to create bilateral troughs at the laminar–lateral mass junction and remove the posterior elements "en bloc."
    - Advantage: no need to place instrument under the lamina and risk cord compression
    - Disadvantage: requires proficiency with the drill and places the lateral mass at risk if the troughs are too lateral
  - A second technique is to use a combination of Leksell and Kerrison instruments (manual laminectomy).
    - Advantage: technique more familiar as it is widely used in the lumbar spine
    - Disadvantage: potential risk of neural injury with instruments placed under lamina in severe stenosis
  - The third technique is to use a footplate craniotome to create bilateral troughs (no significant advantage and may carry higher risks in authors' opinion).
- Perform cervical lateral mass fixation (if necessary) (**Fig. 35.1**).
  - Magerl technique
    - The lateral mass is divided into quadrants.

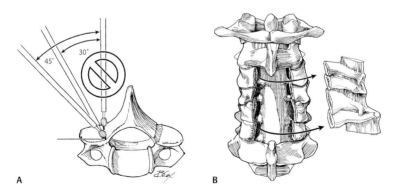

Fig. 35.1 Laminectomy. **(A)** The burr must be directed approximately 30 to 45 degrees in the sagittal plane to avoid burring into the facet joint. Doing so may risk loss of orientation and cause one to burr too deeply, endangering the dural sac or spinal cord. **(B)** En bloc removal of laminae. (From Vaccaro AR, Albert TJ, Spine Surgery: Tricks of the Trade 2nd ed, Thieme; pg. 6, Fig. 2.2B,C.)

- The entry point is at the superior medial quadrant and the trajectory is toward the superior lateral quadrant ("up and out") (**Fig 35.2**).
- Usually achievable for C3-C6
- Roy-Camille technique
  - The entry point is at the midpoint of the lateral mass.
  - The trajectory is 10 degrees lateral in the same axial plane.
  - Typically employed at the C7 level
- If C7 is included in the fixation, pedicle screws are typically used.
  - A laminotomy to palpate the medial edge of the pedicle is useful.
  - The entry point is in line with lateral mass entry points at superior levels.
  - Slight medial angulation is necessary to enter and traverse the pedicle.
- Lateral mass screw size is typically 3.5 or 4.0 mm by 12 to 16 mm.

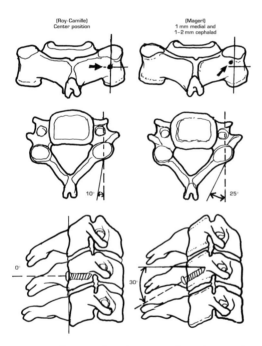

Fig 35.2 The Magerl and Roy-Camille techniques for placement of lateral mass screws in the subaxial cervical spine.

- C7 pedicle screw size is typically 3.5 or 4.0 mm by 16 to 24 mm.
- Insert appropriate-length rods and secure with set screws/caps.
  - Ensure proper application of anti-torque when securing caps to prevent lateral mass fracture/screw pullout.
- Decortication is performed using a high-speed drill; ideally, decorticate facets.
- Bone graft material (autograft plus carrier) is placed along the lateral mass edges bilaterally.
  - Ensure that no graft material is left within the canal or foramen.
- Place subfascial drain and close muscle, fascia, and skin layers.

IV. Complications

- Cerebrospinal fluid (CSF) leak
  - Attempt primary repair using nonabsorbable suture.
  - Alternatively, cover with Gelfoam (Pfizer, New York) and/or fibrin glue.
- Nerve root injury
  - May result either directly during foraminotomy or screw placement or indirectly from stretching/recoiling
  - C5 palsy: Incidence and etiology not well understood. May be due to traction, given that the C5 root is shortest. Often transient but noticeable immediately post–cervical laminectomy.
- Vertebral artery injury
  - Typically results from misplaced lateral mass screw
  - Screw should remain in place and postoperative angiogram used to delineate type of injury (e.g., occlusion, dissection).
- Wound infection

V. Postoperative Care

- Mobilize early with (typically in case of trauma) or without cervical collar.
- Obtain postoperative (PO) upright anteroposterior (AP)/lateral C-spine x-rays.
- Remove drain when output becomes less than 50 ml per 8-hour shift (typically PO day 1 or 2).
- Discharge home when patient meets discharge criteria.

VI. Outcomes

- Class III evidence shows that 70 to 95% of patients show postoperative neurologic improvement after cervical laminectomy and fusion for myelopathy.[1]

VII. Surgical Pearls

- Preoperative cervical kyphosis and loss of lordosis are relative contraindications to posterior laminectomy without instrumentation.
- Focal disc bulges/herniations should be treated via anterior approaches.
- Positioning multiple lateral mass entry points in line facilitates rod placement (often the frustrating step of the procedure).

Common Clinical Questions

1. In the Magerl technique why is the trajectory of lateral mass screws "up and out"?
2. Which nerve root is most prone to indirect injury during posterior cervical laminectormy?
3. Why is preoperative cervical spine alignment an important consideration?

References

1. Anderson PA, Matz PG, Groff MW, et al; Joint Section on Disorders of the Spine and Peripheral Nerves of the American Association of Neurological Surgeons and Congress of Neurological Surgeons. Laminectomy and fusion for the treatment of cervical degenerative myelopathy. J Neurosurg Spine 2009;11(2):150–156

Answers to Common Clinical Questions

1. "Up" to avoid the nerve root and "out" to avoid the vertebral artery
2. C5 nerve root
3. Kyphosis or loss of lordosis may worsen after cervical laminectomy without instrumentation.

36 Cervical Laminoplasty

Sarah I. Woodrow and Allan D. Levi

I. Key Points

- Laminoplasty is a procedure in which the spinal canal is expanded with the integrity of the posterior elements preserved.
- Laminoplasty was developed in Japan in the 1970s as a "tissue-sparing" alternative to laminectomy to minimize its associated risk of instability and progressive kyphotic deformity and thus improve outcomes.[1]

II. Indications

- Multilevel spinal cord compression secondary to one or any combination of the following:
  - Ossification of the posterior longitudinal ligament (OPLL)
  - Cervical spondylosis
  - Congenital canal stenosis
- For consideration in children requiring laminectomies
- Not for isolated neck pain or for patients with a significant kyphotic deformity

III. Technique

- In cases of severe stenosis, awake fiberoptic intubation should be considered to minimize the risk of hyperextension injury and allow for reexamination of patient prior to positioning.
- Place neurophysiologic monitoring leads (include somatosensory evoked potentials [SSEPs], motor evoked potentials [MEPs], and electromyograms [EMGs]) and obtain baseline recordings prior to turning the patient.
- Secure patient's head with or without pins (e.g., Mayfield three-pin headrest [Schaerer Mayfield, Randolph, MA]) and turn the patient prone with the head secured in a neutral to slightly flexed position.
- Tape superior and dorsolateral aspects of both shoulders and secure to the caudal corner of the operating table to aid in radiographic visualization of the lower cervical vertebrae.
- Use fluoroscopy to plan an incision extending from the spinous process of C2 to that of T1 and infiltrate with 1% lidocaine with epinephrine to minimize skin bleeding.

- Make a midline incision and use a subperiosteal dissection to reflect the paraspinal muscles from the caudal end of C2 to the rostral limit of T1.
- Remove the caudal third of the C2 lamina and the rostral third of the T1 lamina using the combination of a high-speed air drill and a 2 mm Kerrison punch, allowing visualization of the underlying dura at these levels.
- Remove the spinous processes from C3 to C7 with a rongeur and morselize the bone for subsequent autografting.
- Perform laminoplasty of lamina C3 to C7 by creating an "open" side and a "hinged" side. The open side is generally the side with the greatest compression and/or the side most clinically symptomatic.
  - Use the high-speed air drill with a small drill bit to create troughs at the level of the lamina-facet junction from C3 to C7 (**Fig. 36.1**).
  - Drill through the outer and inner cortical margins of the lamina on the open side, but only through the outer cortical margin and cancellous bone (and not the inner cortex) on the hinged side.

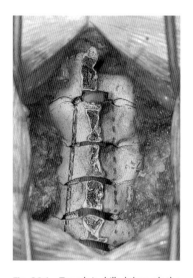

Fig. 36.1 Trough is drilled through the inner and outer cortices at the lamina-facet junction on the left (shown from C3 to C6 only). Partial laminectomy of C2 is shown. Purple crosshatching denotes area of drilling for closed door side.

- Prepare the bone allografts to stabilize the canal expansion.
  - Using rib allografts and the high-speed drill, cut three separate grafts each about 15 to 18 mm in length.
  - Make transverse grooves along the cut surfaces of the rib grafts, approximating the thickness of the cut laminae.
- Prepare to "open the door."
  - Use two small curettes placed into the trough on the open side just deep to the outer cortex.
  - Pull the curettes upward, thereby enlarging the lamina-facet gap and creating a green-stick fracture along the trough on the hinged side. Repeat the process on each successive lamina to expand the canal by about 4 mm (**Fig. 36.2**).
- Place the rib allografts in the gaps that have been created at the C3, C5, and C7 levels (**Fig. 36.3**).
- Place the morselized spinous process autograft over the decorticated bone surfaces of the facet and lamina on the hinged side at C3, C5, and C7 to provide for an intersegmental fusion.
- If the patient suffers from radiculopathy as well as myelopathy, one or more foraminotomies can be performed:
  - Once the lamina has been elevated and the ligamentum flavum excised, drill the mesial third of the facet over the exiting

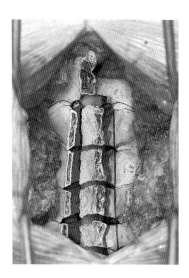

Fig. 36.2 With a trough drilled through the outer cortex only on the contralateral side (closed door side), the laminectomy door is "opened," creating a greenstick-type fracture on the closed side.

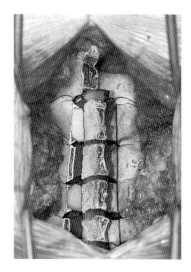

Fig. 36.3 Rib allograft is cut and secured into opening in lamina to expand the spinal canal, typically at C3, C5, and C7.

nerve root and widen the opening as needed with 1 or 2 mm angled Kerrison punches.
- Leave the subfascial drain (e.g., Hemovac [Gohar Shafa, Tehran, Iran]) in situ to minimize hematoma formation.
- Variations in the approach
  - Use spinous processes as autograft instead of the rib allograft
  - Stabilize the rib allograft with mini-plates to the adjacent lamina and facet on the open side or sutures
  - Use titanium spacers to hold open lamina that is affixed to the lamina-facet joint on the open side
  - Perform full-thickness splitting of the lamina in the midline and create bilateral troughs, and then spread the lamina and place allograft spacers (double-door laminoplasty)
  - Should rigid stabilization be required, lateral mass screws can be placed. This is best done after drilling and "opening the door," but prior to graft insertion.

IV. Complications

Early
- Wound infection (2%)
- Dural tear/CSF leak (<1%)
- Hemorrhage (<1%)
- Spinal cord injury (<1%)
- Nerve root injury
- Delayed C5 nerve root injury (2 to 13.3%)

Late
- Postoperative neck pain (40 to 60%)
- Reduced range of motion (20 to 50%)
- New-onset kyphosis (2 to 15%)

V. Postoperative Care

- Mobilize early with cervical bracing.
- Discharge to home once patient is ambulating and tolerating full diet—usually 2 to 3 days postoperatively.

VI. Outcomes

- Clinical outcome studies are drawn largely from the Japanese literature on patients with OPLL and are difficult to compare as a result of patient heterogeneity and different outcome measures used.[2]

- Long-term (5 to 10 years) outcome studies suggest 50 to 70% of patients with either OPLL or cervical spondylitic myelopathy show improvement in their neurologic function following laminoplasty.[3]
- Limited studies comparing this procedure to its corresponding anterior procedure identify similar clinical outcomes, but overall there is a suggestion that outcomes are better than with laminectomy alone.
- Recent studies suggest that clinical outcomes are similar between (1) laminectomy and fusion and (2) laminoplasty, with preserved range of motion and overall lower surgical costs for the latter.

VII Surgical Pearls

- Obtain pre-op x-rays to rule out instability or kyphotic deformity.
- Ensure the provision of drilling gutters at the lamina-facet junction (and not lateral to it) and direct drill medial so as not to disrupt the facet joint
- Lift *gently* when opening the door and ensure that drilling of the closed side (through outer cortex and some cancellous bone) is adequate to avoid creating a true fracture of the lamina. With a true greenstick fracture some tension should remain in the opening to help maintain compression on the rib graft to hold it in place.
- If multiple foraminotomies are required, plan on making the open side the side where more foraminotomies are required.
- Visually inspect the construct and gently stress it once rib allograft is placed to ensure that you have not compromised the canal and that it remains stable.

Common Clinical Questions

1. True or false: Patients with kyphotic deformities and symptoms of myelopathy may benefit from laminoplasty procedures.
2. List three perioperative surgical complications associated with laminoplasty.

References

1. Hale JJ, Gruson KI, Spivak JM. Laminoplasty: a review of its role in compressive cervical myelopathy. Spine J 2006;6(6, Suppl):289S–298S
2. Ratliff JK, Cooper PR. Cervical laminoplasty: a critical review. J Neurosurg 2003;98(3, Suppl):230–238
3. Wang MY, Shah S, Green BA. Clinical outcomes following cervical laminoplasty for 204 patients with cervical spondylotic myelopathy. Surg Neurol 2004;62(6):487–492, discussion 492–493

Answers to Common Clinical Questions

1. False. Kyphotic deformities are a relative contraindication to performing this procedure.
2. Delayed C5 nerve root injury (2 to 13.3%), wound infection (2%), dural tear/CSF leak (<1%), hemorrhage (<1%), spinal cord injury (<1%)

37 Posterior Cervical Foraminotomy

Matthias Setzer, Nam D. Tran, and Frank D. Vrionis

I. Key Points

- The posterior cervical foraminotomy approach (also referred to as laminoforaminotomy) allows nerve root decompression without the need to enter the disc space.
- In contrast to the anterior discectomy approach, posterior cervical foraminotomy is not destabilizing; therefore, there is no need for fusion/implants or harvesting autograft.

II. Indications and Contraindications

Indications
- Cervical neuroforaminal nerve root compression by a (lateral) soft disc herniation or spondylosis (osteophyte) with progressive or intractable cervical radiculopathy
- Cervical nerve root decompression if an anterior approach is not desirable (recurrent surgery, difficult anterior approach, cervicothoracic levels).

Contraindications
- Primary axial neck pain
- Cervical instability at the involved level
- Cervical myelopathy
- Severe kyphosis
- Large central disc herniation
- Central spinal canal stenosis

III. Technique

Patient Positioning
- After induction of general endotracheal anesthesia the patient is positioned in a prone position with the head clamped in a Mayfield head holder (Schaerer Mayfield, Randolph, MA) or in Gardner-Wells tongs with 5 to 10 pounds of traction. The advantages of traction are interspace distraction and stability.
- Alternatively, the patient can be positioned in a (semi)sitting position with the head clamped in a Mayfield head holder. The sitting position reduces venous pressure and reduces intraoperative blood loss. Additionally, the position of the head in rela-

tion to the cervical spine can be better adjusted than in a prone position.
- The (semi)sitting position carries the risk of air embolism and requires the placement of a precordial or intraesophageal Doppler probe and a central venous line for air aspiration in case of an embolism.
- The (semi)sitting position is contraindicated in patients with a patent foramen ovale and the possibility of paradoxical arterial embolism.

Preparation and Draping
- Confirmation and adequate visualization of the correct level with plain x-ray or fluoroscopy in a lateral position is mandatory.

Incision, Soft-Tissue Dissection, and Spine Exposure
Classical Procedure
- Posterior midline incision approximately 3 to 4 cm in length for an open microsurgical approach
- Exposure and incision of the nuchal fascia
- Unilateral, subperiosteal dissection of the muscle layers from the spinous process and lamina to the facet joint with a Bovie cautery (Bovie Medical Corp., Clearwater, FL) and a Cobb elevator. Supra- and interspinal ligaments should be preserved.
- Placement of a retractor and radiographic confirmation of the correct level

Minimally Invasive Procedure
- The proper incision site is marked with a spinal needle and lateral fluoroscopy. The incision is centered slightly rostral to the intended level of decompression.
- The skin incision is made approximately 2 cm lateral to the midline.
- If a retractor system is used (small-blade retractor, tubular retractor), only very small incisions are necessary (1.5 to 2 cm).
- Incise the fascia with a Bovie cautery.
- With the use of a bladed retractor, blunt dissection is performed with a finger down to the level of the lamina.
- If a tubular retractor system is used, a K-wire is positioned on the inferior articular facet of the upper vertebral body under fluoroscopic guidance. In this situation it is imperative that the K-wire engage bone at all times.
- Serial dilators are used to bluntly widen the approach through the muscles, and finally the tubular retractors are placed.
- A final radiographic check is recommended to confirm the correct level.

- The retractor should be placed on the interlaminar space (two-thirds) and on the facet joint (one-third).
- Bring in the draped microscope.

Foraminotomy and Wound Closure
- Expose and mark the cranial and caudal lamina of the appropriate level and check again with fluoroscopy.
- Expose the medial parts of the capsule of the facet joint.
- Perform a laminotomy by removing bone from the lateral parts of the caudal and cranial lamina with a high-speed drill or with a small Kerrison rongeur.
- Open the ligamentum flavum with a nerve hook or a dissector, and resect it with a small Kerrison rongeur.
- Extend the laminotomy cranially and laterally, and expose the lateral edge of the dura and the nerve root. The nerve root is generally displaced dorsally.
- Try to remove free disc material under the nerve root with a nerve hook and a pituitary rongeur.
- If the disc sequestrum is still covered with layers of the posterior longitudinal ligament, it has to be opened with a small dissector or with bipolar forceps.
- Undercut the superior articular process with 1 and 2 mm Kerrison rongeurs until the entire foramen is patent (but preserve at least 50% of the facet) (**Fig. 37.1**).
- Epidural bleeding is controlled with Gelfoam (Pfizer, New York) and Cottonoids (Saramall, Buenos Aires, Argentina).

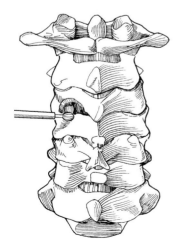

Fig. 37.1 Foraminotomy. The superior articular process can be removed by using a burr to thin it and a 1 mm Kerrison rongeur to remove remaining articular process, leaving the nerve root decompressed. (From Vaccaro AR, Albert TJ, Spine Surgery: Tricks of the Trade 2nd ed, Thieme; pg. 7, Fig. 2.3D.)

- Placement of a wound drain (Hemovac [Gohar Shafa, Tehran, Iran]) is usually not necessary.
- Close fascia with 0 or 2-0 absorbable sutures.
- Use inverted, interrupted 3-0 absorbable sutures for closure of the subcutaneous layer.
- Close the skin with a running, absorbable intracutaneous suture or with staples.

IV. Complications

- Wound dehiscence
- Wound infection and epidural abscess (1.2%)[1]
- Cerebrospinal fluid (CSF) leak (0.6 to 2.5%)[1,2]
- Neurologic deterioration due to injury or manipulation of the nerve root or spinal cord or postoperative epidural hematoma (1.2 to 2.3%)[1,2]
- Air embolism (sitting position) (1.6 to 2.3%)[2,3]
- Persistent radiculopathy indicating residual nerve root compression, epidural scarring, early recurrent disk herniation, or neuropathic pain requiring additional surgery (5.1 to 8%)[1,2]
- Recurrent disk herniation (7.6%)[2]
- Intraoperative hemorrhage caused by epidural veins or as a result of an inadvertent injury to vertebral artery (very rare and usually due to a wrong approach)
- Secondary instability due to excessive resection of the facet joint (4.9%)[1]
- Loss of cervical lordosis (18.5%)[1]

V. Postoperative Care

- Mobilize patient immediately after surgery.
- There is no need for external bracing; patients typically have full range of neck motion.
- Pain control is usually achieved with orally administered opioids.
- Discharge patients when discharge criteria are met (usually on post-op day 1).

VI. Outcomes

- Large series have reported excellent or good outcomes for posterior cervical foraminotomy in 90 to 96% of patients with monoradiculopathy.[1,2,4]

VII. Surgical Pearls

- Removal of more than 50% of the facet significantly compromises torsional stiffness of the cervical spine.[5]
- The entire length of the foramen can be enlarged safely with the use of curettes or a high-speed drill with preservation of more than 50% of the facet by initially working parallel and just inferior to the nerve root and then, as more room is gained, removing the rim just dorsal to the nerve root.
- Minimal bone removal (keyhole exposure) is acceptable, but not at the expense of excessive nerve root retraction or insufficient exposure of the dura with an increased risk of dural laceration.

Common Clinical Questions

1. What are the most common indications for a posterior cervical foraminotomy?
2. What are the two options for performing a posterior cervical foraminotomy?
3. How much of the facet joint can safely be removed without creating instability, and how much of the facet joint is usually removed during a posterior cervical foraminotomy?

References

1. Jagannathan J, Sherman JH, Szabo T, Shaffrey CI, Jane JA. The posterior cervical foraminotomy in the treatment of cervical disc/osteophyte disease: a single-surgeon experience with a minimum of 5 years' clinical and radiographic follow-up. J Neurosurg Spine 2009;10(4):347–356
2. Jödicke A, Daentzer D, Kästner S, Asamoto S, Böker DK. Risk factors for outcome and complications of dorsal foraminotomy in cervical disc herniation. Surg Neurol 2003;60(2): 124–129, discussion 129–130
3. Jadik S, Wissing H, Friedrich K, Beck J, Seifert V, Raabe A. A standardized protocol for the prevention of clinically relevant venous air embolism during neurosurgical interventions in the semisitting position. Neurosurgery 2009;64(3):533–538, discussion 538–539
4. Fehlings MG, Gray RJ. Posterior cervical foraminotomy for the treatment of cervical radiculopathy. J Neurosurg Spine 2009;10(4):343–344, author reply 344–346
5. Zdeblick TA, Zou D, Warden KE, McCabe R, Kunz D, Vanderby R. Cervical stability after foraminotomy. A biomechanical in vitro analysis. J Bone Joint Surg Am 1992;74(1):22–27

Answers to Common Clinical Questions

1. Cervical neuroforaminal nerve root compression by a (lateral) soft disc herniation or spondylosis (osteophyte) with progressive or intractable cervical radiculopathy, and the need for cervical nerve root decompression if an anterior approach is not desirable (recurrent surgery, difficult approach, cervicothoracic levels)

2. The standard procedure with a midline incision and subperiosteal dissection from the midline to the facet joint, and the minimally invasive procedure with a paramedian incision about 2 cm from the midline and blunt dissection through the muscles using small-blade or tubular retractors and serial dilators

3. Removal of more than 50% of the facet significantly compromises torsional stiffness of the cervical spine. During a posterior cervical foraminotomy, typically less than 50% of the facet joint is removed (approximately 30%).

38 Cervical Open Reduction Techniques: Anterior and Posterior Approaches

Harminder Singh, George M. Ghobrial, and James Harrop

I. Key Points

- Cervical facet dislocations result from high-energy traumatic forces transmitted through *flexion/distraction* vectors.
  - A flexion, rotational, and lateral force can result in a unilateral jumped facet.
  - If the mechanism of injury involves *flexion/compression* forces (e.g., diving headfirst into a shallow pool), then facet and vertebral body fractures may be encountered in the form of jumped and/or perched facets.
  - A severe flexion/distraction injury with a compression component is also called a teardrop fracture.
- Rule of thumb: A unilateral jumped facet results in 25% displacement (*anterolisthesis*) of one vertebral body on another (as seen on lateral plain radiographs or computed tomography [CT] scan of the cervical spine); bilateral jumped facets are associated with a 50% anterolisthesis.
- Acute management usually consists of reduction of the dislocated joints and the realignment of fractured cervical segments, through either open surgical intervention or axial cervical traction.
- Re-creating the force vectors of the mechanism of injury can facilitate reduction of the facets or deformity and realign the spine. For example, the cervical spine is flexed and distracted to realign the facets if the mechanism of injury was flexion/distraction.
- The open anterior approach provides for the removal of extruded disc prior to reduction of a dislocated facet. This approach may also be effective for reducing fractures and dislocations.
- Posterior instrumentation reestablishes the posterior tension band and provides the optimal environment for fusion.

II. Indications

Cervical open reduction can restore spinal alignment, decompress the neural elements, and establish rigid internal fixation.
- Cervical open reduction is indicated when:
  - Decompression of neural elements is required

- Closed reduction fails
- Contraindications for closed reduction
  - Patient with altered mental status
  - Skull fracture precluding tong placement
  - A relative contraindication is a rigid spine such as in ankylosing spondylitis.

III. Technique

Anterior Approach
- Neuromonitoring (somatosensory evoked potentials [SSEPs], motor evoked potentials [MEPs]) allows monitoring of spinal cord function during spinal manipulation.
- Localization of the cervical level is possible using fluoroscopy or plain radiographs.
  - Anatomic localizing
    - C5-C6 disc space: level of the cricoid cartilage
    - C3-C4 disc space: 1 cm above level of cricoid cartilage
- If a herniated disc is compressing the neural elements, a complete discectomy is performed prior to anterior reduction.
  - Blunt dissection: Retract carotid sheath laterally and trachea/esophagus medially with retractors to expose anterior spinal column. The anterior longitudinal ligament (ALL) is typically disrupted as a result of trauma.
  - Dissect longus colli laterally with monopolar cautery to expose the cervical vertebrae.
  - In unilateral dislocations, the superior vertebral body will be rotated away from the side of dislocation.
  - The annulus is incised with a scalpel as far laterally as possible to the uncovertebral joints.
  - The disc and posterior longitudinal ligament (PLL) are removed with curettes and with Kerrison and pituitary rongeurs until the dura is visualized. The PLL may be ruptured, particularly with bilateral dislocation.
- Caspar retractors are placed, with pins one level above and below the subluxed and dislocated segments.
  - Angulate pins convergently to place the spine in kyphotic (flexed) posture for distraction.
  - Distract Caspar pins; the superior body will rotate back and become flush with the inferior body (**Fig. 38.1**).
- Once the desired spinal alignment is achieved, a tricortical bone graft harvested from anterior superior iliac crest or allograft is used for arthrodesis.

38 Cervical Open Reduction Techniques

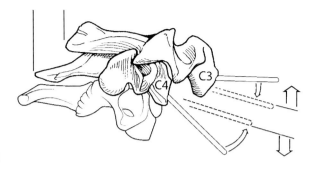

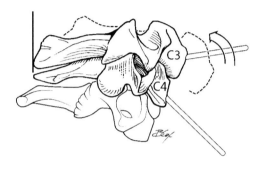

Fig. 38.1 (A,B) Anterior spinal reduction using convergently placed Caspar pins. Distracting the Caspar pins flexes and distracts the spine, unlocking the facets and reducing the spine.

- Anterior plate placement: screws anchoring the plate should be in the middle third of the vertebral body to avoid violation of end plates.

Posterior Approach
- More commonly used when there is disruption of the posterior ligamentous complex and associated facet fractures preventing closed reduction
- Prone position in Mayfield head holder (Schaerer Mayfield, Randolph, MA) or Gardner-Wells tongs, and make a midline incision
- Perform subperiosteal dissection during exposure of laminae and lateral masses.
- Reduction can be performed with direct distraction using two towel clips in opposite directions on the spinous processes using a leveraging mechanism (**Fig. 38.2**).

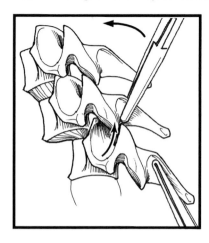

Fig. 38.2 Posterior spinal reduction using two towel clips. The inferior articulating facet of the superior vertebral body is lifted above and over the superior articulating facet of the inferior vertebral body, reducing the spine.

- Alternatively, the superior articulating process of the inferior facet can be drilled away to facilitate reduction.
- Once decompression and reduction are achieved, the spine is locked into place using either lateral mass screws and rods or posterior wiring techniques.
- Decortication of the facets and supplemental bone graft placement in the lateral gutters help with arthrodesis.

IV. Complications

- Wound infection (increased likelihood in trauma population)
- Graft donor site pain from autograft. Allograft bone is an alternative but may have a lower fusion rate.
- Anterior exposure may result in injury to the recurrent laryngeal nerve.
- Esophageal perforation
- Carotid artery and vagal nerve injury due to violation of the carotid sheath
- Horner syndrome: the sympathetic chain lies adjacent and anterior to the longus colli muscles.
- Damage to vertebral artery during posterior fixation
- CSF leak (which may be present from original trauma)
- Delayed fusion increases likelihood of screw loosening, plate migration, graft migration, and ultimately construct breakage.

V. Postoperative Care

- Immobilization for 6 weeks
- Serial radiographic examination: AP, lateral, swimmer's views
- Flexion-extension views for assessment of stability

VI. Outcomes

- Kwon et al did a prospective randomized controlled trial comparing anterior and posterior fixation for unilateral cervical facet injuries and reported equal efficacy between the two techniques.[1]
- Johnson et al reported a 13% incidence of loss of postoperative radiographic alignment during follow-up of cervical facet fracture-dislocations treated with only anterior decompression and fusion.[2]
- Reindl et al reported on 41 consecutive patients with unstable dislocations/subluxations, of whom 8 required anterior reduction after failure of Gardner-Wells traction; in addition, 2 of those 8 failed, requiring posterior surgery as well.[3]
- Fehlings et al reported on 44 consecutive patients treated with posterior cervical fusion for traumatic instability. Long-term follow-up revealed that the cervical spine was successfully stabilized in 93% of cases.[4]

VII. Surgical Pearls

- Best treated anteriorly: large disc herniation with cord compression such that spinal cord can be decompressed prior to distraction
- Best treated posteriorly: hyperflexion injury, including PLL injury, unilateral and bilateral facet dislocation without anterior cervical disc herniation
- Anteriorly, avoid overdistraction of the cervical spine during placement of the interbody graft. Due to the ligamentous laxity prevalent in spinal injury, it is easy to overdistract.
- Posteriorly, be mindful of laminar fractures during exposure. Heat from a Bovie cautery can damage the spinal cord or cause CSF leaks when transmitted through fractured laminae.

Common Clinical Questions

1. When should anterior reduction be utilized when closed reduction is not possible?
2. When should open reduction be performed?
3. Postoperatively after anterior cervical discectomy with fusion, the patient has a hoarse voice and difficulty swallowing. What should the clinician be concerned about?

References

1. Kwon BK, Fisher CG, Boyd MC, et al. A prospective randomized controlled trial of anterior compared with posterior stabilization for unilateral facet injuries of the cervical spine. J Neurosurg Spine 2007;7(1):1–12
2. Johnson MG, Fisher CG, Boyd MC, Pitzen T, Oxland TR, Dvorak MF. The radiographic failure of single segment anterior cervical plate fixation in traumatic cervical flexion distraction injuries. Spine (Phila Pa 1976) 2004;29(24):2815–2820
3. Reindl R, Ouellet J, Harvey EJ, Berry G, Arlet V. Anterior reduction for cervical spine dislocation. Spine (Phila Pa 1976) 2006;31(6):648–652
4. Fehlings MG, Cooper PR, Errico TJ. Posterior plates in the management of cervical instability: long-term results in 44 patients. J Neurosurg 1994;81(3):341–349

Answers to Common Clinical Questions

1. When large anterior disc herniation is present
2. Decompression of neural elements is required. Closed reduction fails. Closed reduction is contraindicated.
3. Injury to the recurrent laryngeal nerve on exposure

39 Resection of Pancoast Tumors

Jean-Paul Wolinsky and Ziya L. Gokaslan

I. Key Points

- T3N0M0 or T4N0M0 tumors (respectively, tumors with chest wall or chest wall and vertebral body invasion, negative nodes, and no metastasis) Pancoast tumors are potentially amenable to curative surgery if complete resection can be achieved.
- Pancoast tumors can be violated, but in contrast to some primary spinal tumors (i.e., chordoma and chondrosarcoma), if total resection is achieved, oncologic goals can still be met.
- Involvement or injury to the C8 and T1 roots or the lower trunk of the brachial plexus can result in significant pain and loss of hand function.

II. Indications

- Isolated lung mass with direct extension into the chest wall, lower trunk of the brachial plexus, and vertebral column
- No evidence of metastatic disease
- Negative mediastinal nodes
- Possibility of complete tumor resection

III. Technique

- Patient is positioned supine and undergoes general endotracheal intubation with a double-lumen tube. Positioning of the endotracheal tube is confirmed via bronchoscopy.
- Mediastinoscopy is performed, confirming that there is no evidence of positive mediastinal lymph nodes. If positive nodes are found, procedure is aborted and surgery is no longer a treatment option.
- If the vertebral artery or subclavian vessels are involved in tumor, they can be bypassed or sacrificed prior to stages 1 and 2 so that they may be resected with the specimen.

Stage 1

Stage 1 can be performed with patient in the lateral position and combined with stage 2, eliminating the need to reposition.

- Patient is taken from the supine position and placed prone on chest rolls and the head secured in a Mayfield head holder (Schaerer Mayfield, Randolph, MA). The cervical-thoracic region is cleaned and prepped in the usual sterile fashion. Prophylactic antibiotics are administered.
- The cervical-thoracic spine is exposed using the standard subperiosteal technique.
- Cervical lateral mass and thoracic pedicle screw instrumentation is inserted.
- Laminectomies are performed at the levels of interest. Nerve roots to be sacrificed are identified, ligated, and sectioned proximal to the dorsal root ganglion.
- Preoperatively, it is determined if the C8 and T1 nerve roots can be preserved, or if they will need to be sacrificed for oncologic reasons. If they are to be preserved, they are identified and traced laterally. The pedicle and the transverse process of T1 are resected. If the chest wall is involved in tumor, but there is no involvement of the vertebral column, then the rib heads are disarticulated from the vertebral body. If the vertebral column is involved in tumor, but the proximal portion of the rib is not, then the proximal portion of the T1 rib is resected. The C8 and T1 nerve roots are traced further laterally, identifying where they come together to form the lower trunk of the brachial plexus. The lower trunk of the brachial plexus is identified and protected during tumor resection. Injury to the C8 or T1 roots or the lower trunk of the brachial plexus can result in significant pain and loss of hand function.
- The lateral aspect of the vertebral column to be resected, contralateral to the tumor, is dissected, and the segmental vessels are ligated and cut.
- The most rostral and caudal disc spaces of the section of the vertebral column to be resected are identified. A Tomita-saw (MANI, Inc., Utsunomiya, Japan) is placed ventral to the thecal sac and posterior to the annulus at both of these disc spaces. The end of the saw, contralateral to the tumor, is tucked lateral to the vertebral column (to be retrieved later, during stage 2). If the most rostral disc space is C7-T1 or higher, this disc will be cut by means of a separate approach, using a standard anterior cervical discectomy technique.
- Two rods are contoured to the shape of the spine to span the cervical and thoracic instrumentation. One rod is secured to

the instrumentation contralateral to the tumor. The second rod is retained for stage 2. The wound is then temporarily closed.

Stage 2
- The patient is repositioned in the lateral decubitus position (tumor side up) on a bean bag. After the patient is properly positioned and secured to the table, the head is secured via a Mayfield head frame.
- The chest and posterior wound are cleaned, prepped, and draped.
- The posterior wound is reopened.
- The bronchus ipsilateral to the tumor is occluded and the lung deflated.
- A posterior-lateral thoracotomy is performed at the interspace below the section of chest wall involved with tumor. The skin incision is extended medially to intersect with the midline spinal incision. The paraspinous musculature is mobilized off of the transverse processes and ribs. The rostral aspect of the thoracotomy incision is elevated as a myocutaneous flap.
- The chest wall is then cut, starting at the level of the thoracotomy and extending rostrally, lateral to the extent of tumor involvement, until the rostral aspect of the tumor margin is passed. The intercostal nerves, arteries, veins, and musculature are sectioned with the chest wall.
- A formal lung lobectomy is performed proximal to the tumor, isolating the tumor from the lung.
- The contralateral Tomita-saws are retrieved ventral to the vertebral bodies, and using the saws, the discs are cut.
- The specimen is now completely mobilized and can be delivered en bloc. Pancoast tumors can be violated, and unlike the case for primary spinal tumors (i.e., chordoma and chondrosarcoma), if total resection with negative margins is achieved, the oncologic goals can still be met.
- The vertebral column defect is reconstructed, and arthrodesis is then performed.
- Two thoracostomy tubes are placed and tunneled out through separate incisions.
- A thoracoplasty is constructed, and the thoracotomy and posterior incisions are closed in the standard fashion.

IV. Complications
- Cerebrospinal fluid (CSF) leak and meningopleural fistula: These should be closed primarily, and the closure should be reinforced with fibrin glue. Postoperatively, the patient's tho-

racostomy should be transitioned to water seal as early as possible. Postoperative positive airway pressure (BiPAP) may decrease the chance of a meningopleural fistula. Postoperative lumbar drainage should be considered. Postoperative suspected CSF leaks can be verified by analyzing the pleural fluid for β_2 transferrin.
- Thoracic duct injury and chyle leak/chylothorax: Primary ligation of the thoracic duct to control the leak should be attempted. High-volume thoracostomy output suggests the possibility of a thoracic duct injury.
- Esophageal injury: Primary closure at the time of injury should be undertaken. Treat an injury in the postoperative period with a high degree of suspicion as such injuries carry significant morbidity and mortality.
- Pseudarthrosis
- Instrumentation failure
- C8, T1, lower trunk injury
- Bronchopleural fistula
- Vascular injury

V. Postoperative Care

- Intensive care unit (ICU)
- Thoracostomies to 20 cm H_2O suction until there is no evidence of pneumothorax, H_2O seal for 24 hours, then discontinue one thoracostomy every 24 hours.
- Incentive spirometry

VI. Outcomes

- Two-year and 5-year survival rates of patients undergoing complete resection with negative margins are 62% and 40%, respectively, compared with 29% and 12% for patients with positive margins.[1-3]

VII. Surgical Pearls

- Ligate nerves proximal to dorsal root ganglion to decrease the chances of chronic dysesthetic pain.
- When dissecting around the vertebral body, contralateral to the tumor, stay in the plane between the vertebral body and the segmental vessels to keep the vasculature protected during the resection.
- Suspected thoracic duct injuries can be better visualized 30 minutes after administering cream through a nasogastric tube. The chyle will become milky rather than clear, and can be seen better.

Common Clinical Questions

1. Lung tumor lesions involving the vertebral column are usually treated for palliation. Is the Pancoast tumor treated in this way?
2. Is mediastinoscopy an important element in the workup of a Pancoast tumor?
3. Can the C8 and T1 nerve roots be sacrificed without significant consequences?

References

1. York JE, Walsh GL, Lang FF, et al. Combined chest wall resection with vertebrectomy and spinal reconstruction for the treatment of Pancoast tumors. J Neurosurg 1999;91(1, Suppl):74–80
2. Gandhi S, Walsh GL, Komaki R, et al. A multidisciplinary surgical approach to superior sulcus tumors with vertebral invasion. Ann Thorac Surg 1999;68(5):1778–1784, discussion 1784–1785
3. Bolton WD, Rice DC, Goodyear A, et al. Superior sulcus tumors with vertebral body involvement: a multimodality approach. J Thorac Cardiovasc Surg 2009;137(6):1379–1387

Answers to Common Clinical Questions

1. Pancoast tumors without nodal involvement or metastasis, even if they demonstrate invasion into the chest wall (T3M0N0) or vertebral column (T4M0N0), if they can be completely resected, are associated with a significant improvement in survival.
2. Positron emission tomography (PET), computed tomography (CT), and bone scans are useful tools for the staging of metastasis. Mediastinoscopy is useful in verifying that a patient does not have positive lymph nodes. Positive lymph nodes on mediastinoscopy will render a patient no longer N0, in which case surgery for treatment is no longer an option.
3. Sacrifice of the C8 or T1 nerve root will result in significant loss of hand function and can also be a source of chronic pain.

40 Cervical-Thoracic Junction Technique

Matthew B. Maserati and David O. Okonkwo

I. Key Points

- The cervical-thoracic junction (CTJ) is an anatomically and biomechanically unique region of the vertebral column that is particularly susceptible to traumatic injury, intervertebral disk and zygapophyseal joint degeneration, and iatrogenic (postsurgical) deformity.[1,2]
- Reconstruction and fixation at the CTJ must be carefully planned, with key anatomic and biomechanical principles taken into account.
  - The CTJ is a transitional zone between the mobile, lordotic cervical spine and the relatively rigid, kyphotic thoracic spine.
  - Posterior element morphology transitions from large lateral masses and small pedicles in the cervical spine to larger pedicles and indistinct lateral masses in the thoracic spine, with implications for posterior fixation.
- Several surgical approaches exist for accessing pathology at the CTJ, and the choice of the most appropriate approach requires a comprehensive preoperative workup.
  - Thorough history with attention to pulmonary status, overall cardiac health, prior neck surgery or radiation therapy (ear, nose, and throat [ENT]evaluation of vocal cords and recurrent laryngeal nerve function should be considered for these patients), and prior thoracic surgery
  - Physical examination with attention to signs of myelopathy but also to body habitus and sagittal balance to identify any relevant deformity such as thoracic hyperkyphosis
  - Multimodality radiographic evaluation
    - Standing anteroposterior (AP) and lateral radiographs with swimmer's view (consider placing a radiopaque marker in the manubrial notch)
    - Magnetic resonance imaging (MRI) for assessment of the neural elements and discoligamentous structures
    - Computed tomography (CT), especially in trauma and for assessment of posterior element morphology when posterior fixation is planned (thin cuts and three-dimensional reconstructions may further aid preoperative planning)
    - Consider a vascular study (e.g., CT angiography) to delineate vertebral artery anatomy

– The superior mediastinum is unfamiliar territory for most spine surgeons. It contains critical structures such as the thoracic duct, azygos vein, great vessels and their branches, the sympathetic chain, and the pleural apices, thus carrying the potential for catastrophic visceral injury.

II. Indications

- Fractures
    - Unstable traumatic fracture/dislocation
    - Osteoporotic fracture causing neurologic deficit, deformity, or persistent pain refractory to less invasive treatments
- Neoplasms
    - Vertebral/epidural metastases
    - Intradural-extramedullary tumors
    - Intramedullary tumors
- Infection
    - Osteomyelitis/discitis meeting criteria for surgery
    - Spinal tuberculoma (Pott disease)
- Deformity
    - Post-laminectomy kyphosis
    - Chin-on-chest deformity
    - Degenerative kyphoscoliosis
    - Posttraumatic kyphosis
- Symptomatic herniated nucleus pulposus in the upper thoracic spine (C7-T3)
    - Radiculopathy (after 6 to 8 weeks of failed conservative therapy)
    - Neurologic deficit from spinal cord compression

III. Technique

- Three principal approaches to the CTJ
    - Anterior
    - Anterolateral
    - Posterior
- Anterior approach[2,4]
    - Options
        - Suprasternal (i.e., conventional low cervical or "Smith-Robinson") approach: use preoperative mid-sagittal cervical-thoracic MRI or CT to determine the lowest vertebra and intervertebral disc accessible without sternotomy.
        - Transclavicular (not discussed here; see Kurz et al[5])
        - Transmanubrial/sternal splitting (**Fig. 40.1**)

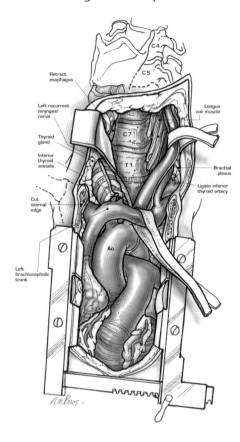

Fig. 40.1 Sternal splitting approach and exposure. (From Haher R, Merola A, Surgical Technique for the Spine, Thieme; pg. 74, Fig. 15-2B.)

- Advantages
  - Permits direct visualization of ventral pathology
  - Ideal for approaching a midline ventral lesion causing cord compression, and for performing an anterior release for correction of deformity
- Disadvantages
  - Superior mediastinum is unfamiliar anatomy and may require the assistance of an access surgeon, particularly for transsternal approach.
  - Risks injury to recurrent laryngeal nerve, thoracic duct, and sympathetic chain (**Fig. 40.2**)
  - Sternal splitting adds significant morbidity.
- Anterolateral (transthoracic) approach[2]
  - Advantages
    - Permits visualization of anterior pathology from anterior vantage point

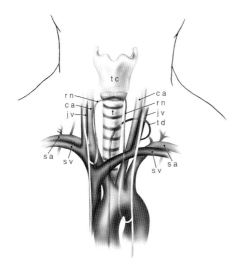

Fig. 40.2 Surgical anatomy relevant to an anterior cervical discectomy. Subclavian artery (sa), subclavian vein (sv), carotid artery (ca), jugular vein (jv), recurrent laryngeal nerve (rn), thoracic duct (td), trachea (t), and thyroid cartilage (tc) (with permission from Barrow Neurological Institute).

- Permits anterior column reconstruction with less risk to neural elements
- Disadvantages
  - Typically requires the assistance of an access surgeon
  - Violation of thoracic cavity and attendant pulmonary morbidity
- Posterior approaches[2,6,7]
  - Options
    - Straight midline approach (cervical-thoracic laminectomy, with possible addition of pedicle screw fixation)
    - Lateral extracavitary approach
    - Transpedicular approach
    - Costotransversectomy
    - Pedicle subtraction/Smith-Peterson osteotomy
  - Advantages
    - Does not require the assistance of an access surgeon
    - Dissection is entirely extrapleural
    - Single approach allows for both decompression and stabilization
  - Disadvantages
    - Ventral pathology may be obscured by the spinal cord and nerve roots.
    - Does not permit correction of a fixed kyphotic deformity
    - Muscle atrophy and/or proximal junctional instability may result from overly aggressive dissection during exposure.

- Anterior column reconstruction through posterior approach places the neural elements at risk.
- Special considerations in performing posterior fixation at the CTJ
  - Screws in this region are under significant stress and at greater risk of pullout or breakage.[1,2,6]
    - Avoid stopping a construct at the CTJ (C6-T2).
    - Consider bicortical fixation.
  - Rods must be carefully contoured with attention to differences between the patient's preoperative curvature and the desired final result.[6]
    - Ensure that sagittal balance and horizontal gaze are preserved or restored.
    - Limit the prominence of the rod ends (particularly in thinner patients).
  - The transition from lateral mass screws in the low cervical spine to pedicle screws in the thoracic spine complicates rod contouring and placement.[6]
    - Consider cervical pedicle screw fixation.
    - Use polyaxial screws for fixation at—and immediately adjacent to—the CTJ.
    - Dual-diameter rods are available to accommodate the larger heads of lower thoracic pedicle screws.
    - For some long constructs and difficult deformity cases, cross-connectors may be used to connect noncollinear rods.

Anterior (Transmanubrial) Approach[1,2]

- Place patient in supine position on radiolucent table.
  - Consider electrophysiologic monitoring such as somatosensory and motor evoked potentials (SSEPs, MEPs), particularly in cases of spinal cord compression and/or myelopathy.
  - Preoperative reduction with traction may be beneficial in cases of severe kyphosis (obtain initial baseline SSEPs and MEPs prior to attempting reduction).
- Sterile prep and drape.
- Incision (**Fig. 40.1**)
  - May use T-shaped incision on the anterior chest wall or an oblique supraclavicular incision beginning just anterior to the (left) sternocleidomastoid muscle and extending inferomedially over the sternum for a variable length depending on the level of the pathology.
    - Manubrium typically corresponds to T2-T3 level (correlate with preop imaging).

- Left-sided approach may facilitate avoidance of recurrent laryngeal nerve injury.
- Divide platysma and perform sharp dissection to define sternocleidomastoid and strap muscles superiorly.
  - Transection of the omohyoid muscle may permit additional retraction.
- Identify the manubrium inferiorly and perform subperiosteal dissection posteriorly, taking care to protect the brachiocephalic veins.
- Using a sternal saw or high-speed drill, split the manubrium.
  - Take care to preserve muscular attachments.
- Perform blunt dissection of the potential space medial to the carotid sheath and lateral to the strap muscles, down to the prevertebral fascia.
  - Take care to avoid injury to the thoracic duct (typically on the left and at C7-T1, but may extend up to C6 in some cases).
- Confirm pathologic level using fluoroscopy or plain radiography.
- Perform decompression (discectomy, corpectomy) and stabilization.
  - Use long-handled, angled instruments to overcome the long distance from the anterior chest wall to the anterior thoracic spine, and to avoid line-of-sight issues.
  - Options for anterior column reconstruction
    - Iliac crest autograft ("gold standard" but associated with donor site morbidity)
    - Allograft strut
    - Polyetheretherketone (PEEK) or titanium cage (avoid titanium in osteoporotic patients due to large discrepancy in modulus of elasticity and possibility of settling)
    - Typically supplement with anterior plate fixation
- Fill wound with saline and watch for bubbles (the presence of bubbles indicates transgression of the apical visceral pleura and necessitates placement of a chest tube through a separate incision).
- Leave a drain in the prevertebral space.
- Close in layers (wire manubrium).

IV. Complications

- Minor
  - Superficial wound dehiscence
  - Injury to strap muscles (exacerbating preexisting respiratory compromise)

- Nonunion of the clavicle/manubrium
- Traction injury to the recurrent laryngeal nerve
– Major
  - Injury to carotid sheath
  - Injury to azygos vein
  - Injury to thoracic duct (chyle leak)
  - Injury to great vessels in the mediastinum
  - Injury to the sympathetic chain (Horner syndrome)
  - Injury to pleural apices (hemopneumothorax)
  - Perforation of trachea or esophagus
  - Deep wound infection
  - Cerebrospinal fluid (CSF) leak
  - Injury to spinal cord or exiting nerve roots

V. Postoperative Care

- Consider monitoring patient in the intensive care unit, particularly in cases of lengthy operative time, significant blood loss, and preoperative pulmonary or cardiac compromise.
- Perioperative hypotension should raise concern of great vessel injury after an anterior approach.
- For anterior approaches, monitor drain output for evidence of chyle leak.
- Consider maintaining patient in cervical-thoracic orthosis for 8 to 12 weeks in patients with poor bone quality or when fixation is otherwise felt to be suboptimal.

VI. Outcomes

- No long-term studies or large series have been reported.
- Small series report anterior approach–related mortality of 0 to 40%, but comprise different patient populations with widely varying pathology and premorbid status.[1,2]
- Posterior approaches are probably associated with decreased morbidity.

VII. Surgical Pearls

- Preoperative workup is critical, with special attention paid to body habitus and sagittal balance, cardiopulmonary comorbidities, and appropriate imaging, including the anterior chest wall (when anterior approach is being considered).

- Assistance of an access surgeon is advisable for work in the superior mediastinum.
- Avoid stopping a construct at the CTJ and consider bicortical screws for greater strength.
- Anterior column reconstruction is essential, since it is responsible for 80% of load bearing.
- Posterior approaches are probably associated with less morbidity but place the neural elements at increased risk when pathology is wholly ventral, or when one is placing an anterior graft.

Common Clinical Questions

1. What elements of the patient history and physical examination are uniquely important when one is considering a surgery at the cervical-thoracic junction?
2. What are the advantages and disadvantages of the anterior approach to the cervical-thoracic junction?

References

1. An HS, Vaccaro A, Cotler JM, Lin S. Spinal disorders at the cervicothoracic junction. Spine (Phila Pa 1976) 1994;19(22):2557–2564
2. Mummaneni PV, Lenke L, Haid RW. Fixation options for the cervicothoracic junction. In Spinal Deformity: A Guide to Surgical Planning and Management. St. Louis, MO: Quality Medical; 2007
3. Comey CH, McLaughlin MR, Moossy J. Anterior thoracic corpectomy without sternotomy: a strategy for malignant disease of the upper thoracic spine. Acta Neurochir (Wien) 1997;139(8):712–718
4. Sharan AD, Przybylski GJ, Tartaglino L. Approaching the upper thoracic vertebrae without sternotomy or thoracotomy: a radiographic analysis with clinical application. Spine (Phila Pa 1976) 2000;25(8):910–916
5. Kurz LT, Pursel SE, Herkowitz HN. Modified anterior approach to the cervicothoracic junction. Spine (Phila Pa 1976) 1991;16(10, Suppl):S542–S547
6. Chapman JR, Anderson PA, Pepin C, Toomey S, Newell DW, Grady MS. Posterior instrumentation of the unstable cervicothoracic spine. J Neurosurg 1996;84(4):552–558
7. Fessler RG, Dietze DD Jr, Millan MM, Peace D. Lateral parascapular extrapleural approach to the upper thoracic spine. J Neurosurg 1991;75(3):349–355

Answers to Common Clinical Questions

1. Body habitus, sagittal contour at the cervical-thoracic junction, cardiac and pulmonary status, prior neck or cardiothoracic surgery, and prior radiation therapy to the neck or superior mediastinum
2. The advantages include direct visualization of ventral pathology, anterior release for correction of kyphotic deformity, and the ability to reconstruct the anterior column with less risk to the neural elements. Disadvantages include the need for an access surgeon due to the unfamiliar anatomy of the superior mediastinum; potential injury to the recurrent laryngeal nerve, sympathetic chain, and thoracic duct; and significant additional morbidity if sternal splitting is required.

41 Thoracic Pedicle Technique

Ryan J. Halpin and Tyler R. Koski

I. Key Points

- Transpedicular instrumentation allows for anterior and posterior column spinal fixation for a more rigid construct that is biomechanically superior to the use of thoracic hooks.
- Thoracic pedicles are smaller and more variable in size than pedicles of the lumbar spine.[1]
- Sagittal pedicle height gradually increases from upper to lower thoracic spine.
- Transverse pedicle width decreases from the upper thoracic spine to the mid-thoracic spine (T5-T6) before gradually increasing through the lumbar spine.
- The transverse pedicle angle decreases from T1 to T12.
- Straightforward screw trajectories are associated with higher pullout strengths than anatomic trajectories, although anatomic trajectories may allow for a larger pedicle screw diameter.[2]
- Extrapedicular screws are biomechanically inferior to intrapedicular screws but are an excellent alternative when anatomy dictates their use.[3]

II. Indications

- Reduction and stabilization of traumatic fractures
- Stabilization for tumor resection, infection, or spinal inflammatory disease (i.e., ankylosing spondylitis)
- Correction of spinal deformity such as kyphosis or scoliosis

III. Technique

- The authors use a free hand technique[4] and prefer to place the pedicle screw parallel to the superior end plate with appropriate medial angulation. Fluoroscopy and image guidance may be used at the discretion of the surgeon.
- Exposure
  - Soft tissues are meticulously cleared from the posterior elements of the levels to be fused, and the levels above and below, including their facet capsules, are spared.
  - Exposure extends from the spinous process, lamina, and facet medially to the tips of the transverse processes laterally.

- Facetectomy
    - The facet capsules are cleared of soft tissue to expose the "plateau" ridge of the thoracic lamina above the "valley" of the superior facet. At the intermediate levels the inferior facet may be removed with an osteotome to assist with visualization of the superior facet.
- Starting point (**Fig. 41.1**)
    - Cortical burr holes are made in the thoracic lamina ridge (plateau) 1 to 2 mm lateral to the midpoint of the superior facet (valley).
    - Starting points are generally more lateral at the upper thoracic spine and become more medial toward the mid-thoracic spine (T7) before once again becoming more lateral in the distal thoracic spine.
    - Look for a cortical "blush" after the burring, which suggests entry into the cancellous portion of the pedicle.

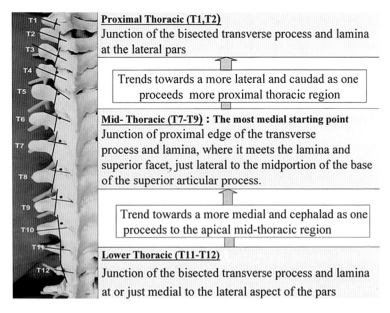

Fig. 41.1 Pedicle screw starting points with 3.5 mm acorn-tipped burr. The posterior elements are burred to create a posterior cortical breach roughly 5 mm in depth. (From Kim YJ et al, Free hand pedicle screw placement in the thoracic spine: is it safe? Spine. 2004;29(3):333-342. Reprinted with permission.)

- Pedicle probe
  - We use a 35 mm pedicle probe having a blunt 2 mm tip with a slight curve.
  - The probe is initially pointed laterally to avoid medial wall violation and inserted to a depth of 15 to 20 mm. A hole probe is then used to assess for a floor, and all four walls (superior, inferior, medial, and lateral) are assessed for breaches.
  - The probe is then reinserted with the curve pointed medially into the vertebral body at an appropriate depth based on computed tomography (CT) scan (average of 30 mm in the upper levels and 40 to 45 mm in lower levels). The probe is removed and the hole probe is inserted to again assess the four walls and the floor for violations of the cortex.
- Tapping
  - The tract is then under-tapped using a tap diameter 1 mm smaller than that of the planned screw. If the tract is small or if there is any concern about deviation, the tract may be tapped using a cannulated tap over a K-wire.
  - After the tap is removed, the hole is probed again for breaches. The depth of the hole probe is measured and compared with the preoperative length of the planned screw before a decision is made on the appropriate screw length.
- Screw placement
  - The screw is slowly placed into the pedicle tract with close attention paid to make sure it does not deviate from the planned trajectory.
- Screw confirmation
  - Screw placement can be assessed using intraoperative anteroposterior (AP) and lateral x-ray, fluoroscopy, or CT scanning.
  - Triggered electromyography (EMG) from intercostal and abdominal muscles can be used to test screws prior to placing the rods, although this method is not as reliable as it is for the lumbar spine
- Salvage techniques
  - New tracts in different trajectories can be made using the same technique as described above. K-wires and cannulated taps may be used to avoid entry into the original tract, and care must be taken when placing the tap or screw over the K-wire to prevent the K-wire's advancement due to binding.
  - Extrapedicular screws can be placed by starting more laterally and using a "in-out-in" technique through the transverse process and then back into the vertebral body.
  - Pedicle, infralaminar, and transverse process hooks and sublaminar wires can also be utilized if necessary.

IV. Complications

- Medial breach rates range from 0.04 to 24%. Breaches as great as 2 to 4 mm (similar to the volume taken up by a thoracic hook) may be tolerated without injury to the spinal cord, which lies 2 to 4 mm medial to the pedicle at some levels.[4]
- Lateral breach rates range from 0.4 to 29% and may result in injuries to the aorta, segmental vessels, lung parenchyma, or visceral structures, or pneumothorax.
- Anterior cortical breaches range from 0 to 8% and have the potential to cause injuries to the esophagus, aorta, or vena cava.
- Both proper screw placement and the ability to detect a breach in the pedicle using a probe have been shown to be dependent on the level of training of the surgeon. Medial breaches are more difficult to detect than lateral breaches. Breaches of the anterior cortex are easiest to detect.

V. Postoperative Care

- Follow-up imaging is done at the discretion of the surgeon. The authors prefer early postoperative CT scanning to evaluate placement if an intraoperative CT scan was not performed.

VI. Outcomes

- Multiple clinical and biomechanical studies have shown that properly placed pedicle screw constructs are superior to hook or hybrid constructs in terms of rigid fixation, the ability to correct coronal and sagittal deformities, and preventing loss of correction.
- Experienced spine surgeons report malpositioning of screws at rates of 1.5 to 6.2%. CT scans detect pedicle perforation at higher rates than x-rays.[4]
- Neurologic, vascular, and visceral injuries are rare (<1%) but can be devastating.

VII. Surgical Pearls

- A thin-cut CT scan is helpful for reviewing the anatomy of thoracic pedicles and their relationship to neurovascular structures prior to surgery.
- Pedicle screws may be augmented by injections of polymethylmethacrylate (or hydroxyapatite, calcium phosphate, or carbonated apatite) in patients who are at risk for screw pullout (i.e., those with osteoporosis).

- Extrapedicular screws (using the "in-out-in" technique) are a viable option when the pedicles are too small to accept a screw or for revision instrumentation cases.
- Limit soft-tissue exposure to the levels being fused and avoid disrupting the facet capsules at the levels above and below the fusion.
- Any change in resistance upon insertion of the pedicle probe should raise suspicion of a tract violation, and the tract should be probed immediately. Medial breaches are located in the first 10 to 15 mm of the tract.

Common Clinical Questions

1. Extrapedicular thoracic screws (i.e., those that use the "in-out-in" technique):
   A. Are biomechanically stronger than intrapedicular screws
   B. Are biomechanically equivalent to intrapedicular screws but carry a higher risk of injury
   C. Are biomechanically weaker than intrapedicular screws
   D. Cannot be used as a salvage technique for a missed screw

2. True or false: Tapping the screw tract is not a useful technique in the thoracic spine due to the small pedicle size.

3. True or false: CT scanning is the most accurate indicator of appropriate screw positioning.

References

1. Gray's Anatomy 1918 Edition. Public Domain
2. Lehman RA Jr, Polly DW Jr, Kuklo TR, Cunningham B, Kirk KL, Belmont PJ Jr. Straight-forward versus anatomic trajectory technique of thoracic pedicle screw fixation: a biomechanical analysis. Spine (Phila Pa 1976) 2003;28(18):2058–2065
3. White KK, Oka R, Mahar AT, Lowry A, Garfin SR. Pullout strength of thoracic pedicle screw instrumentation: comparison of the transpedicular and extrapedicular techniques. Spine (Phila Pa 1976) 2006;31(12):E355–E358
4. Kim YJ, Lenke LG, Bridwell KH, Cho YS, Riew KD. Free hand pedicle screw placement in the thoracic spine: is it safe? Spine (Phila Pa 1976) 2004;29(3):333–342, discussion 342

Answers to Common Clinical Questions

1. C. Extrapedicular screws are biomechanically weaker than intrapedicular screws. They are useful as a salvage technique for a missed screw as well as when pedicles are too small to accept an intrapedicular screw.

2. False. Under-tapping is useful in the thoracic spine. Under-tapping by 1 mm is biomechanically superior to under-tapping by 0.5 mm or tapping at an equal diameter to the planned screw.

3. True. CT is more accurate in detecting misplaced screws than x-ray or magnetic resonance imaging (MRI).

42 Lateral Extracavitary Approach

Beejal Y. Amin and Muwaffak Abdulhak

I. Key Points

- The posterolateral approach allows for circumferential neural decompression under direct visualization with extrapleural/extravisceral dissection.
- Single-stage ventral and dorsal column support can be achieved using the same incision.

II. Indications[1,2]

- Thoracic disc herniations or osteophytes
- Thoracic fractures
- Anterolateral decompression for neoplasms
- Osteomyelitis with anterior column compromise
- Lesions located between T3 and L2

III. Preoperative Preparation[2]

- Sagittal magnetic resonance imaging (MRI) should include "scout radiographs" because of the ability they provide to count to the precise spinal level of interest.
- Anteroposterior (AP) chest x-ray confirms presence of 12 ribs.
- Spinal angiogram is useful in case of lesions between T6 and L2 to identify the radiculomedullary artery of Adamkiewicz.
- Computed tomography (CT) scan can be helpful for studying the bony anatomy.

IV. Technique[1–3]

- The patient is intubated and general anesthesia is administered.
- Antiembolism stockings and Foley catheter are placed.
- Large-bore peripheral and central catheters are necessary given the possibility of rapid blood loss during the procedure.
- Patient is placed in the prone position on a spinal table.
  - The patient must be well secured to the table to allow for safe lateral tilting during surgery.
  - Arms are tucked at the sides or above the head and all pressure points are padded.
- Spinal cord monitoring is optional.

- Incision is made in the midline with a "hockey stick"–shaped curve.
  - Incision is carried through the subcutaneous tissue to the thoracolumbar fascia.
  - Self-retaining retractors are placed, and the fascia is opened vertically over the spinous processes.
  - Exposure of the spinous process, lamina, facets, costotransverse junction, and rib at each level is performed.
- The curved portion of the skin incision is made just caudal to the last level to be instrumented and is angled 8 cm laterally to allow adequate soft tissue retraction.
- The fascial incision is curved laterally to expose the lateral border of the erector spinae muscles.
- The erector spinae muscles are dissected off the ribs and reflected medially.
  - The muscle group can be tented up with a Penrose drain.
- Reconfirm the spinal level and rib of interest with AP fluoroscopy.
- Remove the rib 7 to 10 cm lateral to the costovertebral junction.
  - Rongeuring the tip of the corresponding transverse process may facilitate this procedure.
  - Special attention should be given to ensure the pleura is not punctured.
- Identify the neurovascular bundle and follow it medially to the vertebral foramen.
  - If necessary, ligate the intervening intercostal vessels and nerves.
  - The nerve should be sectioned proximal to the dorsal root ganglion prior to closure to prevent anesthesia dolorosa.
- The sympathetic chain is encountered and displaced ventrally in a subperiostal fashion.
- A localization radiograph is taken with a spinal needle placed into the disc space.
- Visualization of the vertebral body and pedicle is enhanced by tilting the operating table 15 to 20 degrees away from the surgeon.
- The foramen is enlarged with the use of curettes until the lateral aspect of the thecal sac is exposed.
  - Consider starting with a midline laminectomy in case of severe ventral thecal sac compression.
  - Epidural bleeding can be controlled with a hemostatic agent and Cottonoids (Saramall, Buenos Aires, Argentina); electrocautery should be avoided adjacent to the thecal sac.

- The rostral portion of the pedicle just inferior to the disc space is removed.
- The annulus of the disc is incised just ventral to the posterior longitudinal ligament.
- Disc material and bone ventral to the thecal sac are broken down into the cavity with the use of curettes or thin, flat instruments.
- After removal of adjacent discs, corpectomy can be completed with a high-speed drill.
  - The adequacy of ventral decompression is determined by use of dental mirror.
- Anterior stabilization can be achieved with the placement of an anterior graft into the corpectomy site.
  - The use of expandable cages is recommended to provide anterior support.
- The operating table is tilted back to the neutral position.
- AP/lateral x-rays can aid in assessing the position of the anterior graft and facilitate placement of posterior instrumentation.
- The wound is closed in a multilayered fashion (**Fig. 42.1**).

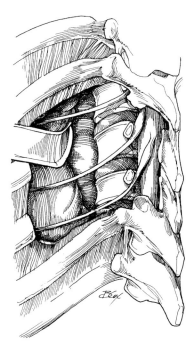

Fig. 42.1 Lateral view of the retracted paraspinal muscle bundle medially and the myocutaneous flap laterally, the lateral dural sac and exiting nerve roots, and the lateral vertebrae.

V. Complications[1,2]

- Pneumothorax
- Hemothorax
- Pleural effusion
  - Significant pleural fluid collections are best treated with tube thoracostomy rather than thoracentesis.
- Dural tear
- Spinal cord injury
- Anesthesia dolorosa

VI. Postoperative Care

- Aggressive pulmonary toilet is necessary to prevent postoperative pneumonia.
- Surgical drains and chest tubes are typically discontinued at 48 to 72 hours.
- External orthosis is recommended following instrumentation cases for up to 12 weeks.

VII. Outcomes[2]

- Reported series showed 70% improvement in myelopathy from thoracic disc herniation.
- Eighty percent improvement is reported in neurologic condition from traumatic lesions of thoracic spine.
- Morbidity rate is significant and reported to be as high as 55% in one series.[2]

VIII. Surgical Pearls

- The intercostal nerve should be divided proximal to the dorsal root ganglion to prevent anesthesia dolorosa.
- Meticulous dissection of the rib and rib head to avoid pleural injury along with gentle retraction of the lung may help minimize pulmonary morbidity.

Common Clinical Questions

1. Where should the nerve be sacrificed in relation to the dorsal root ganglion?
   A. Proximal to the dorsal root ganglion
   B. Distal to the dorsal root ganglion
2. The benefits of the lateral extracavitary approach include:
   A. Circumferential neural decompression can be achieved under direct visualization.
   B. Single-stage ventral and dorsal column support can be achieved using the same incision.
   C. Both A and B

References

1. Larson SJ, Holst RA, Hemmy DC, Sances A Jr. Lateral extracavitary approach to traumatic lesions of the thoracic and lumbar spine. J Neurosurg 1976;45(6):628–637
2. Resnick DK, Benzel EC. Lateral extracavitary approach for thoracic and thoracolumbar spine trauma: operative complications. Neurosurgery 1998;43(4): 796–802, discussion 802–803
3. Capener N. The evolution of lateral rhachotomy. J Bone Joint Surg Br 1954;36-B(2):173–179

Answers to Common Clinical Questions

1. A (to prevent anesthesia dolorosa)
2. C

43 Transpedicular Approach

Frank La Marca, Paul Park, and Juan M. Valdivia

I. Key Points

- Alternative posterior approach for anterior decompression avoids the morbidity associated with anterior (i.e., transthoracic, thoracoabdominal) approaches for neural decompression.
- Less extensive dissection required compared with other anterior approaches
- Particularly effective technique for soft thoracic disc herniations or intrapedicular lesions
- Not ideal for large calcified central thoracic disc herniations

II. Indications

- Soft central or lateral thoracic disc herniations, anterolateral calcified thoracic disc hernations
- Reduction of retropulsed fragment(s) in vertebral burst fracture
- Resection and/or biopsy of intravertebral/intrapedicular lesions
- Decompression of anterolateral spinal canal in the setting of tumor

III. Technique

- Patient is in prone position on Jackson table with gel rolls or frame.
- Neurophysiologic monitoring (transcranial motor evoked potentials and somatosensory evoked potentials should be considered)
- Fluoroscopy: Obtain multiple views for correct localization. Either count from the sacrum or obtain anteroposterior (AP) views counting ribs, having confirmed 12 rib-bearing segments preoperatively. For extremely obese patients, a marker can be placed preoperatively by interventional radiology with subsequent imaging to confirm marker as a viable reference point.
- Midline incision: ipsilateral erector spinae muscles dissected to expose lamina, facet complex, transverse process
- If instrumentation is required, exposure is increased to encompass the targeted segments.
- In the thoracic spine, the medial portion of the transverse process overlies the pedicle.

43 Transpedicular Approach

- If necessary, AP fluoroscopy can be used to localize the pedicle margins.
- The pedicle inferior to the targeted disc space is targeted (i.e., the T8 pedicle for a T7-T8 disc herniation).[1,2]
- At a minimum, a laminotomy is created adjacent to the targeted pedicle.
- The posterior cortex of the pedicle is opened with a high-speed drill. Sequential passage of curettes and/or high-speed drill is used to create a channel through the cancellous pedicle. The walls of the pedicle can be thinned to an "eggshell" thickness with the drill. Once the vertebral body is reached, a down-going curette can be used to safely fracture the medial wall of the pedicle laterally, exposing the lateral margins of the dura. The medial portion of the adjacent facet is resected and the superior wall of the pedicle is removed to expose the disc space.
- A Woodson elevator is used to carefully palpate the ventral epidural space to identify the lesion.
- For disc herniations, the disc space is entered just lateral to the dura. Disc material is removed with rongeurs. The high-speed drill is then used to create a cavity encompassing the disc space as well as the adjacent vertebral bodies (**Fig. 43.1**). The drill is angled to extend the cavity medially, maintaining a thin margin of disc annulus or posterior vertebral wall between the drill tip and the ventral dura. A small down-going curette is then used

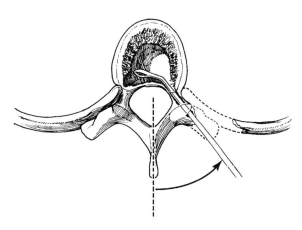

Fig. 43.1 To allow access to the interior of the vertebral body, it may be necessary to resect the rib, rib head, and transverse process. (From Vaccaro AR, Albert TJ, Spine Surgery: Tricks of the Trade 2nd ed, Thieme; pg. 89, Fig. 25.2.)

to gently push the disc herniation into the cavity, allowing removal with rongeurs.[3]
- Note that the ventral dura is not well visualized with this technique. For more centralized masses, an instrument such as a down-going curette is used to localize the mass by palpation. The curette is then used to push the mass into the cavity (**Fig. 43.1**).
- For retropulsed bone or tumor, more of the vertebral body is removed to create the cavity into which the epidural mass is pushed.
- For larger masses, a bilateral transpedicular approach can be used.
- With bilateral approaches, fusion should be considered.

IV. Complications

- Infection
  - Discitis
- Durotomy
  - Pseudomeningocele formation
- Transient/permanent neurologic injury
  - Spinal cord injury if excessive retraction is applied to the dura during the decompression
- Inadequate visualization of the ventral epidural space, resulting in suboptimal anterior decompression

V. Postoperative Care

- Consider neurologic intensive care unit for close monitoring, particularly for patients with preexisting neurologic deficit or significant comorbidities.
- Routine postoperative imaging is not required.
- Urgent MRI is needed if new neurologic deficit is present.

VI. Outcomes

- In properly selected patients, neurologic outcomes for symptomatic thoracic disc herniations treated by the transpedicular approach are similar to outcomes for the transthoracic approach.

VII. Surgical Pearls

- Review axial and sagittal images on computed tomography (CT) to understand the pedicular anatomy; may use three-dimensional reconstruction.

- When anatomy is distorted due to prior surgery or fusion mass, fluoroscopy and pedicle marker may be used to localize the pedicle as for pedicle screw placement.
- If anterior decompression is unsafe due to scarring with anterior dura or fragment indenting spinal cord, consider opening dura for adequate visualization of spinal cord in relation to the anterior pathology.
- Anterior unintended durotomy or cerebrospinal fluid (CSF) leak can be treated locally with Duragen (Integra Life Sciences Corp., Plainsboro, NJ) or Dura-Guard (Synovis, St. Paul, MN) and a sealant agent
- Postoperative lumbar drain should be considered with durotomy.

Common Clinical Questions

1. What is the main disadvantage of the transpedicular approach for anterior decompression?
2. A large central calcified disc herniation is best approached via which technique?
3. Is fusion necessary after a transpedicular approach?

References

1. Vaccaro A, Albert T. Spine Surgery: Tricks of the Trade. New York: Thieme Medical Publishing; 2009
2. Vanichkachorn JS, Vaccaro AR. Thoracic disk disease: diagnosis and treatment. J Am Acad Orthop Surg 2000;8(3):159–169
3. Bilsky MH. Transpedicular approach for thoracic disc herniations. Neurosurg Focus 2000;9(4):e3

Answers to Common Clinical Questions

1. Inadequate visualization of the ventral midline dura
2. Transthoracic
3. For a unilateral transpedicular approach, fusion is typically not necessary.

44 Costotransversectomy

Dean B. Kostov and Adam S. Kanter

I. Key Points

- Conservative management of thoracic disc herniation with radiculopathy is the preferred primary management.
- The presence or progression of myelopathy due to thoracic disc pathology is accepted as an indication for surgery.
- Costotransversectomy is best suited for ipsilateral noncalcified central pathology and is contraindicated for contralateral decompression and large central calcified disease.
- Costotransversectomy provides a well-tolerated surgical corridor to address ventral and ventrolateral pathology via a posterior approach, but care must be taken in working around the neural structures.
- Excellent choice for patients who cannot tolerate anterior approaches via thoracotomy

II. Indications

- Thoracic disc herniation[1–4]
- Drainage of spinal abscess/infections (originally described for tubercular abscess by Ménard)
- Spinal decompression of ventral and ventrolateral space-occupying lesions[2–4]
- Resection of paraspinal nerve sheath tumors[2,3]
- Correction of kyphotic deformity[2]

III. Technique (Fig. 44.1)

- Position patient prone or partial lateral. Incision can be paramedian, T-shaped, straight, or curvilinear with convexity toward the midline to allow for greater access.
- The incision is carried through skin, trapezius, and/or latissimus dorsi (for lower approaches) and erector spinae with medial retraction to expose the ribs and transverse process of the caudal vertebrae of the level of interest.
- Subperiosteal dissection of the perichondrium around the rib is performed, protecting the pleura and neurovascular bundle (use a semisharp subperiosteal dissector such as a Doyen rib raspatory).

44 Costotransversectomy

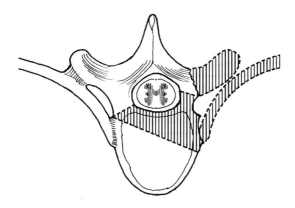

Fig. 44.1 Cross-section of the costotransversectomy approach. The shaded area depicts bone that may be removed using this approach to expose the spinal canal. (From Vaccaro AR, Albert TJ, Spine Surgery: Tricks of the Trade 2nd ed, Thieme; pg. 86, Fig. 24.3.)

- After sharp division of the costotransverse ligament, the transverse process is removed at the junction with the lamina using rongeurs or a high-speed drill.
- Transection of the rib about 3 to 5 cm (depending on the exposure needed) from the costotransverse junction and disarticulation of the rib from the costovertebral joint is then performed.
- Partial laminectomy and facetectomy are carried out to identify the lateral margin of the dura using a high-speed drill and/ or small Kerrison rongeurs.
- The pleura may be protected ventrally with a malleable retractor, and a rib spreader may be used to increase exposure depending on number of levels indicated.
- Careful dissection along the superolateral border of the pedicle can be performed to safely expose the vertebral body or identify the disc space, depending on the goals.
- Discectomy should be performed laterally first, followed by the creation of a cavity centrally that can be used to push mediodorsal pathology inward to facilitate safe removal without manipulation of the spinal cord. This cavity may be enlarged to include partial vertebral resection as needed.
- If vertebral column resection is to be performed, then a midline approach with or without T-shaped extension is best to allow for safe instrumentation.
- If the spine is to be destabilized due to vertebral column resection, posterior instrumentation with gradual reduction of kyphosis using temporary rods should be done first.

- During closure, the field should be flooded with irrigation and a Valsalva maneuver performed to identify any pleural compromise. If pleura is violated, primary repair should be attempted with or without placement of a chest tube.
- The wound should be closed in layers and drains placed as needed.

IV. Complications

- Highly dependent on pathology and procedure performed
- Neurologic decline (5.5%), neurovascular bundle compromise, hemothorax
- Pneumothorax (as high as 25%), injury to pleura, lung contusion, atelectasis[2-4]
- Dural tear, symptomatic or asymptomatic pseudomeningocele
- Infection
- Injury to great vessels lying anterior to vertebral body
- Injury to radiculomedullary arterial branches, leading to spinal cord infarct

V. Postoperative Care

- Chest x-ray should take place in recovery room to evaluate for pneumothorax.
- Patient should be placed in a monitored unit with continuous pulse oxymetry performed.
- Incentive spirometry and pulmonary toilet are key in the postoperative period.
- Pain should be adequately controlled to prevent guarding and shallow breathing.
- Early mobilization with standard spinal postoperative care (e.g., deep vein thrombosis [DVT] prophylaxis)

VI. Outcomes

- Improvement in weakness ranging from 30 to 58%
- Improvement in radiculopathy or local pain ranging from 42 to 91%
- Spasticity and myelopathy improvement has been reported as high as 95%.
- Comparing costotransversectomy with anterior or combined approaches for treatment of oncologic disease, the perioperative complication profile is similar, but a posterior approach may be better tolerated in patients with multiple medical comorbidities.

VII. Surgical Pearls

- The spinal cord should never be manipulated to gain exposure.
- If the goal of surgery is anterior column resection, then posterior instrumentation should be placed with a temporary rod prior to destabilization of the vertebral column
- Following the neurovascular bundle back will lead to the neural foramen, and the removal of the rib head leads to the disc space of interest.
- If more exposure is needed one should remove more rib, allowing a greater lateral corridor, rather than trying to work via a more posterior approach.

Common Clinical Questions

1. With central thoracic disc herniations, what side is preferred for performing a costotransversectomy approach if indicated?
2. What is the origin of the major arterial supply to the spinal cord from T8 to the conus, and where is it located?
3. During positioning, what is a useful anatomic landmark for the T7 vertebral level?

References

1. Greenberg MS. Handbook of Neurosurgery. 6th ed. New York: Thieme Medical Publishers; 2006:322–323, 516–521
2. Vaccaro AR. Spine Surgery: Tricks of the Trade. 2nd ed. New York: Thieme Medical Publishers; 2006:83–87
3. McCormick WE, Will SF, Benzel EC. Surgery for thoracic disc disease. Complication avoidance: overview and management. Neurosurg Focus 2000;9(4):e13
4. Wiggins GC, Mirza S, Bellabarba C, West GA, Chapman JR, Shaffrey CI. Perioperative complications with costotransversectomy and anterior approaches to thoracic and thoracolumbar tumors. Neurosurg Focus 2001;11(6):e4

Answers to Common Clinical Questions

1. The left side is preferred to avoid the great veins (the aorta is much more resilient).
2. The artery of Adamkiewicz, located on the left in 80% of patients, and arising between T9 and T12 in 75% of the population
3. The inferior tip of the scapula

45 Thoracoscopic Approach
Timothy D. Uschold and Steve W. Chang

I. Key Points
- Working angles and trajectories to the thoracic spine are comparable between the thoracoscopic and open anterolateral (thoracotomy) approaches. Posterior elements, contralateral roots, and the contralateral pedicle cannot be accessed.
- Thoracoscopy allows access to the entire thoracic spine (T1 to T12) and eliminates the need for an approach surgeon. Similar access may be obtainable with mini-open techniques.
- Thoracoscopy requires a unique skill set, knowledge of anatomy, and familiarity with unusual instruments. Proficiency typically requires considerable laboratory preparation.
- Single-lung ventilation via a double-lumen endotracheal tube is required for thoracoscopic access. Patients with significant obesity, cardiac dysfunction, and/or pulmonary comorbidities may require specialist referral for preoperative clearance.

II. Indications
- Microdiscectomy for symptomatic thoracic herniation
- Sympathectomy: primarily utilized for palmar hyperhidrosis after failure of medical management. Craniofacial hyperhidrosis, axillary hyperhidrosis, reflex sympathetic dystrophy, and palmar ischemic phenomena are less common indications.[1]
- Osteomyelitis/discitis, epidural abscess, nerve sheath tumor, vertebral biopsy, corpectomy, costovertebral joint pain, vertebral reconstruction, and spinal deformity[2]
- Contraindications: malignant tumors requiring en bloc resection, intradural pathology. Due to high rates of intradural migration and calcification, open thoracotomy is favored for giant (occupying >40% of canal diameter) midline herniated discs.[3]

III. Technique
- The patient is turned to the lateral decubitus position, an axillary roll is placed, and the upper arm is gently raised and supported via an armboard. After the patient is secured to the operating table, the bed is rotated to assist gravity retraction of the lung.

- Single-lung ventilation ensues after reconfirmation of position of the endotracheal tube.
- The surgeon stands facing the patient's chest. Various portal configurations are acceptable depending on the level of interest. Working portals are biased toward the anterior axillary line (usually equidistant from the level of interest), and the endoscopic portal is biased toward the posterior axillary line.
- A 1 cm incision is made along the superior costal margin. Blunt dissection with a hemostat and/or finger, as in chest tube placement, is used to pierce the parietal pleura. Working portals are placed under direct vision with the endoscope. Minor adhesions are lysed using a combination of blunt and sharp dissection.[4]
- Sympathectomy for palmar hyperhidrosis:
  - One or two working portals are required (typically the third and/or fourth intercostal spaces), and the endoscope is placed at the fifth intercostal space.
  - The second rib is identified inferior to the apical fat pad and the brachiocephalic and subclavian vessels. The sympathetic chain is then transected at the second and third rib heads with bipolar cautery followed by scissors. The ends are gently dissected and separated.[1]
- Discectomy
  - Based on the necessary exposure, the parietal pleura overlying the rib heads and/or bodies is incised with cautery. The pleura can be reflected with elevators, cautery, or further sharp dissection. Segmental vessels are mobilized, ligated, coagulated, and transected when necessary (**Fig. 45.1**).
  - A dissector is used to separate the neurovascular bundle from the inferior costal margin and to dissect the superior margin free from pleura and muscular attachment. The costovertebral joint is disarticulated using a levered Cobb elevator. The distal rib is transected, and the rib head is removed. The exposed pedicle is resected with Kerrison rongeurs. The dura and exiting root are now visualized.
  - A cavity is drilled into the disc space and adjacent bodies, and the disc fragment is removed with careful curettage directed away from the thecal sac.
- Closure
  - A chest tube connected to standard suction (-20 cm H_2O) is directed toward the lung apex through a working portal and secured in an airtight fashion. The thoracic wall is inspected with the endoscope. The remaining working portals are closed, and the atelectatic lung is reinflated under direct vision.

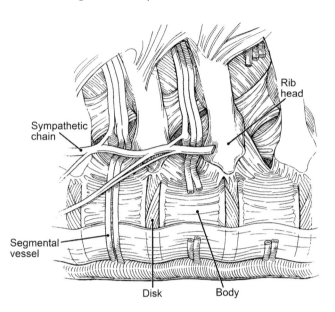

Fig. 45.1 Thoracic anatomy demonstrating relationship of vertebral bodies to ribs, sympathetic chain, and segmental vessels (used with permission from Barrow Neurological Institute).

- Chest tubes may be removed before the patient leaves the operating room. Alternatively, chest tubes can be left in place until output diminishes to less than 100 cc/day, transitioned to water seal, and removed later.[4]

IV. Complications

- Durotomy: Repair methods include hemoclips or fascial harvest for onlay graft with fibrin sealant, and temporary lumbar cerebrospinal fluid (CSF) diversion. Chest tubes should be placed to water seal. Occult CSF leaks may be identified with a Valsalva maneuver.
- Wrong-level procedure: Localization can typically be achieved by identifying anatomic landmarks with the endoscope and confirmed by fluoroscopy. Ribs articulate with the disc space above the corresponding vertebral body (e.g., the T5 rib leads to the T5 pedicle and T4/T5 disc space). A radiopaque fiducial may be placed preoperatively in the pedicle of interest.
- Persistent pneumothorax or atelectasis
- Miscellaneous complications: neurovascular compression syndromes (positioning), intercostal neuralgia (typically tran-

sient), gustatory sweating (sympathectomy), Horner syndrome (sympathectomy involving stellate ganglion), and chylothorax

V. Postoperative Care

- An upright anteroposterior radiograph is obtained in the recovery room and the next morning to evaluate for persistent pneumothorax.
- Aggressive pulmonary toilet, incentive spirometry, and nebulizer use are promoted to prevent atelectasis.

VI. Outcomes

- Sympathectomy
  - Increase of more than 1°C in palmar temperature monitoring, an indirect marker of vasodilation, is a useful intraoperative prognostic for success.[1]
  - Uniform reports of 96 to 100% relief of palmar hyperhidrosis. Rate of compensatory hyperhidrosis (e.g., legs, back, trunk) ranges from 50 to 61% in large series. No useful predictors of compensatory hyperhidrosis.[4]
- Discectomy
  - Advantages reported over thoracotomy in terms of pulmonary complications, operative pain, wound complications, chest tube duration, intercostal neuralgia and rib resection, and decreased length of hospital stay

VII. Surgical Pearls

- To avoid inadvertent injury to lung parenchyma or to vascular or neural structures, the working tips of all instruments should be visualized at all times with the endoscope.
- A larger cavity drilled into the disc and body, if necessary, may be useful during discectomy. All movements should be directed away from the thecal sac.
- Disc calcification is not a contraindication to thoracoscopic microdiscectomy (unless giant) but may require more extensive drilling (e.g., diamond burr) to protect the thecal sac against levered resection during curettage.
- Portal incisions should be planned to facilitate conversion to open thoracotomy if needed.
- Use of an angled endoscope may be useful for confirming decompression of the anterior thecal sac and root(s), especially in the setting of suspected residual disc.

Common Clinical Questions

1. Describe characteristics of a herniated disc least appropriate for thoracoscopic microdiscectomy.
2. What are the success rate and most common side effect of thoracoscopic sympathectomy for palmar hyperhidrosis at T2/T3?
3. Name three surgical or postoperative strategies to prevent severe complications related to CSF leakage during thoracoscopic surgery.

References

1. Han PP, Gottfried ON, Kenny KJ, Dickman CA. Biportal thoracoscopic sympathectomy: surgical techniques and clinical results for the treatment of hyperhidrosis. Neurosurgery 2002;50(2):306–311, discussion 311–312
2. Han PP, Kenny K, Dickman CA. Thoracoscopic approaches to the thoracic spine: experience with 241 surgical procedures. Neurosurgery 2002;51(5, Suppl):S88–S95
3. Hott JS, Feiz-Erfan I, Kenny K, Dickman CA. Surgical management of giant herniated thoracic discs: analysis of 20 cases. J Neurosurg Spine 2005;3(3):191–197
4. Dickman CA, Rosenthal DJ, Perin NI. Thoracoscopic microsurgical discectomy. In Dickman CA, Rosenthal DJ, Perin NI. Thoracoscopic Spine Surgery. New York: Thieme; 1999: 221–244

Answers to Common Clinical Questions

1. Midline, giant, calcified herniated nucleus pulposus
2. Nearly 100% with symptomatic improvement. Compensatory hyperhidrosis is the most common side effect.
3. Lumbar drain placement, fascial graft repair with fibrin sealant, attempt primary repair of durotomy with hemoclips and chest tubes placed to water seal

46 Pedicle Subtraction Osteotomy/ Smith Petersen Osteotomy

Frank La Marca, Paul Park, and Juan M. Valdivia

I. Key Points

- For correction of mainly symptomatic fixed sagittal imbalance (pedicle subtraction osteotomy [PSO]) and nonfixed sagittal imbalance (Smith-Petersen osteotomy [SPO])[1]
- An asymmetric PSO can also be used for correction of coronal imbalance.
- Can aid in the correction of coronal balance via posterior column release (SPO) or three-column release (PSO)
- Can be performed on the thoracic or lumbar spine

II. Indications

- Uncompensated spinal kyphoscoliosis (thoracic and/or lumbar) with or without progression
- Correction of fixed kyphosis requiring more than 30 degrees of correction (PSO) at one spinal segment
- Correction of nonfixed deformity requiring 5 to 10 degrees of correction (SPO) per spinal segment

III. Technique

Pedicle Subtraction Osteotomy

- 1. Position on Jackson frame with extended chest bolster.
- 2. Neurophysiologic monitoring should be used (transcranial motor evoked potentials, somatosensory evoked potentials, electromyography) to minimize neurologic injury during correction
- 3. Place two to three levels of bilateral pedicle screws cephalad and caudal to the target vertebral segment (i.e., commonly L2 or L3 in the lumbar spine).
- 4. Remove transverse process and rib head (if in thoracic spine).
- 5. For 360 degree extrapedicular vertebral body exposure, dissect soft tissues and vascular structures from vertebral body with placement of malleable retractors to maintain separation.[2]
- 6. Perform Gill laminectomy of the target vertebral body and partial laminectomies of the adjacent segments (**Fig. 46.1A**).
- 7. Decancellate and resect pedicle while contralateral temporary rod is in place.

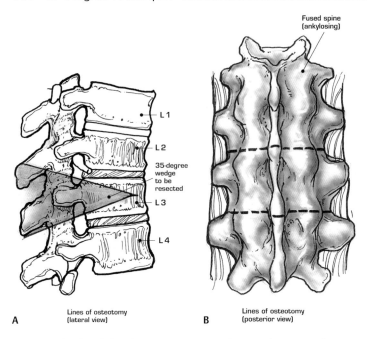

Fig. 46.1 (A,B) Pedicle subtraction osteotomy. (From Haher R, Merola A, Surgical Technique for the Spine, Thieme; pg. 234, Fig. 50-3A,C.)

- 8. Resect (chisel or drill) a posterior wedge out of vertebral body (**Fig. 46.1B**).[3]
- 9. Repeat steps 5 and 6 on the contralateral side.[2]
- 10. Resect remaining posterior vertebral body cortex; impact bone into cavity previously created during wedge resection of vertebral body with angled bone tamp or down-going curette.[2]
- 11. Use fluoroscopy to confirm adequate resection in addition to visual inspection.[3]
- 12. Compress across pedicle screws to close down osteotomy (**Fig. 46.1B**).
- 13. Evaluate neurophysiologic monitoring and/or wakeup test to ensure absence of neurologic compromise.

Smith-Petersen Osteotomy
- 1. Position on Jackson frame with extended chest bolster.
- 2. Consider use of multimodal neurophysiologic monitoring to minimize neurologic complications during deformity correction.
- 3. Place pedicle screw instrumentation across targeted segments.

46 Pedicle Subtraction Osteotomy/Smith Petersen Osteotomy

- 4. Remove interspinous ligaments with rongeur.
- 5. Spinous processes are removed at each targeted segment in a 45 degree angle in addition to removal of the upper and lower lamina edges.
- 6. Bilateral facetectomies are performed with osteotomes and/or a high-speed drill[4] (**Fig. 46.2A**).
- 7. Remove ligamentum flavum.
- 8. Compress across the screw heads to close the osteotomy[4] (**Fig. 46.2B**).
- 9. The patient may be placed in extension to assist in closure of the osteotomy.[4]

IV. Complications

- Neurologic injury due to iatrogenic spinal stenosis upon closure of the osteotomy
- Spinal subluxation during osteotomy
- Durotomy

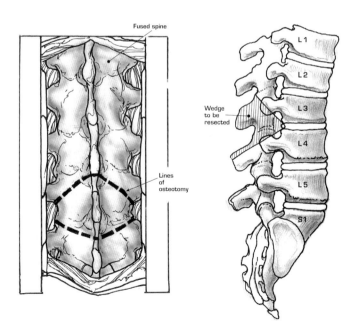

Fig. 46.2 (A,B) Smith-Petersen osteotomy. (From Haher R, Merola A, Surgical Technique for the Spine, Thieme; pg. 228, Fig. 49-1A,B.)

- Hypotension due to excessive blood loss during osteotomy; avoid hypotension especially during correction maneuvers as spinal cord ischemia may result
- Epidural hematoma
- Vascular injury
- Pseudarthrosis

V. Postoperative Care

- Immediate neurologic evalution upon wakeup
- Admission to neurologic intensive care for close monitoring
- Maintenance of blood pressure
- Consider postoperative computed tomography (CT) scan to evaluate adequacy of bone resection and juxtaposition of osteotomy margins.

VI. Outcomes

- With PSO, average curve improvements are 61 degrees in scoliosis cases, 56 degrees in global kyphosis cases, and 51 degrees in angular kyphosis cases.[4]
- Clinical and radiographic outcomes are superior with PSO in the lumbar spine rather than in the thoracic. The lower the PSO is performed, the less angulation is required for sagittal balance correction.[1]
- In properly selected patients, sagittal balance can be restored with PSO or multiple SPO safely.

VII. Surgical Pearls

- Ensure that bone resection is adequate and wide enough laterally in both PSO and SPO to prevent interference upon osteotomy closure or compression of neurologic structures.
- Use thrombin powder or bioabsorbable bone wax to minimize bleeding during PSO without compromising fusion rates. Aprotinin is also an option, although controversy exists over possible associated complications.
- Do not resect the anterior vertebral wall entirely during PSO, as it will serve as a hinge during pedicle screw compression and osteotomy closure and prevent vertebral segment subluxation.
- Posterior laminectomy resection should be complete and include any epidural scar removal to assess dural sac adequately after osteotomy closure and ensure there is no spinal canal compression.

– During SPO closure, place patient in extension to lengthen the anterior spinal column and facilitate osteotomy closure and to minimize strain on the pedicle screw construct.

Common Clinical Questions

1. How many degrees of correction can be achieved with PSO as opposed to SPO?
2. What is the main advantage of a PSO/SPO procedure?
3. In regard to the anterior and middle columns, what is the main difference between PSO and SPO?

References

1. Dorward IG, Lenke LG. Osteotomies in the posterior-only treatment of complex adult spinal deformity: a comparative review. Neurosurg Focus 2010;28(3):E4
2. Bridwell KH, Lewis SJ, Rinella A, Lenke LG, Baldus C, Blanke K. Pedicle subtraction osteotomy for the treatment of fixed sagittal imbalance. Surgical technique. J Bone Joint Surg Am 2004;86-A(Suppl 1):44–50
3. Bridwell KH, Lewis SJ, Lenke LG, Baldus C, Blanke K. Pedicle subtraction osteotomy for the treatment of fixed sagittal imbalance. J Bone Joint Surg Am 2003;85-A(3):454–463
4. La Marca F, Brumblay H. Smith-Petersen osteotomy in thoracolumbar deformity surgery. Neurosurgery 2008;63(3, Suppl):163–170

Answers to Common Clinical Questions

1. Up to 30 degrees per level with PSO compared with 10 degrees per level with SPO
2. Correction of sagittal imbalance and reestablishment of lordosis or correction of kyphosis
3. PSO is a closing wedge osteotomy involving the three columns, and thus shortens the middle and posterior columns. SPO, in contrast, uses the middle column as a pivot, thus lengthening the anterior column and shortening the posterior column.

47 Transthoracic Approach

Brian Kwon and David H. Kim

I. Key Points

- The transthoracic approach places the major vessels of the thoracic cavity at risk and threatens injury to the lungs and heart.
- An injury to the spinal cord at this level may result in paraplegia.
- Mark levels carefully, and make frequent use of radiographs or fluoroscopy.

II. Indications

- Thoracic myelopathy resulting from spinal cord compression[1]
  - Herniated nucleus pulposus (HNP), stenosis, or ossification of the posterior longitudinal ligament (OPLL)
  - Cervical and lumbar pathology ruled out
- Infections
  - Discitis or osteomyelitis
- Trauma
- Tumors
- Not for axial thoracic spine pain

III. Technique

- Position lateral decubitus.[2]
- Alert anesthesia staff to use double-lumen endotracheal tube so that deflation of lung can be performed if necessary.
- Confirm level(s)
  - If using open technique, manually palpate ribs (enlist help of thoracic surgeon).
  - Live fluoroscopy: use fixed markers, such as spinal needles placed into facet joints (to mark pedicles or ribs).
  - Count ribs on anteroposterior (AP) view (take note of males with missing twelfth rib).
  - Lower thoracic vertebrae can be counted from sacrum.
  - Confirm as many times as necessary (thoracic vertebrae look alike!).
- Make skin incision over disc or vertebral body based on imaging.
  - Semilinear or linear
- Upper thoracic discs (T2 to T5) may require mobilization of scapula.

- Cut latissimus dorsi, serratus anterior, and teres major muscles *midsubstance*—allows scapula to be deflected cephalad and dorsally.
- For lower thoracic discs (T9 to T12), hemidiaphragm may need to be released from the vertebrae.
- Resect rib for visualization (**Fig. 47.1A–C**).
  - Preserve nerve root if possible; otherwise sacrifice by ligating a *segment* of nerve to prevent painful neuromas. Tell patient about post-op paresthesia.
  - Excellent source of structural or morselized autograft
- Can get to discs and vertebrae via transpleural or retropleural approach
  - Incise parietal pleura.
  - Lifts off lateral side of vertebral body
- Deflate lung.
- Ligate segmental vessels close to azygous vein/aorta.

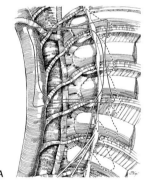
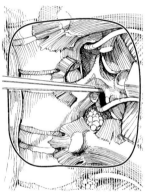
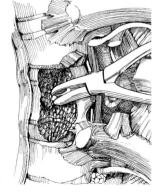

Fig. 47.1 (A,B) A window is made through the parietal pleura over the vertebral body. (C) The corpectomy is performed all the way to the contralateral pedicle. (From Anterior thoracic decompression. In: Spine Surgery: Tricks of the Trade 2nd ed. Vaccarro AR, Albert TJ, eds. Thieme; pg. 108, Figs. 31.2, 31.3.)

- Necessary for corpectomies
- Follow nerve root into foramen.
- Rib head resection is necessary above T9-T10.[3]
  - May not be necessary at T11 or T12
  - Helpful to see pedicle, the primary landmark for performing discectomy

IV. Complications

- Spinal cord injury
  - Spinal neuromonitoring necessary
  - Direct spinal cord trauma
  - Vascular insufficiency
    - Note ligation of multiple segmental vessels for multilevel surgery.
- Lung injury
  - From retractors, burr, other equpment
- Vascular injury
- Thoracic duct injury
  - On the right in lower thoracic spine (T9 to T12), on the left in upper thoracic spine (T4 and above)
- Pneumothorax
- Post-op neuritis

V. Postoperative Care

- Chest tube, for transpleural approach
  - Placed outside operative incision
- Bracing optional

VI. Outcomes

- Generally good for neurologic outcomes depending on the severity of preoperative myelopathy
  - Can use Japanese Orthopedic Association score or Nurick grade
- Pain outcomes less predictable

VII. Surgical Pearls

- Mark levels carefully with good intra-op imaging.
- Can follow rib, rib head, and nerve root to disc space

Common Clinical Questions

1. Which of the following is *not* an appropriate indication for transthoracic spine surgery?
   A. Infection
   B. Tumor
   C. Trauma
   D. Back pain

2. Complications of transthoracic spine surgery include (choose all that apply):
   A. Spinal cord injury
   B. Incisional hernia
   C. Neuralgia
   D. Chylothorax

3. True or false: Thoracic vertebrae can be easily differentiated from one another.

References

1. Bohlman HH, Zdeblick TA. Anterior excision of herniated thoracic discs. J Bone Joint Surg Am 1988;70(7):1038–1047
2. Currier BL, Eismont FJ, Green BA. Transthoracic disc excision and fusion for herniated thoracic discs. Spine (Phila Pa 1976) 1994;19(3):323–328
3. Moro T, Kikuchi S, Konno S. Necessity of rib head resection for anterior discectomy in the thoracic spine. Spine (Phila Pa 1976) 2004;29(15):1703–1705

Answers to Common Clinical Questions

1. D. Back pain or axial pain is not an appropriate indication. Surgical outcomes for axial pain are less reliable and, given the inherent risks of thoracic spine surgery, such pain is not a good indication for it.

2. A, C, D. Spinal cord injury can occur from direct trauma to the cord or ischemia due to hypotension or ligation of the segmental vessel from which the anterior spinal artery arises. Neuralgia results from ligation of thoracic nerve root. Thoracic duct injury can occur in lower, right-sided thoracic approaches.

3. False. Thoracic vertebrae look very similar and because of the overlying rib cage, anatomic differences cannot be used to confirm operative level.

48 Retroperitoneal Approaches to the Thoracolumbar Spine

Camilo A. Molina, Ziya L. Gokaslan, and Daniel M. Sciubba

I. Key Points

- Of utmost importance to performing any ventrolateral approaches to the lumbar spine is extensive knowledge of the regional anatomy, including the abdominal wall, peritoneal contents, retroperitoneal contents, and ventrolateral musculature and neural elements.
- Conventional open anterior (transperitoneal) approaches to the lumbar spine require mobilization of the sympathetic plexus and great vessels, which is associated with a significant incidence of complications. Retroperitoneal approaches to the lumbar spine minimize the incidence of such complications by avoiding mobilization of the large bowel, sympathetic plexus, and great vessels.
- The indications to perform a particular type of approach are more dependent on the localization of the pathology, the balance between advantages and disadvantages, and the surgeon's knowledge of the approach than on the pathology itself. For example, the indications to perform an interbody fusion range from preoperative segmental instability to iatrogenic instability due to wide decompressions, but do not dictate a specific approach. In other words, the indications for a minimally invasive interbody fusion are the same as for an open interbody fusion. However, the relative localization of the instability, the skill of the surgeon, complication risks, and the health status of the patient indicate the preferential use of a particular approach over another (i.e., retroperitoneal versus transperitoneal).
- In general, left-sided approaches are more practical than right-sided approaches because it is less difficult to separate the aorta from the spine than to separate the more delicate inferior vena cava, particularly in cases of retroperitoneal fibrosis that occur in patients previously treated with radiation therapy due to neoplasms.

II. Conventional Open Retroperitoneal Access

- Indications
  - Open retroperitoneal access provides a wide anterior exposure to the spine, allowing for the treatment of spine patholo-

gies of degenerative, traumatic, and neoplastic origins. The most widely used approach is to perform anterior lumbar interbody fusions to treat a variety of spine pathologies that develop due to degenerative and neoplastic spine diseases, such as *degenerative disc disease, trauma-related internal disc disruption, pseudarthrosis, decompression for neural stenosis,* and *spine deformity.*[1–3] This approach can also been employed to perform anterior access lumbar corpectomies[1,2,4]; it is also a common avenue for treating epidural spinal neoplasms and cases of complex spine deformity.
- Surgical technique varies with the level accessed.
  - Lumbosacral (L2 to S1)[1]
    - A paramedian incision traversing the subcutaneous tissue to expose the external oblique muscle is made, preferably on the left to avoid the more prominent common iliac vein on the right. The external oblique muscle is then incised at the medial aponeurotic region, after which the rectus sheath is opened. The rectus muscle is then mobilized mediolaterally to preserve segmental innervation of the abdominal wall.
    - Following mobilization of the rectus muscle, the retroperitoneal space is developed at the level of the semilunar line. This is done by dissecting the peritoneum in a lateromedial direction, freeing it from the superficial posterior rectus sheath (superior to the semilunar line). The peritoneal sac is then bluntly dissected off the psoas muscle, allowing for retroperitoneal access to the lumbar spine (it is important to identify and follow the ipsilateral ureter to identify the left iliac vein and artery).
    - Exposure is then assisted by a self-retaining retractor (Omni-Retractor, Omni, St. Paul, MN). The left iliac artery and vein are retracted medially and segmental vessels divided laterally. It is crucial to avoid injury to vascular and lymphatic structures (**Fig. 48.1**).
    - Following completion of the procedure, hemostasis should be confirmed and the self-retractor blades removed one by one to ensure a dry field. The wound is then irrigated and the abdominal wall reconstructed in plane-by-plane fashion.
  - Thoracolumbar (T12 to L2): thoracoabdominal approach[1]
    - The patient is secured in the lateral decubitus position. Approach is mostly via the left side.
    - An obliquely oriented thoracoabdominal incision is made and extended from the tenth or eleventh rib to the abdominal wall.
    - The rib is dissected free from its bed via division of subcutaneous tissues, serratus anterior, latissimus dorsi, and intercostal

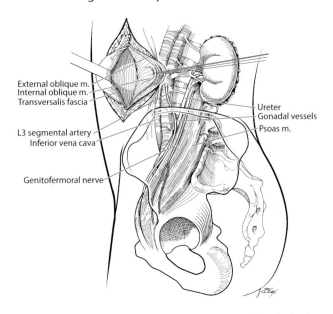

Fig. 48.1 Lateral view of the retroperitoneal approach to the lumbar spine.

muscles. The rib should be exposed at its superior border to avoid the neurovascular bundle below. The rib dissection is followed obliquely to the abdominal wall by dividing the external and internal oblique muscles. However, this distance should be limited to minimize postoperative muscular dysfunction. The transversalis layer is visible deep to the split costal margin and can be divided to expose the peritoneum.

- The peritoneum is ventrally dissected of overlying structures (diaphragm and psoas muscle) to open the retroperitoneal space.
- The diaphragm is taken down, leaving a distal cuff for repair, avoiding the more central region to prevent damage to the phrenic nerve. The lung is gently compressed cranially with a moist lap pad. The parietal pleura is now visualized and can be opened to access the anterior thoracolumbar spine.
- For access to the anterior disc space, segmental vessels to the vertebral bodies are dissected and divided. These vessels must be handled with the utmost care as they pose a significant risk for hemorrhage and are a vital supply to both intra- and extraspinal structures. Some advocate preoperative angiography of the artery of Adamkiewicz to assist surgical

approach and diminish the risk of paraplegia. Care should also be employed to prevent injury to retroperitoneal lymphatics (cisterna chyli and thoracic duct) and the development of large lymphoceles.
- Following completion of the procedure, if the diaphragm was incised, a large-bore chest tube is applied and the diaphragm repaired with nonabsorbable sutures. The thoracic cavity is then closed by employing rib-approximating sutures and repairing the intercostalis musculature. The anterior abdominal wall, serratus anterior, and latissimus dorsi muscles are reapproximated and reconstructed plane by plane via running nonabsorbable sutures.
- Management of vascular anatomy
  - Vascular concerns related to such approaches include managing the aorta, inferior vena cava, iliac vessels, iliolumbar vein, and segmental vessels.
  - With regard to the major vessels in the thoracolumbar and lumbar regions, the aorta usually is more toward the left side of the spinal column and the inferior vena cava is more toward the right side. Such anatomy should be reviewed and confirmed preoperatively. Most surgeons prefer to approach the patient from the left, as aortic damage is easier to repair than damage to the vena cava. However, if pathology is eccentric to one side, the surgeon should be prepared to approach from either side.
  - Iliac vessels, which are the caudal extensions of the aorta and inferior vena cava, usually are not encountered with a lateral approach unless L5 is involved with the pathology.
  - The iliolumbar vein is an important direct tether in a left-sided dissection at L4-L5 or lower. This lumbar vein crosses from the inferior vena cava to approximately the level of the L5 body. Any dissection that exposes L4-L5 to the left of the left common iliac vein and inferior vena cava requires the identification, ligation, and division of the iliolumbar vein. Start at the L4-L5 disc and dissect distally to the L5 body until the iliolumbar vein is visualized.
  - Segmental arteries and veins lie at the lateral aspect of the vertebral bodies within the "valleys" of the lateral spine. Such vessels must be identified and ligated prior to exposure of the lateral vertebral body with subperiosteal dissection. If a segmental artery is sectioned with a Bovie cautery device (Bovie Medical Corp., Clearwater, FL), it may retract toward the aorta and continue bleeding. Therefore, early identification and ligation are paramount with exposure.

- Complications
  - Retroperitoneal fibrosis, rectus muscle hematoma, pancreatitis, femoral nerve palsy, ureteral injuries, lymphoceles, pseudomeningocele, latissimus dorsi rupture, impotence, and retrograde ejaculation[2,5,6]
  - Acutely developing lymphoceles can be remedied by oversewing the lymphatic chain with a nonabsorbable suture.
- Outcomes
  - Advantages of a conventional open retroperitoneal approach relative to a posterior approach include higher rates of fusion due to the ability to place larger interbody fusion devices, the ability to perform more complete disc excisions, and a reduced incidence of nerve damage. Furthermore, this approach is associated with decreased pulmonary complications and length of hospital stay.
  - A conventional retroperitoneal approach is also associated with better outcomes in comparison with an anterior transperitoneal approach. For example, in addition to avoidance of large-vessel and bowel injury, the retroperitoneal approach is associated with a decreased incidence of retrograde ejaculation for exposures of L4-L5.

III. General Postoperative Care for Retroperitoneal Approaches

- Retroperitoneal approaches do not typically require bowel rest in the postoperative period, unlike the transperitoneal approach. Nonetheless, although infrequent, bowel injury can occur via a retroperitoneal approach and is primarily identified by ileus and/or peritoneal irritation. Therefore, caution must be taken to identify and assess patients demonstrating signs of peritoneal irritation or dysfunction such as an absence of flatus.
- Patients should be monitored for the development of deep vein thrombosis (DVT) and potential pulmonary embolisms (PEs). Patients are at high risk for developing DVT or PEs due to the significant manipulation of the deep veins (particularly the iliac vein), which commonly leads to the formation of venous thrombi.

IV. Surgical Pearls

- As a general rule in any spine surgery, segmental vessels obstructing the target structure must be ligated on the anterior portion of the vertebral body to preserve optimal collateral circulation to the neuroforamen and spinal cord.

- In mobilizing or traversing the psoas muscle, two things should be considered. First, it is beneficial to stay on the anterior third of the psoas muscle to prevent nerve root injury. Second, it is important to visualize and protect the genitofemoral nerve running on the surface of the psoas muscle. This prevents complications such as retrograde ejaculation or paresthesias of the anterior thigh.

Common Clinical Questions

1. Retroperitoneal approaches are preferentially done on the left side of the patient for all the following reasons *except:*
   A. It is generally safer to mobilize the aorta than the inferior vena cava
   B. The common iliac vein may be more prominent on the right side
   C. The presence of the liver may minimize exposure
   D. The left ureter is less susceptible to injury than the right ureter

2. Complications of retroperitoneal exposure include all of the following *except:*
   A. Retroperitoneal fibrosis
   B. Appendicitis
   C. Ureteral injury
   D. Femoral nerve palsy

3. To obtain adequate exposure, an essential component of the thoracoabdominal approach is:
   A. Incising the diaphragm along along the costal margin and leaving a cuff attached to the rib
   B. Transecting the psoas to allow full retraction of the muscle
   C. Dissection of the lumbar plexus from the overlying psoas muscle
   D. Avoiding sacrifice of segmental arteries

References

1. Gumbs AA, Bloom ND, Bitan FD, Hanan SH. Open anterior approaches for lumbar spine procedures. Am J Surg 2007;194(1):98–102
2. Gumbs AA, Shah RV, Yue JJ, Sumpio B. The open anterior paramedian retroperitoneal approach for spine procedures. Arch Surg 2005;140(4):339–343
3. McAfee PC, Bohlman HH, Yuan HA. Anterior decompression of traumatic thoracolumbar fractures with incomplete neurological deficit using a retroperitoneal approach. J Bone Joint Surg Am 1985;67(1):89–104
4. Payer M, Sottas C. Mini-open anterior approach for corpectomy in the thoracolumbar spine. Surg Neurol 2008;69(1):25–31, discussion 31–32
5. Patel AA, Spiker WR, Daubs MD, Brodke DS, Cheng I, Glasgow RE. Retroperitoneal lymphocele after anterior spinal surgery. Spine (Phila Pa 1976) 2008;33(18):E648–E652
6. Peng CW, Bendo JA, Goldstein JA, Nalbandian MM. Perioperative outcomes of anterior lumbar surgery in obese versus non-obese patients. Spine J 2009;9(9):715–720

Answers to Common Clinical Questions

1. D
2. B
3. A

49 Open and MIS Lumbar Microdiscectomy

Ali A. Baaj and Mark S. Greenberg

I. Key Points

- Conservative therapy is the initial and primary treatment modality for radiculopathy caused by a herniated nucleus pulposus (HNP) in the lumbar spine.
- Lumbar microdiscectomy is a safe and effective procedure when the indication is appropriate.
- Cauda equina and conus syndromes caused by HNP in the lumbar spine constitute neurosurgical emergencies and require immediate evaluation.

II. Indications

- Symptomatic HNP
  - Radiculopathy (after 6 to 8 weeks of failed conservative therapy)
  - Cauda equina syndrome
  - Conus syndrome
- Not for isolated axial low back pain
- No instability on preoperative dynamic plain radiographs

III. Technique

Open

- The patient is placed in the prone position.
  - Use of a Wilson frame may widen the interlaminar space and assist in access.
- Fluoroscopy is used for localization.
- A 2 to 3 cm midline incision is made with a number 10 scalpel.
- A subperiosteal dissection of tissue from spinous process and lamina on the ipsilateral side is performed.
  - Supraspinous and interspinous ligaments should be preserved.
- The medial facet joint is the lateral limit of the dissection.
- A retractor (e.g., Williams or Taylor) is placed.
- The inferior lamina of the superior level and superior lamina of the inferior level are identified and confirmed with fluoroscopy.
- Using a high-speed drill, a laminotomy (usually) is performed by drilling the inferior part of the superior level.
  - For inferior fragment migration, some of the superior lamina from the inferior level may need to be removed.

- Ligamentous flavum is removed with curette and Kerrison punch.
- The operative microscope is brought in.
- The nerve sleeve and dura are gently retracted medially (**Fig. 49.1**).
- The posterior longitudinal ligament (PLL) and annulus fibrosus are incised with a number 11 blade, medial to lateral (always incise away from dura).
- Disc material is removed with a pituitary rongeur.
  - The surgeon must have an understanding of where the anterior longitudinal ligament (ALL) is to prevent inadvertent penetration into the retroperitoneal vessels with the pituitary rongeur.
- The disc space is irrigated and loose disc tissue is removed.
- An instrument (e.g., Woodson or dental dissector) is passed beneath the dura to ensure there is no residual fragment.
- A nerve hook is used to probe under the PLL superior and inferior to the disc space to check for residual.
- The fascia is closed with 0 or 2-0 absorbable suture.
- The subcutaneous layer is closed with inverted, interrupted 3-0 absorbable suture.
- The skin is closed with running suture, staples, or skin adhesive.

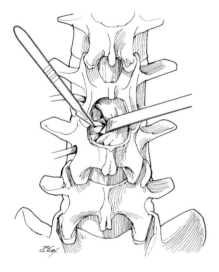

Fig. 49.1 Dorsal view of laminotomy defect showing thecal sac, traversing nerve root (retracted medially), and herniated disc.

Minimally Invasive Technique
- After correct positioning and localization, a 12 to 16 mm incision is made 10 mm lateral to the midline on the appropriate side.
- The thoracodorsal fascia is incised with blade or cautery, and serial dilators are positioned with the use of fluoroscopy.
- The final dilator and working tube should be docked over the interlaminar space with visualization of the inferior lamina of the superior level.
- The operative microscope is brought in.
- Soft tissue is dissected and drilling is performed until ligamentum flavum is reached.
  - If drilling is done too laterally, the pedicle or facet joint is at risk; confirm location with fluoroscopy if needed.
- The ligament is removed and discectomy is performed as in the open approach.
- If a wider decompression is needed, the working tube may be repositioned to allow access to more lamina, and even the contralateral foramen.

IV. Complications
- Cerebrospinal fluid (CSF) leak (5 to 8%)[1]
  - Attempt primary repair using nonabsorbable suture (typically challenging).
  - Alternatively, cover with Gelfoam (Pfizer, New York) and/or fibrin glue.
- Nerve root injury (1%)
- Wound infection (1%)
- Vascular injury (<1%)
  - Suspected injury to the iliac vessels anteriorly (e.g., bright red blood from disc space or sudden, unexplained drop in blood pressure) requires immediate wound closure, repositioning of patient to supine, and immediate vascular surgery consult.

V. Postoperative Care
- Mobilize early; no need for bracing.
- Discharge to home when patient meets discharge criteria (typically, ambulating, tolerating a diet, voiding, and receiving adequate pain control from oral medications—usually same day or on post-op day 1).

VI. Outcomes

- There is an 85% chance of a good (minimal symptoms) or excellent (asymptomatic) outcome.[2]
- First recurrence is usually treated with repeat microdiscectomy. Further recurrence may necessitate fusion.
- Multiple randomized trials have been plagued by crossovers between cohorts, and the most definitive statement that can be made is that decisions for surgery versus conservative treatment based on symptoms, duration, and patient preference results in similar good outcomes in both treatment groups.[3]

VII. Surgical Pearls

- Ensure the HNP is the pain/symptom generator based on exam and imaging.
- Minimal disruption of medial facet (don't confuse the facet for the lamina during the initial approach)
- Overly aggressive drilling of facet may lead to instability.
- Ensure you are not in a nerve root axilla when performing discectomy.
- Preoperative dynamic films may be necessary to rule out instability
- May need hemilaminectomy or complete laminectomy if treating large central disc (e.g., for cauda equina or conus syndrome).

Common Clinical Questions

1. What is the best way to avoid drilling into the facet joint or pedicle during MIS discectomy?
2. When evaluating for recurrent lumbar herniated disc, what radiologic examination is most appropriate?
3. When evaluating a recurrent lumbar herniated disc, what radiologic exam is helpful in ruling out instability?

References

1. German JW, Adamo MA, Hoppenot RG, Blossom JH, Nagle HA. Perioperative results following lumbar discectomy: comparison of minimally invasive discectomy and standard microdiscectomy. Neurosurg Focus 2008;25(2):E20
2. Hoffman RM, Wheeler KJ, Deyo RA. Surgery for herniated lumbar discs: a literature synthesis. J Gen Intern Med 1993;8(9):487–496
3. Weinstein JN, Tosteson TD, Lurie JD, et al. Surgical vs nonoperative treatment for lumbar disk herniation: the Spine Patient Outcomes Research Trial (SPORT): a randomized trial. JAMA 2006;296(20):2441–2450

Answers to Common Clinical Questions

1. Obtain anteroposterior/lateral fluoroscopy shots intraoperatively to confirm location.
2. MRI with and without contrast
3. Flexion-extension x-rays

50 Lumbar Foraminotomy (MIS)

Ali A. Baaj and Juan S. Uribe

I. Key Points

- Removing more than one-third of the medial facet joint when performing a foraminotomy could lead to instability.
- The combination of a high-speed drill and small-caliber Kerrison rongeur should be utilized to safely perform a foraminotomy.
- Foraminal stenosis and nerve root compression are the result of hypertrophy/degeneration of the superior articulating facet of the lower vertebra.

II. Indications

- Focal lateral recess and/or foraminal stenosis

III. Technique

- The patient is placed in the prone position.
  - A Wilson radiolucent frame is adequate if no fixation is planned.
- Fluoroscopy is utilized for localizing the level of the foramen.
- A paramedian 2 to 3 cm incision is made 1 cm lateral to the midline.
- The fascia is incised with a monopolar cautery.
- Serial dilators and a nonexpandable tube retractor are placed under fluoroscopic visualization.
  - The optimal arrangement is to dock the dilator/tube retractor on the inferior aspect of the lamina of the superior level. For example, for a L4/L5 foraminotomy, the tube is positioned on the inferior aspect of the L4 lamina.
  - This approach is similar to that of minimally invasive surgery (MIS) for microdiscectomy
- The operative microscope is brought over the field.
  - This is optional, but the microscope provides for better illumination and visualization through the tubular retractor.
- The inferior aspect of the lamina is drilled until the underlying ligamentum flavum is visualized.
- With the use of nerve hooks, curettes, and Kerrison rongeurs, the ligamentum flavum is resected.
- The traversing nerve root is typically visualized at this point.

- The medial facet is undermined until the medial pedicle is palpated with a Woodson or ball-ended probe.
- With a number 2 Kerrison, the foramina above and below the pedicle are widened and hypertrophied ligament is resected until the shoulder of the exiting root is visualized.
- A ball-ended probe should pass easily in the foramina to confirm adequate decompression.
- The space is irrigated and the fascial, subcutaneous, and skin layers are closed in standard fashion.
  - Subfascial drains are not typically used.

IV. Complications[1]

- Cerebrospinal fluid (CSF) leak (<5%)
  - Technically challenging to repair primarily through the MIS tube
- Nerve root injury (<1%)
- Wound infection (<1%)

V. Postoperative Care

- Mobilize early without brace.
- Discharge to home when patient meets discharge criteria.
  - Typically same day or postoperative day 1

VI. Outcomes

- The presumed benefits of MIS foraminotomy include reduced blood loss, less tissue damage, and shorter hospital stays. However, no randomized trial has compared traditional open with MIS foraminotomy.

VII. Surgical Pearls

- Leaving the ligamentum flavum intact until all the "bony work" is completed protects the dura during drilling and when the Kerrison punches are in use.
- Aggressive drilling of the facet to remove more than one-third may lead to facet joint instability.
- Patients whose history and exam findings of radiculopathy correlate with the foraminal stenosis seen on imaging will likely have the best outcomes from this procedure.

Common Clinical Questions

1. What is the roof of the intervertebral foramen composed of?
2. Which nerve root exits below the L4 pedicle?
3. How do you ensure you're not drilling pedicle?

References

1. Christie SD, Song JK. Minimally invasive lumbar discectomy and foraminotomy. Neurosurg Clin N Am 2006;17(4):459–466

Answers to Common Clinical Questions

1. The superior articulating facet of the inferior vertebra
2. The L4 nerve root
3. Take an anteroposterior fluoroscopy shot intraoperatively or go more medial and expose the ligament/dura medially.

51 Lumbar Laminectomy

Armen Deukmedjian, Ali A. Baaj, and Juan S. Uribe

I. Key Points

- An adequate lumbar laminectomy affords good central decompression and lateral gutter decompression, and sets the stage for foraminotomies at the corresponding spinal levels.
- Removing more than one-third of the medial facet joints during a laminectomy could accelerate degeneration and cause instability, necessitating a subsequent fusion.

II. Indications

- Focal or multilevel lumbar central and lateral recess stenosis

III. Technique

- Place patient in the prone position.
    - A Wilson frame is adequate if no instrumentation is planned; otherwise an OSI table is generally used.
- Localize with fluoroscopy.
- Make a midline incision at the appropriate level and perform a subperiosteal dissection to detach the erector spinae muscles from the lamina.
- Stop at the medial aspect of the facet joint. Do not disturb the facet joint capsule.
- Use a Horsley or Leksell rongeur to remove the spinous process(es).
- Use a drill with an AM-8 bit to complete the laminectomy; alternatively, use Kerrison and Leksell rongeurs.
    - The facets are often hypertrophied, and the medial one-third can be drilled or removed with Kerrison rongeurs.
- Know your landmarks and be careful to avoid drilling the facet joint, pedicle, or pars.
- Remove the ligamentum flavum with Kerrison rongeurs to complete the decompression.
- Use a ball-ended probe to inspect the foramina (**Fig. 51.1**).
    - Use the number 2 Kerrison if necessary to perform the foraminotomy.
- Use a subfascial drain if the wound is extensive.
- Ensure a tight fascial closure and close the skin in the standard fashion.

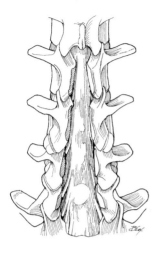

Fig. 51.1 Dorsal view of lumbar spine showing decompressed thecal sac and nerve roots with laminectomy taken to the medial facets laterally.

IV. Complications

- Cerebrospinal fluid leak (CSF) leak (0.3 to 13%; increases to about 18% in redo operations)[1]
  • Should be repaired using nonabsorbable suture
- Neurologic deficit (0.3%)[1]
- Wound infection (1 to 5%)[2]
- Spondylolisthesis[3]
- Death (0.06%)[1]

V. Postoperative Care

- Mobilize early without brace.
- Remove drain when output drops below 50 ml per 8-hour shift (typically postoperative day 1).
- Discharge home when patient meets discharge criteria.

VI. Outcomes

- Review of literature reveals 60 to 70% with good to excellent results.[1-4]
- Reoperation in 10 to 30% for recurrent/adjacent-level stenosis, spondylolisthetic stenosis, or instability[1,3-5]

VII. Surgical Pearls

- With advanced degenerative disease, obtain preoperative dynamic films to rule out a dynamic spondylolisthesis.

- Leaving the ligamentum flavum until all the "bony work" is completed protects the dura during drilling and use of the Kerrison punches.

Common Clinical Questions

1. Why are preoperative dynamic x-rays sometimes obtained before a lumbar laminectomy?
2. During lumbar laminectomy, what location is associated with the highest likelihood of a CSF leak?

References

1. Greenberg M. Handbook of Neurosurgery. 7th ed. New York: Thieme Medical Publishers; 2010:448–450
2. Turner JA, Ersek M, Herron L, Deyo R. Surgery for lumbar spinal stenosis. Attempted meta-analysis of the literature. Spine (Phila Pa 1976) 1992; 17(1):1–8
3. Caputy AJ, Luessenhop AJ. Long-term evaluation of decompressive surgery for degenerative lumbar stenosis. J Neurosurg 1992;77(5):669–676
4. Tuite GF, Stern JD, Doran SE, et al. Outcome after laminectomy for lumbar spinal stenosis. Part I: Clinical correlations. J Neurosurg 1994;81(5):699–706
5. Katz JN, Lipson SJ, Larson MG, McInnes JM, Fossel AH, Liang MH. The outcome of decompressive laminectomy for degenerative lumbar stenosis. J Bone Joint Surg Am 1991;73(6):809–816

Answers to Common Clinical Questions

1. To rule out spondylolisthesis
2. The superior aspect of the lamina, or in the lateral recess if there is significant stenosis

52 Posterior and Transforaminal Lumbar Interbody Fusion (PLIF/TLIF) (Open)

Devin Vikram Amin and Adam S. Kanter

I. Key Points
- Arthrodesis across one or more vertebral disc spaces is indicated in conditions that produce spinal instability.
- Bilateral posterior lumbar interbody fusion (PLIF) may be performed at L5-S1 with less potential for neural injury due to the enlarged capacity of the neural canal at this level.
- A primary advantage of the transforaminal lumbar interbody fusion (TLIF) procedure over PLIF is the reduction in nerve root retraction, and thus in neural complications.

II. Indications
- Spondylolisthesis grade I or II
- Reoperation for pseudarthrosis
- Degenerative disc disease causing discogenic low back pain
- Recurrent disc herniation with mechanical back pain, or recurrent radiculopathy
- Lumbar deformity with coronal or sagittal plane imbalance
- Neural foraminal stenosis from disc space collapse

III. Technique
Transforaminal Lumbar Interbody Fusion
- Exposure of the disc space
  - Expose the vertebral spinous process and lamina of the levels above and below the operative disc space using lateral x-ray to confirm the anatomic level. In the case of a L4-L5 TLIF, the medial facet joint (inferior articular process) of the L4/L5 interspace on the primary symptomatic side is removed.
  - This is performed with a high-speed drill or osteotome to create a sagittal cut in the lamina and a transverse cut through the pars interarticularis directly over the exiting nerve root at the inferior aspect of the pedicle of the index neural foramen.
  - The joint capsule and ligamentum flavum can be detached with monopolar electrocautery. A Leksell rongeur is used to remove the medial facet, which is morselized for fusion autograft. The superior (or lateral) facet of the caudal level is then

removed with a Kerrison rongeur until the superior aspect of the next pedicle is encountered. Care must be taken to avoid injury to the exiting nerve root within the foramen at this level.
- The shoulder of the traversing nerve root is visualized exiting the thecal sac at the level of the disc space. The medial and superior borders of the caudal pedicle limit the amount of the superior facet that can be removed. A high-speed drill can be used to shave bony osteophytes to optimize the trajectory into the disc space and minimize nerve root retraction during interbody graft placement.

- Discectomy
  - The discectomy is performed by incising the annulus with a scalpel and then using curettes and pituitary rongeurs to remove the nucleus pulposus and cartilaginous end plates, thus exposing the bony surface of the vertebral end plates for fusion.
  - Preservation of the bony end plates will serve to prevent graft subsidence into the cancellous portion of the vertebral body.
- Interbody grafting
  - An interbody graft of the appropriate size is packed with autograft or other fusion substrate[1] and carefully impacted into the disc space.[1] A nerve retractor is placed against the traversing nerve root shoulder to protect it during graft placement.
  - The interbody graft should not protrude beyond the dorsal aspect of the adjacent vertebrae.
- Pedicle screw placement
  - The pedicle screw entry point is indicated by the mamillary process: the junction of the transverse process, superior facet, and pars interarticularis. The lateral to medial trajectory varies generally from 5 to 20 degrees from L1 to L5 (i.e., 5 degrees at L1 and increasing at 5 degree increments per caudal level).
  - The rostral to caudal trajectory should parallel the pedicle as directed by palpation with a Woodson-Adson or similar instrument if a decompression has been performed, or alternatively, using intraoperative fluorscopy or image guidance.
  - Once the pedicle screws have been placed, a lordotic rod is inserted and the cap screws are tightened with compression across the screw heads. This restores lordosis and compresses the interbody graft to prevent graft migration and facilitate fusion.
- Closure
  - A multilayer closure is performed using absorbable sutures in the lumbodorsal fascia and subdermis. Staples or nylon suture is used to close the skin.

- If a surgical drain has been left in the wound, it is secured to the skin with suture and the wound is covered with an appropriate dressing.

Posterior Lumbar Interbody Fusion
- The PLIF procedure is similar to TLIF with respect to exposure, discectomy, and closure.
- The key difference is that the approach to the disc space is more medial and a portion of the facet remains, necessitating neural element retraction for discectomy and interbody graft placement (**Fig. 52.1**).[2]
- Laminectomy is routinely performed with a high-speed drill and rongeurs, following which the ligamentum flavum is resected to expose the thecal sac. Bilateral foraminotomies are routinely performed with a Kerrison rongeur to ensure adequate nerve root decompression, but the distal aspects of the roots themselves are not typically exposed as in the TLIF procedure.
- Once visualization has been accomplished, a dural retractor is used to medialize the neural elements and expose the underlying disc space.
- The discectomy, graft placement, and pedicle screw construct techniques are similar to those for the TLIF technique. Careful attention must be paid during intervertebral work to limit medial retraction of the neural elements. [3]

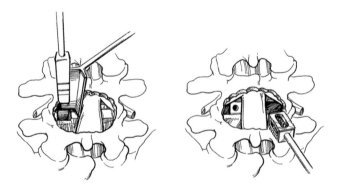

Fig. 52.1 An implant filled with cancellous bone graft is inserted into the rectangular channel. Note the teeth of the cage that engage the vertebral bone. (From Fessler R, Sekhar L, Atlas of Neurosurgical Techniques, Thieme; pg. 686, Fig. 95-3B.)

IV. Complications

- Dural tear (5 to 14%) can occur at any stage of the procedure, but most commonly occurs during the thecal sac and nerve root exposure.[4]
- Nerve root injury secondary to retraction has been reported in up to 13% of cases, with resultant radiculopathy, typically transient.
- Vascular injury during the discectomy, typically from breach of the anterior longitudinal ligament, requires packing of the disc space, emergency closure, and vascular consult for laparotomy and/or interventional repair of the injured vessel.
- Infection (1 to 5%), typically with skin flora

V. Postoperative Care

- Mobilize early; consider deep vein thrombosis (DVT) prophylaxis if patient is not ambulating on post-op day 1.
- Pain management with patient-controlled administration of narcotics augmented with muscle relaxants, and transition early to oral medications
- Discontinue wound drain based on output (e.g., less than 100 ml in 24 hours).

VI. Outcomes

- Clinical success rate is typically 75% for relief of mechanical back pain and radiculopathy.
- Fusion rates around 90% have been reported in multiple series.[5]

VII. Surgical Pearls

- Strict dissection along the periosteum minimizes blood loss.
- PLIF procedures may be more suited to the L5 to S1 disc space.
- Nerve root retraction can be reduced or eliminated with the more lateral to medial trajectory of the TLIF procedure.
- The introduction of pedicle screw and rod constructs has reduced the incidence of pseudarthrosis from TLIF and PLIF procedures.

Common Clinical Questions

1. A patient with known tethered cord would be better suited for which lumbar interbody fusion procedure?
2. The pars interarticularis is transected completely in which lumbar interbody fusion procedure?
3. The lateral to medial trajectory is greatest for pedicle screws inserted at which lumbar level?

References

1. Mummaneni PV, Rodts GE Jr. The mini-open transforaminal lumbar interbody fusion. Neurosurgery 2005;57(4, Suppl):256–261
2. Khoo LT, Palmer S, Laich DT, Fessler RG. Minimally invasive percutaneous posterior lumbar interbody fusion. Neurosurgery 2002;51(5, Suppl):S166–S1
3. Cole CD, McCall TD, Schmidt MH, Dailey AT. Comparison of low back fusion techniques: transforaminal lumbar interbody fusion (TLIF) or posterior lumbar interbody fusion (PLIF) approaches. Curr Rev Musculoskelet Med 2009;2(2):118–126
4. Greenberg MS. Handbook of Neurosurgery. 6th ed. New York: Thieme Medical Publishers; 2006:744–748.

Answers to Common Clinical Questions

1. TLIF. The degree of neural element retraction is less with the TLIF procedure, which reduces the risk of traction on the conus medullaris.
2. TLIF. A complete medial facetectomy is part of the TLIF technique.
3. L5. The angle increases from 5 to 20 degrees as the lumbar level increases from L1 to L5.

53 Minimally Invasive Transforaminal Lumbar Interbody Fusion (MIS TLIF)

Michael Y. Wang

I. Key Points

- Minimally invasive transformational lumbar interbody fusion (MIS TLIF) can be utilized to achieve lumbar spinal decompression, fixation, and fusion.
- The intent behind this approach, which is still unproven, is to reduce soft-tissue injury, blood loss, recovery time, and length of hospital stay associated with open TLIF.
- It is important to recognize the anatomic landmarks at the interpedicular space, referred to as a Kambin triangle: medial (traversing root), lateral (exiting root), and base (inferior pedicle)

II. Indications

Harms first described the transforaminal lumbar interbody fusion (TLIF) technique for circumferential fusion in 1982 using an interbody spacer and a supplemental pedicle screw construct.[1] This procedure was a departure from the traditional posterior lumbar interbody fusion (PLIF) in that the TLIF required only a unilateral facetectomy and a single interbody cage. TLIF then became popular due to the lower rates of nerve root injury given the reduced surgical manipulation of neural elements, and it was also found to be effective for revision surgery because the midline dural sac did not have to be exposed.

A minimally invasive approach for accomplishing the TLIF procedure was subsequently developed.[2] This technique utilized the advantages of expandable working tubes and percutaneous pedicle screw technology to reduce the soft-tissue injury that has been documented to result from open surgery.[3] Although no class I evidence exists to demonstrate the superiority of MIS TLIF over open TLIF, comparative studies suggest a trend toward reduced postoperative pain, hospital length of stay, infection rates, and blood loss.[4] MIS TLIF can generally be applied in all situations where an open TLIF can be used.

- Single- or two-level degenerative disc disease with correlative clinical symptoms
- Spondylolisthesis less than Meyerding grade III

- Recurrent lumbar disc herniation
- Spondylosis with radiculopathy and back pain
- Focal spinal deformity concentrated at less than three intersegmental levels
- Synovial cysts exhibiting spinal instability

III. Technique

There are several variations of the MIS TLIF technique. Here a standard approach is described that has been successfully utilized by numerous surgeons.

- The patient is positioned prone on a Jackson operating room table, which offers several advantages. The location of the incision is targeted under fluoroscopy, and two paramedian skin incisions are made between 3 and 4 cm lateral to the midline. Sharp incision of the fascia allows for blunt finger dissection between the longissimus and multifidus muscles along a modified Wiltse plane (**Fig. 53.1**).[5] This not only minimizes trauma to muscular tissues but also minimizes intraoperative bleeding and creates a natural plane that allows for efficient maintenance of the trajectory of the retractors. The approach, if unilateral, is taken from the side where decompression is most necessary.

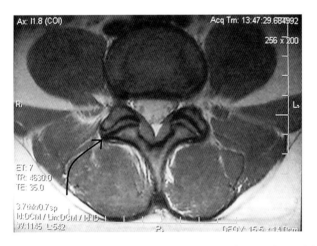

Fig. 53.1 Axial magnetic resonance image (MRI) showing the modified Wiltse plane between the longissimus and multifidus muscles. High MRI signal can be seen along this plane between the muscles, giving direct access to the facet joints.

- Tubular dilator retractors are then placed through this plane and the level confirmed with fluoroscopy. Monopolar cautery is then used to clear any muscle tissue over the facet joint, making sure to expose the lateral aspect of the joint.
- Once the surgeon has confirmed the location of the pars and the lower pedicle, a quarter-inch osteotome or high-speed burr is used to remove the facet joint. Either a partial or complete facetectomy can be performed, with greater bone removal for cases with more medial compression. Care must be taken not to drill into the pedicle. After facet removal the lateral aspect of the ligamentum flavum is visualized. This is resected until the lateral thecal sac is seen (**Fig. 53.2**). Autograft bone is saved for later grafting purposes.
- Further decompression can then be performed as needed, with removal of ipsilateral ligamentum flavum, decompression under the pars, or contralateral decompression. This is best achieved by angling the retractors more medially. Alternatively, bilateral decompression can be accomplished through dual ports placed on each side.
- After palpation of the caudal pedicle and confirmation of the location of the exiting and traversing nerve roots, the annulus is incised, followed by aggressive intervertebral disc removal and end plate preparation, as with the open technique. This is followed by intervertebral cage placement.
- The neural elements are reinspected. If a posterolateral fusion is desired, the dura is covered with Gelfoam (Pfizer, New York)

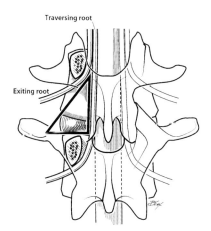

Fig. 53.2 A Kambin triangle.

and the lateral facets and transverse processes are decorticated with a drill. This is followed by bone graft application.
- Supplemental pedicle screw placement can then be accomplished either using a mini-open technique (through the retractor with visualization) or percutaneously before or after the decompression. For the mini-open method, the screw placement is very similar to open TLIF. Various methods are used for percutaneous targeting, including (1) AP only, (2) the owl's-eye en face approach, (3) biplanar fluoroscopy, and (4) image guidance. All percutaneous methods involve placement of a joshed needle into the pedicle, followed by the use of a cannulated awl and tap to create a screw entry tract. Finally, screw placement and rod tunneling are used to connect the construct components.
- A drain is not typically used.

IV. Complications

- Cerebrospinal fluid (CSF) leakage is uncommon with these procedures because the dural exposure is limited to those areas that are to be decompressed directly. Dural repair can be difficult. Some surgeons have advocated leaving the durotomy unrepaired and applying a collagen sponge locally, which suggests that the limited dead space reduces the risk of CSF leakage postoperatively.
- Incomplete neural decompression is more problematic than in open surgery given the small working corridor. Care must be taken to visualize critical landmarks to ensure that any compression (such as at a far lateral disc) is adequately addressed. The critical landmarks include the caudal pedicle, pars interarticularis, and lateral ligamentum flavum.
- Nerve root injury is best avoided by maintaining an appreciation of the medial-lateral location in which the surgeon is working. Careful identification and control of the exiting and traversing nerve roots prior to discectomy is critical.
- Cage misplacement occurs most frequently when inadequate disc material has been removed or the bony end plate has been violated. Care in end plate preparation is essential to minimize graft settling. In addition, it is desirable that the cage cross the midline, and this can be confirmed with fluoroscopy.
- Screw misplacement is most commonly the result of poor targeting technique. Thus, close familiarity with one technique

for ensuring that the pedicle is not breached is essential. The anteroposterior (AP) targeting techniques are excellent for preventing neural injuries.
- Pseudarthrosis can be minimized but never totally prevented. Proper end plate preparation, cage sizing, and the use of osteobiologic adjuvants will limit this complication. In addition, attention to postoperative nutrition, bracing, and external electrical bone stimulation are helpful.

V. Postoperative Care

Care after surgery is the same as with open TLIF. Patients should be rapidly mobilized with physical therapists, with external bracing as a treatment option. Muscle spasm occurs more commonly with MIS procedures and is best treated with muscle relaxants and benzodiazepines, as opposed to narcotics.

VI. Outcomes

Proper patient selection is vital for achieving excellent outcomes. Although MIS TLIF has not been conclusively shown to be superior to open TLIF, several reports suggest this pattern. In a well-selected population, radiculopathy will show meaningful improvement in 80 to 95% of cases; axial back pain will improve in 70 to 85% of cases.

VII. Surgical Pearls

- In cases where substantial muscle creeps under the edges of the retractor, consider pharmacologic paralysis. Also consider removing the retractor and making a longer fascial opening, followed by placement of a deeper retractor.
- When performing a contralateral neural decompression, leave the ipsilateral ligamentum flavum intact at first. This will push the thecal sac ventrally, keeping it out of the way while the contralateral work is being performed.
- Intervertebral disc can be removed efficiently using an insert-and-rotate scraper. These devices allow entry into collapsed disc spaces and also effectively remove any disc herniations causing neural compression.
- Self-distracting cages, usually with a "bulleted" nose, will allow the placement of larger interbody cages, as it is difficult to use pedicle screw manipulation of a laminar spreader to open the disc space in MIS surgery.

Common Clinical Questions

1. MIS TLIF is utilized because it is believed to result in all of the following *except*:
   A. Decreased soft-tissue damage
   B. Higher fusion rates
   C. Shorter hospital stays
   D. Reduced blood loss
2. One of the critical maneuvers to reduce neural injury is:
   A. Remove more facet bone so that less nerve retraction is needed
   B. Use of intraoperative intravenous steroids
   C. Stronger pedicle screw fixation
   D. Repair of dural tears
3. When placing intervertebral cages in a MIS TLIF it is important to:
   A. Make sure the cage is higher than 13 mm
   B. Make sure the cage is longer than 27 mm
   C. Use only nondegradable interbody devices
   D. Cross the midline

References

1. Harms J, Rolinger H. A one-stager procedure in operative treatment of spondylolistheses: dorsal traction-reposition and anterior fusion (author's transl). Z Orthop Ihre Grenzgeb 1982;120(3):343–347
2. Schwender JD, Holly LT, Rouben DP, Foley KT. Minimally invasive transforaminal lumbar interbody fusion (TLIF): technical feasibility and initial results. J Spinal Disord Tech 2005;18(Suppl):S1–S6
3. Kawaguchi Y, Matsui H, Tsuji H. Back muscle injury after posterior lumbar spine surgery. Part 2: Histologic and histochemical analyses in humans. Spine (Phila Pa 1976) 1994;19(22):2598–2602
4. Dhall SS, Wang MY, Mummaneni PV. Clinical and radiographic comparison of mini-open transforaminal lumbar interbody fusion with open transforaminal lumbar interbody fusion in 42 patients with long-term follow-up. J Neurosurg Spine 2008;9(6):560–565
5. Wiltse LL, Bateman JG, Hutchinson RH, Nelson WE. The paraspinal sacrospinalis-splitting approach to the lumbar spine. J Bone Joint Surg Am 1968;50(5):919–926

Answers to Common Clinical Questions

1. B
2. A
3. D

54 Percutaneous Pedicle Screw Placement

Michael Y. Wang

I. Key Points

- Numerous methods can be used for implanting percutaneous pedicle screws, such as image guidance, en face targeting, and biplanar fluoroscopy.
- Percutaneous screws can be safely placed in the thoracolumbar spine using a simple method based primarily on anteroposterior (AP) x-rays.
- Percutaneous screw-rod constructs are a truly minimally invasive surgical (MIS) technique for segmental fixation.

II. Indications

Percutaneous placement of transpedicular screws with connecting rods can find application in virtually any setting where open screw fixation might be utilized in the thoracolumar spine. For a fusion setting, this can be employed in conjunction with interbody fusion for stabilization,[1] such as after an anterior lumbar interbody fusion (ALIF), lateral interbody fusion, transforaminal lumbar interbody fusion (TLIF), or transsacral fusion. In addition, a speculum retractor can be used to expose the lateral masses for posterolateral fusion bed preparation in conjunction with percutaneous fixation. Also, percutaneous fixation can be used for stabilization or "internal bracing" in the absence of a bony arthrodesis.[2] Thus, whether a fusion is intended or not, percutaneous screw-rod fixation can be used to confer spinal stability for degenerative, traumatic, neoplastic, and infectious pathologies.

III. Technique

There are various methods for targeting the pedicles of the lumbar or thoracic spine. These include (1) frame-based or frameless image-guided navigation,[3] (2) biplanar fluoroscopy in the AP and lateral views, (3) "en face" or "direct down the pedicle" imaging,[4] (4) a mini-open technique with tactile feedback, and (5) an AP-based targeting method.[5] This chapter will describe the AP-based targeting method.

- 1. The patient is positioned prone on a radiolucent operating table. Care is taken to ensure that there are no obstructions to the fluoroscopic image at the level(s) of interest, as the technique is heavily dependent on intraoperative imaging.

54 Percutaneous Pedicle Screw Placement

- 2. An absolutely precise AP view is registered at the level of screw placement. This is done by first ensuring that the axial rotation of the fluoroscope aligns the spinous process equidistant between the right and left pedicles (**Fig. 54.1**). Either the fluoroscope can be moved or the bed rotated to register this image, but the surgeon must compensate for any rotation depending on the method used. The sagittal (Ferguson) angle is then adjusted so that the anterior and posterior cortical rims of the upper end plate of the vertebral body are superimposed into a single line. This ensures that the x-ray beam is completely aligned with the sagittal plane of the pedicles (and thus an ideal screw trajectory).
- 3. The skin is then marked so that a cutaneous entry point can be made 1 to 2 cm lateral to the lateral border of the pedicle. A Jamshidi needle (MedSurge, Chennai, India) is then inserted through the skin and directed slightly medially to contact the bone surface. The needle is then docked at the junction of the transverse process and facet joint near the mamillary process (the attachment of the multifidus muscle).
- 4. Once the Jamshidi needle has been docked on this ideal pedicle screw starting point, the needle is marked 2 cm above the skin surface with a surgical marker (**Fig. 54.2**). The needle is then hammered into the pedicle to a depth of 2 cm (where the marking meets the skin surface). The trajectory will be medialized to match the patient's anatomy (10 to 30 degrees). If a proper AP image has been obtained, making the Jamshidi needle parallel to the horizon and parallel to the upper end plate will place the needle in the proper sagittal orientation.
- 5. So long as the medial wall of the pedicle is not breached at a depth of 2 cm, there will be no medial pedicle wall violation; the needle will have passed the depth of the pedicle (and spinal

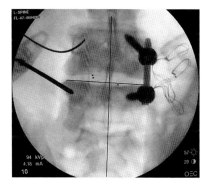

Fig. 54.1 AP projection on the L5 vertebral body. Note that the upper end plate of the L5 body is visualized as a single line and that the spinous process is equidistant between the two pedicles.

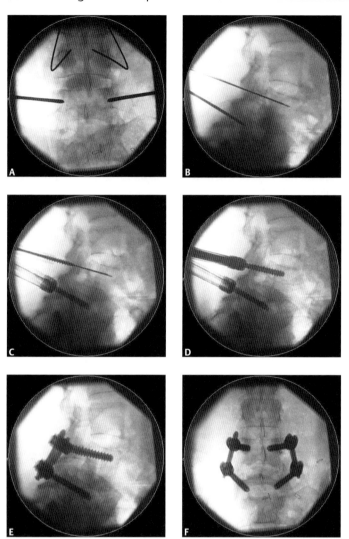

Fig. 54.2 **(A)** AP view targeting the lower vertebral body. Note the rotation in relation to the body above (where the spinous process is not in the midline). Docking at the junction of the facet joint and transverse process is followed by 2 cm of medial needle advancement. **(B)** The needle is confirmed on lateral fluoroscopy as having passed the spinal canal, ruling out pedicle wall violation. **(C)** An insulating sheath is used to minimize soft-tissue trauma while an awl and tap are advanced over the K-wire. **(D)** Final screw positioning with extension tabs attached to guide rod insertion. Final construct as visualized on **(E)** lateral and **(F)** AP views.

canal) following 2 cm of advancement. Once the Jamshidi needle has been placed, the inner stylet is removed and a Kirschner wire (K-wire) is inserted into the vertebral body.
- 6. The procedure is then conducted at other vertebral levels with adjustments in fluoroscopic targeting for each level. After all of the K-wires have been placed, the fluoroscope is moved to a lateral position. The K-wires are then used to guide an awl and tap for pedicle preparation as with open surgery. Final pedicle screw placement is then performed followed by K-wire removal.
- 7. During the procedure, care is taken to ensure that the K-wires do not violate the anterior vertebral body and enter the retroperitoneum, which could cause vascular or hollow viscus injury. In addition, care must be taken not to lose control of the wires or have them pull out prematurely.
- 8. Following screw placement a percutaneous rod is advanced subfascially through the screw extensions to connect the segmental levels (**Fig. 54.3**). Rod insertion can occur through one of the end screw incisions or through a separate incision distal to the screws.
- 9. It is helpful to have at least some bend in the rod, as "steering" the rod medially or laterally is made easier by rotating the rod along its long axis to turn the tip medially or laterally.

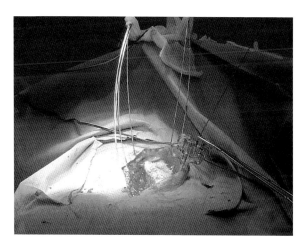

Fig. 54.3 Jamshidi needles and K-wires in place. Note the use of a long skin incision with placement of instrumentation through the exposed fascia and the use of a needle driver to control the K-wire during manipulation.

Finally, set screws are placed through the screw extensions to lock the rod to the individual screws.

IV. Complications

The complications associated with percutaneous screw placement are akin to those encountered with open surgical instrumentation procedures. In addition, there are risks associated with loss of control of the K-wires, which can result in inadvertent entry into the retroperitoneum.

Difficulties can be encountered with initial pedicle cannulation or with rod passage and screw-rod connection. Use of the AP-based technique results in a low rate of pedicle violation as long as high-quality fluoroscopic images are utilized for targeting the Jamshidi needles. Rod passage and connection techniques are often specific to the implant manufacturers and the instruments available for rod and screw manipulation, so they are not described here.

V. Postoperative Care

Care after surgery is the same as with open instrumentation. Patients should be rapidly mobilized with physical therapists, with external bracing as a treatment option. Muscle spasm occurs more commonly with MIS procedures and is best treated with muscle relaxants and benzodiazepines as opposed to narcotics.

VI. Surgical Pearls

- In many instances all of the surgery can be accomplished by a single surgeon standing on the side opposite the fluoroscope. This improves surgical workflow and minimizes the risk of contaminating the sterile field. Because of the highly imaging-dependent nature of the method described here, standing on the same side as the pedicle screw insertion (which is typical for open surgery) is much less important.
- When a rod is passed across the thoracolumbar junction it is usually preferable to pass the rod from cranial to caudal.
- Because the screw head heights and orientation are not immediately visible, the surgeon should be prepared to pass a prepared rod initially, and then remove it and recontour or resize the implant to achieve the optimal construct. Forcing the screw and rod to mate may result in screw pullout.

Common Clinical Questions

1. Percutaneous pedicle screws can be safely inserted using all of the following techniques *except*:
   A. AP-guided imaging
   B. Pure freehand technique
   C. Biplanar fluoroscopy
   D. Image guidance
2. When using the AP-based technique for percutaneous pedicle cannulation, how far is the Jamshidi needle advanced before passing the medial pedicle wall?
   A. 1 cm
   B. 2 cm
   C. 3 cm
   D. 4 cm
3. Bending the rod allows what to be accomplished more easily?
   A. Cutting the rod to size
   B. Reducing spondylolistheses
   C. Rod-screw mating
   D. Medial and lateral maneuvering

References

1. Schwender JD, Holly LT, Rouben DP, Foley KT. Minimally invasive transforaminal lumbar interbody fusion (TLIF): technical feasibility and initial results. J Spinal Disord Tech 2005;18(Suppl):S1–S6
2. Jeanneret B, Jovanovic M, Magerl F. Percutaneous diagnostic stabilization for low back pain. Correlation with results after fusion operations. Clin Orthop Relat Res 1994;304(304):130–138
3. Wang MY, Kim KA, Liu CY, Kim P, Apuzzo ML. Reliability of three-dimensional fluoroscopy for detecting pedicle screw violations in the thoracic and lumbar spine. Neurosurgery 2004;54(5):1138–1142, discussion 1142–1143
4. Magerl F. Verletzungen der Brust- und Lendenwirbelsaule. Langenbecks Arch Chir 1980;352:428–433
5. Harris EB, Massey P, Lawrence J, Rihn J, Vaccaro A, Anderson DG. Percutaneous techniques for minimally invasive posterior lumbar fusion. Neurosurg Focus 2008;25(2):E12

Answers to Common Clinical Questions

1. B
2. B
3. D

55 Minimally Invasive Lateral Retroperitoneal Trans-Psoas Interbody Fusion (e.g., XLIF, DLIF)

Edwin Ramos, Ali A. Baaj, and Juan S. Uribe

I. Key Points

- Success with this technique relies heavily on[1]
  - Careful patient positioning
  - Gentle retroperitoneal dissection
  - Meticulous psoas splitting with electromyographic (EMG) monitoring
  - Fusion bed preparation with release of contralateral annulus
  - Appropriate-size interbody implant placement

II. Indications[2]

- Axial low back pain caused by
  - Degenerative disc disease
  - Spinal stenosis (mild to moderate only) with significant back pain component
  - Grade 1 to 2 spondylolisthesis
  - Adjacent-segment disc degeneration
  - Interbody fusion as stand-alone or adjunct in treatment of degenerative scoliosis
- Postdiscectomy space collapse with neuroforaminal stenosis (indirect decompression)
- Total disc replacement
- Thoracolumbar corpectomies
  - Burst fractures
  - Tumors
  - Treatment of deformity with sagittal plane imbalance

III. Technique

- Patient positioning
  - The patient is placed on a radiolucent bendable table in true 90 degree lateral decubitus position with the top of the crest just inferior to the table break.
  - Usually the left side is up, unless the crest is higher on that side or there has been previous surgery on that side.
  - Flex the table to increase the distance between the iliac crest and the ribs. This allows access to the disc space (important at L4-L5 to clear the crest and above L3 to clear the lower ribs).

- Localize the skin incision with lateral fluoroscopy by centering crossed K-wires over the disc's mid-position. For multilevel approaches, a single longitudinal incision with individual transverse fascial openings for each level is adequate.
- Retroperitoneal access (single skin/fascia incision technique)
  - Work perpendicular to the floor while dissecting through the muscle fibers to avoid entry into the peritoneal cavity, which is anteriorly displaced in the lateral position.
  - Entry into the retroperitoneal cavity is confirmed by the appearance of bright yellow fat and a loss of resistance by the muscle tissues. Finger dissection is then performed so that the surgeon can feel the psoas muscle deep in the cavity and the transverse processes posteriorly.
- Trans-psoas approach and retractor placement
  - A series of tubular dilators are placed with EMG monitoring. Directional EMG monitoring (Neurovision, NuVasive, San Diego, CA) allows not only proximity to motor nerves but also the location of these nerves in relation to the dilator (**Fig. 55.1**). It is essential to guide the dilators with the finger to the psoas muscle to avoid inadvertent entry into the peritoneal cavity.
  - Lateral fluoroscopy will guide dilator placement into the middle (or just posterior to the middle) of the disc space while bluntly splitting the fibers of the psoas. A K-wire is placed through the initial dilator and into the disc space to hold it in place. EMG monitoring is performed with each dilator prior to the introduction of a larger dilator.

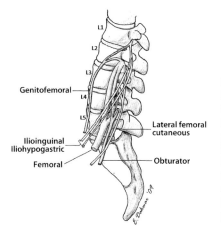

Fig. 55.1 Lateral view of the lumbar plexus. Understanding this anatomy is critical for successful implementation of the lateral transpsoas approach. (From Uribe JS et al. Defining the safe working zones using the minimally invasive lateral retroperitoneal transpsoas approach: an anatomical study, Journal of Neurosurgery Spine, Aug 2010. Reprinted with permission.)

- The retractor is then placed and a shim needle is introduced to the disc space under AP fluoroscopy to secure it.
- Preparation of the disc space
  - The disc space is incised with a knife just anterior to the shim, with a small rim of disc kept just in front of it to keep the retractor from sliding anteriorly.
  - A Cobb elevator is passed along both end plates and through the contralateral annulus under fluoroscopic guidance.
  - A series of instruments (curettes, pituitaries, rasps) are used to clean the space and prepare the end plates.
- Interbody spacer and instrumentation are then placed.
- The retractor is removed slowly in the open configuration to allow the psoas muscle to be inspected for bleeding.
- The external oblique fascia is closed with interrupted absorbable suture and the skin is closed in a subcuticular fashion.

IV. Complications[1,3,4]

- Hip flexor weakness, thigh numbness, quadriceps weakness, genitofemoral neuralgia
- Abdominal viscera perforation
- Rupture of anterior longitudinal ligament
- Great vessel injury
- Kidney-ureteral injury
- Graft subsidence
- Psoas/retroperitoneal hematoma
- Abdominal wall paresis
- Rhabdomyolysis

V. Postoperative Care

- For single-level lumbar cases the patient is mobilized in the immediate post-op period without a brace. No drains are placed.
- The patient is usually discharged on postoperative day 1 for single-level cases.
- In case of significant leg weakness or a drop in hematocrit, a computed tomography (CT) or magnetic resonance imaging (MRI) scan is indicated to rule out a psoas hematoma.

VI. Outcomes

- If thigh numbness (12 to 75%) occurs (from retraction against the femoral nerve—anterior femoral cutaneous), it usually resolves by the time of the 3-month follow-up without treat-

ment. This is more common at L4-L5 level due to the proximity of the femoral nerve to the surgical field.[1]
- Hip flexor weakness correlates with trauma to the psoas muscle. It is rarely a neurogenic injury. Gentle placement of the dilators and retractor limits the incidence of this.
- Quadriceps weakness is likely due to injury of the femoral nerve.
- Arthrodesis rates and clinical outcomes are similar to those for other interbody techniques[1-4]; however, since the technique is in its infancy, long-term outcomes are still uncertain.

VII. Surgical Pearls

- Do not proceed with surgery unless perfect AP and lateral projections of the disc space have been prepared. This is best accomplished by careful patient positioning, not by adjusting the fluoroscopy machines.
- Minimize the amount of lateral flexion of the patient and flex the ipsilateral hip during positioning. This may decrease the amount of tension on the lumbar plexus.
- Guide the initial dilator with finger dissection through the retroperitoneal space to prevent visceral injury.
- Ideally no nerves will be encountered during EMG stimulation. In other than ideal situations, place the nerve posterior to the retractor, where it can be safely retracted away from the surgical field without the risk of root avulsion or stretch injury.

Common Clinical Questions

1. Which nerve runs over the psoas muscle and is likely to be affected by a lateral approach at L2-L3?
2. What is the most likely explanation for post-op hip flexor weakness?
3. Retraction against which nerve at the L4-L5 level is responsible for post-op anterior thigh numbness?

References

1. Dakwar E, Cardona RF, Smith DA, Uribe JS. Early outcomes and safety of the minimally invasive, lateral retroperitoneal transpsoas approach for adult degenerative scoliosis. Neurosurg Focus 2010;28(3):E8
2. Ozgur BM, Aryan HE, Pimenta L, Taylor WR. Extreme Lateral Interbody Fusion (XLIF): a novel surgical technique for anterior lumbar interbody fusion. Spine J 2006;6(4):435–443
3. Knight RQ, Schwaegler P, Hanscom D, Roh J. Direct lateral lumbar interbody fusion for degenerative conditions: early complication profile. J Spinal Disord Tech 2009; 22(1):34–37
4. Tormenti MJ, Maserati MB, Bonfield CM, Okonkwo DO, Kanter AS. Complications and radiographic correction in adult scoliosis following combined transpsoas extreme lateral interbody fusion and posterior pedicle screw instrumentation. Neurosurg Focus 2010;28(3):E7

Answers to Common Clinical Questions

1. The genitofemoral nerve
2. Psoas muscle bruising as opposed to damage to femoral nerve branches to the psoas
3. The femoral nerve (sensory fibers via the anterior femoral cutaneous nerve)

56 Anterior Lumbar Interbody Fusion (ALIF)

Krzysztof B. Siemionow and Kern Singh

I. Key Points

- Anterior lumbar interbody fusion (ALIF) offers several potential advantages over other surgical approaches.
  - The ability to perform a complete or subtotal discectomy
  - Large surface area for fusion and structural grafting
  - Favorable fusion environment (compression)
  - Effective for anterior releases, particularly in the setting of high-grade deformity
  - Posterior muscle sparing
  - Indirect foraminal decompression

II. Indications

- Spondylolisthesis (typically grade I or II)
- Degenerative disc disease causing mechanical low back pain
- Postdiscectomy collapse with neural foraminal stenosis
- Treatment of posterior pseudarthrosis
- Treatment of post-laminectomy kyphosis
- Treatment of coronal and/or sagittal imbalance

III. Technique

- Place the patient supine on a regular operating table or a flat Jackson table.
- A bump under the sacrum will allow for increased lumbar lordosis.
- Slight Trendelenburg position will allow the abdominal contents to displace cephalad away from the surgical field.
- The operative level is identified with lateral fluoroscopy. This localizes the skin incision (critical for mini-ALIF approaches).
- A left transverse or longitudinal paramedian incision is made.
- The anterior rectus sheath is identified and divided in line with the skin incision.
- Blunt dissection is used to mobilize the rectus and to identify its lateral border.
- The lateral edge of the rectus abdominis muscle is retracted toward the midline, exposing the posterior rectus sheath (above the arcuate line) or, less commonly, the arcuate line and the preperitoneal space (below the arcuate line).

- The posterior rectus sheath–arcuate line is carefully divided in a superior-to-inferior direction and the preperitoneal space identified.
- Using blunt dissection, the peritoneum is mobilized off of the anterior and lateral abdominal wall and retroperitoneal blunt dissection is used to identify the psoas muscle.
- Hand-held retractors are advanced.
- The ureter, peritoneum, and abdominal contents are mobilized across the midline.
- The psoas muscle is released and then retracted laterally, allowing direct visualization into the disc space.
- With blunt dissection medial to the psoas muscle, the index disc space is identified and confirmed with a marker and fluoroscopy.
- Retractors are placed around the lateral annulus, first on the right side, retracting the abdominal contents and the iliac vein (**Fig. 56.1**).

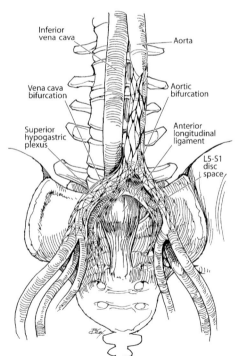

Fig. 56.1 Key anterior retroperitoneal structures.

- Once the disc space is confirmed, an annulotomy is made with either a knife or electrocautery.
- A Cobb elevator and curette are used to remove the cartilaginous end plates, carefully preserving the subchondral bone/end plate.
- Pituitary rongeurs are used to remove the disc fragments.
- An interbody graft (allograft, titanium, or polyetheretherketone [PEEK]) is appropriately sized to gently distract the disc space and contact the ring apophysis.
- The anterior rectus sheath is closed with nonabsorbable sheath. The posterior sheath does not require repair.

IV. Complications[1,2]

- Iliac vein injury
- Ileus
- Retrograde ejaculation occurs secondary to injury to the superior hypogastric plexus (sympathetic chain). The superior hypogastric plexus provides innervation to the internal vesical sphincter. The reported incidence of retrograde ejaculation after ALIF varies widely in the literature, ranging from 0.4 to 5.9% of male patients.[3,4]
- Ureteral injury
- Deep vein thrombosis
- Abdominal hernia
- Rectus muscle paresis

V. Postoperative Care

- Patients are mobilized on the first postoperative day.
- Diet is advanced as tolerated starting on the first postoperative day.
- Discharge to home when patient meets discharge criteria (typically, ambulating, tolerating a diet, voiding, and adequate pain control on oral medications).

VI. Outcomes

- Satisfactory clinical outcomes can be anticipated in 70% of patients.[5]
- Fusion rates vary from 85 to 95% in most series and depend on whether autograft or bone morphogenetic protein (BMP) is used.[6]
- Interbody subsidence is an expected phenomenon and occurs in as many as 85% of cases, particularly stand-alone grafts.[7]

VII. Surgical Pearls

- Localize with fluoroscopy prior to making a skin incision.
- Trendelenburg position allows the abdominal contents to move cephalad out of the operative field. This position also decreases venous bleeding.
- Avoid the use of monopolar cautery around the sympathetic chain prior to the annulotomy.
- Take care not to violate the subchondral end plates.

Common Clinical Questions

1. What is retrograde ejaculation and how can the risk be minimized?
2. At what level does the aorta bifurcate, and why is that important for anterior spinal procedures?
3. List four indications for anterior lumbar interbody fusion.

References

1. Jarrett CD, Heller JG, Tsai L. Anterior exposure of the lumbar spine with and without an "access surgeon": morbidity analysis of 265 consecutive cases. J Spinal Disord Tech 2009;22(8):559–564
2. Brau SA. Mini-open approach to the spine for anterior lumbar interbody fusion: description of the procedure, results and complications. Spine J 2002;2(3):216–223
3. Sasso RC, Burkus JK, LeHuec JC. Retrograde ejaculation after anterior lumbar interbody fusion: transperitoneal versus retroperitoneal exposure. Spine (Phila Pa 1976) 2003;28(10):1023–1026
4. Tiusanen H, Seitsalo S, Osterman K, Soini J. Retrograde ejaculation after anterior interbody lumbar fusion. Eur Spine J 1995;4(6):339–342
5. Madan SS, Boeree NR. Comparison of instrumented anterior interbody fusion with instrumented circumferential lumbar fusion. Eur Spine J 2003;12(6):567–575
6. Burkus JK, Transfeldt EE, Kitchel SH, Watkins RG, Balderston RA. Clinical and radiographic outcomes of anterior lumbar interbody fusion using recombinant human bone morphogenetic protein-2. Spine (Phila Pa 1976) 2002;27(21):2396–2408
7. Choi JY, Sung KH. Subsidence after anterior lumbar interbody fusion using paired stand-alone rectangular cages. Eur Spine J 2006;15(1):16–22

Answers to Common Clinical Questions

1. Retrograde ejaculation occurs secondary to injury to the superior hypogastric plexus, a part of the sympathetic chain, which provides innervation to the internal vesical sphincter. Avoid using monopolar cautery around the sympathetic chain. Consider using a posterior approach in young males. When it occurs, retrograde ejaculation results in a normal sexual climax followed by the lack of ejaculate. Sperm typically is not propelled forward and ends up in the bladder.

2. In two-thirds of cases, the aorta bifurcates at L4/L5. Approaches to the L4/L5 intervertebral disc are more challenging and require mobilization of the iliac vessels.

3. Spondylolisthesis (usually grade I or II), treatment of pseudarthrosis, postdiscectomy collapse with neuroforaminal stenosis, and treatment of lumbar deformity with coronal and/or sagittal imbalance

57 Axial Lumbar Interbody Fusion (AxiaLIF)

Elias Dakwar and Juan S. Uribe

I. Key Points

- Minimally invasive presacral approach for intervertebral discectomy and fusion
  - Originally described for L5-S1 and extended to include L4-L5
  - Relies on indirect decompression
  - Not intended to be used as a stand-alone, requires supplemental fixation such as transfacet pedicle screws or pedicle screw-rod fixation

II. Indications

- Degenerative disc disease
- Radiculopathy
- Spondylolisthesis (grade I or II)
- Revision
  - Pseudarthrosis
  - Extension of long fusion to sacrum

III. Contraindications

- Aortic bifurcation below L5-S1 or aberrant midline vessel anterior to S1
- Previous pelvic or retroperitoneal surgery
- Inflammatory bowel disease
- Sacral agenesis
- Severe sacral lordosis
- Spondylolisthesis exceeding grade II

IV. Preoperative Management

- Imaging
  - Magnetic resonance imaging (MRI) of the lumbar spine (computed tomography [CT] if MRI is contraindicated) including the tip of the coccyx to evaluate the trajectory, aberrant or anomalous vascular structures, and presacral fat pad
- Bowel prep performed the day before surgery
  - GoLYTELY (Braintree Laboratories, Braintree, MA), 4 L
  - MiraLax (Merck, Whitehouse Station, NJ), 64 oz

- Mag Citrate (Metagenics, San Clemente, CA)
– Antibiotics
  - Make sure to include anaerobic and gram (negative) coverage.

V. Technique[1]

– Setup: biplanar fluoroscopy and radiolucent bed
– Position: prone with the knees below the level of the hips using Jackson table or OSI table (Mizuho OSI, Union City, CA) with sling for the legs
– A 20 French catheter is inserted into the rectum and 10 ml of air is insufflated to improve visualization of the rectum during fluoroscopy.
– The anus is isolated with an occlusive dressing and the sacrococcygeal region is prepped and draped in the usual sterile fashion.
– A 15 mm skin incision is made 1 cm lateral to the tip of the coccyx and 2 cm caudal to the left or right paracoccygeal notch. Be sure to continue the incision through the underlying fascia (**Fig. 57.1**).
– Blunt finger dissection is used to develop the presacral space and push the rectum anteriorly.

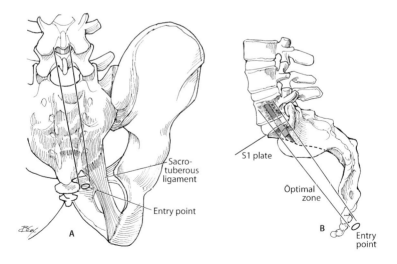

Fig. 57.1 (A,B) Schematic diagram depicting the optimal trajectory and entry point for presacral access to the L5-S1 axial lumbar interbody fusion.

- A dissecting tool is advanced along the anterior midline of the sacrum using an oscillating movement to sweep the presacral fat away from the floor of the pelvis, and it is then docked at the S1-S2 junction.
- Once the trajectory is confirmed by fluoroscopy, a guide pin is placed into the sacrum (**Fig. 57.1**).
- A series of dilators are then carefully placed until the working cannula is securely docked into the sacrum.
- The guide pin is then removed and a drill is passed into the sacrum and disc space.
- A series of disc space cutters and wire brushes are used to perform the discectomy.
- Once the discectomy is performed, bone graft material is inserted into the disc space through the cannula. It is important to place the bone graft prior to drilling into the body of L5 so that bone graft material is not packed into that defect.
- An appropriate-size three-dimensional (3D) axial titanium rod is placed through the sacrum into the disc space and into the L5 vertebral body. The axial rod has a differential pitch that creates distraction across the disc space as it is rotated.
- Once satisfactory placement of the axial rod is achieved, the working cannula is removed, and the wound is irrigated and closed in the standard fashion. Dermabond liquid dressing (Ethicon, a Johnson & Johnson company, New York) is placed over the incision as an occlusive dressing.

VI. Postoperative Care

- Mobilize patient early with or without brace, according to surgeon preference.
- No procedure-related restrictions
- Discharge to home when patient meets discharge criteria, including tolerating regular diet, ambulating, voiding, and adequate pain control on oral medications.

VII. Potential Complications

- Bowel perforation[2]
- Vascular injury
  - Transverse sacral veins or middle sacral artery
- Infection

VIII. Outcomes

- Limited outcomes
- Fusion rate, 91%; Oswestry Disability Index (ODI), decrease of 26 points; Visual Analogue Scale (VAS), decrease of 7 points at one-year follow-up[3,4]

IX. Surgical Pearls

- True anteroposterior (AP) and lateral fluoroscopy images with continuous imaging throughout the procedure to ensure proper trajectory and safe access

Common Clinical Questions

1. True or false: Axial lumbar interbody fusion relies on indirect decompression.
2. True or false: Axial lumbar interbody fusion is safe to perform in patients with a grade III or IV spondylolisthesis.

References

1. Marotta N, Cosar M, Pimenta L, Khoo LT. A novel minimally invasive presacral approach and instrumentation technique for anterior L5-S1 intervertebral discectomy and fusion: technical description and case presentations. Neurosurg Focus 2006;20(1):E9
2. Botolin S, Agudelo J, Dwyer A, Patel V, Burger E. High rectal injury during trans-1 axial lumbar interbody fusion L5-S1 fixation: a case report. Spine (Phila Pa 1976) 2010; 35(4):E144–E148
3. Aryan HE, Newman CB, Gold JJ, Acosta FL Jr, Coover C, Ames CP. Percutaneous axial lumbar interbody fusion (AxiaLIF) of the L5-S1 segment: initial clinical and radiographic experience. Minim Invasive Neurosurg 2008;51(4):225–230
4. Asgarzadie F. Khoo L, Cosar M, Marotta N, Pimenta L: One Year Outcomes of Minimally-Invasive Presacral Approach and Instrumentation Technique for Anterior Lumbosacral Intervertebral Discectomy and Fusion, in 22nd Annual CNS mtg, 2007

Answers to Common Clinical Questions

1. True
2. False

58 Facet Screw Fixation/Fusion
Ben J. Garrido and Rick C. Sasso

I. Key Points
- Pedicle screw fixation historically has been the gold standard for lumbar fusion stabilization. However, criticisms of the pedicle screw construct—including higher complication rates, bulky hardware, increased pain, and excessive wide soft-tissue dissection—have led to a more innovative, minimally invasive fixation technique. Translaminar facet screws have been found to be biomechanically advantageous, significantly increasing the stiffness and stability in compression, extension, flexion, bending, and torsion of spinal motion segments.[1,2]
- Facet screws were first described by King in 1948 as short screws placed horizontally across the facet joint. Boucher's modifications in 1959 included an increased screw length directed more vertical into the pedicle. Today's technique includes Magerl's 1984 modification, involving a longer screw with an entry point at the base of the contralateral spinous process, increasing its effective fixation strength by expanding the working length at both sides of the facet.[3]
- This technique involves a minimally invasive approach without significant soft-tissue dissection. Improved outcomes—including biomechanical stability, decreased complication rates, reduced reoperation rates, lower operative times, minimal blood loss, and improved patient-perceived outcomes—have been demonstrated.[4]
- The use of image navigation with this posterior stabilization technique has been validated as a safe, feasible, economical and efficient method associated with low screw misplacement rates and excellent operative field viewing.[4]

II. Indications
- In conjunction with anterior interbody fusion for symptomatic discogenic pain unresponsive to at least 6 months of aggressive nonoperative treatment where posterior elements are present, intact
- Primary circumferential lumbar fusion with less than grade II spondylolisthesis
- Repair of pseudarthrosis after stand-alone anterior lumbar interbody fusion (ALIF)

III. Technique

- The patient is placed in the prone position on a radiolucent Jackson table frame.
- Image navigation rather than fluoroscopy used to localize incision.
- A small posterior midline incision is made at the appropriate level.
- A subperiosteal dissection along the spinous process and lamina to the targeted facet is performed bilaterally. The cephalad juxtalevel facet joint is not exposed. Supraspinous and interspinous ligaments should be preserved.
- The facet joint is the lateral limit of the dissection.
- A retractor is placed, allowing visualization of both the start point and contralateral caudal facet joint.
- A small, 2 cm incision is made lateral to the midline incision to allow a blunt bullet or drill guide to obtain the appropriate trajectory. Dock at the spinolaminar junction and target the contralateral facet/pedicle.
- Create a pilot hole with a starting awl, leaving enough room for the contralateral translaminar facet screw along the width of the spinolaminar junction. Place the first screw at the cephalad, superior aspect of the spinolaminar confluence and the second contralateral screw caudal to it in line with the lamina.
- Using a high-speed drill with a long 2.85 mm bit and image navigation (if available), drill to the contralateral facet/pedicle using tactile progression through the anatomical bony trajectory. Take care not to breach ventrally into the canal, and ideally stay within the lamina. Measure for screw length off the calibrated drill.
- While maintaining the drill guide in fixed position, use power to insert a 4.0 mm screw along the same drilled hole.
- Complete the tightening off power. Avoid overtightening the screw or fracturing the spinous process.
- Repeat the preceding steps for the contralateral translaminar facet screw.
- Obtain final imaging studies (**Fig. 58.1**).
- Decorticate posterior bony elements/lamina and add bone graft substitute.
- Close the fascia with 0 absorbable suture.
- Close the subcutaneous layer with inverted, interrupted 2-0 absorbable suture.
- Close the skin with running suture or skin adhesive.

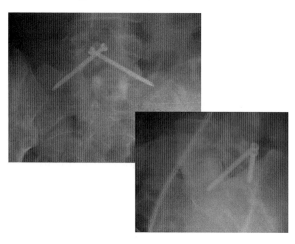

Fig. 58.1 Anteroposterior and lateral views demonstrating facet screw trajectory.

IV. Complications

- Spinous process fracture
- Ventral trajectory breach with either screw or drill
- Nerve root injury
- Wound infection
- Pseudarthrosis

V. Postoperative Care

- Mobilize early without bracing.
- Discharge home when patient meets discharge criteria (typically, ambulating, tolerating a diet, voiding, and adequate pain control on oral medications).

VI. Outcomes

- Reported reoperation rate is 5%, versus 24 to 37.5% for pedicle screw constructs, a statistically significant difference.[4]
- Operative time and blood loss have been shown to be significantly lower in the translaminar facet screw cohort compared with the pedicle screw population.[4]
- Patient-recorded outcomes include a significant decrease in postoperative Visual Analogue Scale (VAS) pain scores for both translaminar facet screw and pedicle screw constructs.[4]

VII. Surgical Pearls

- Obtain adequate visualization of the starting point, trajectory, and contralateral caudal facet joint.
- Plan accordingly for the placement of both screws and the ideal position prior to drilling.
- Establish an appropriate starting point at the confluence of the spinous process and lamina. Do not start high on the spinous process.
- Perform final screw tightening off power and do not overtighten or strip the screw, or fracture posterior bony elements.

Common Clinical Questions

1. Which of the following is a characteristic of the translaminar facet screw?
   A. Requires a wide soft-tissue dissection
   B. Not a minimally invasive technique
   C. Combines an increased working length with greater fixation strength
   D. Can be used with bilateral pars defects
2. Translaminar facet screws have been associated with:
   A. Longer operative times
   B. Lower rates of reoperation compared with pedicle screws
   C. Greater operative blood loss
   D. Inferior biomechanical properties relative to pedicle screws

References

1. Heggeness MHO, Esses SI. Translaminar facet joint screw fixation for lumbar and lumbosacral fusion. A clinical and biomechanical study. Spine (Phila Pa 1976) 1991;16(6, Suppl):S266–S269
2. Ferrara LA, Secor JL, Jin BH, Wakefield A, Inceoglu S, Benzel EC. A biomechanical comparison of facet screw fixation and pedicle screw fixation: effects of short-term and long-term repetitive cycling. Spine (Phila Pa 1976) 2003;28(12):1226–1234
3. Magerl FP. Stabilization of the lower thoracic and lumbar spine with external skeletal fixation. Clin Orthop Relat Res 1984;189(189):125–141
4. Best NM, Sasso RC. Efficacy of translaminar facet screw fixation in circumferential interbody fusions as compared to pedicle screw fixation. J Spinal Disord Tech 2006;19(2): 98–103

Answers to Common Clinical Questions

1. C
2. B

59 Interspinous Process Decompression
Ravi Ramachandran and Peter G. Whang

I. Key Points
- Lumbar stenosis refers to compression of the thecal sac, which may result in lower extremity pain/numbness (i.e., neurogenic claudication).
- Interspinous devices (ISDs) are designed to perform an "indirect" decompression by maintaining flexion of a stenotic segment, which increases the dimensions of the spinal canal and foramina.
- Appropriate candidates for ISD should experience clear relief of their claudication with lumbar flexion (i.e., sitting).
- This technique may give rise to reduced surgical morbidity and more rapid rehabilitation compared with laminectomy with or without arthrodesis.

II. Indications
- Symptomatic neurogenic claudication secondary to spinal stenosis with or without spondylolisthesis (confirmed by computed tomography [CT] or magnetic resonance imaging [MRI]) that has failed to respond to conservative treatments (e.g., physical therapy, medications, or epidural injections)
- Limiting lumbar extension may also target various sources of low back pain by unloading the posterior disc and facet joints.[1]
- Contraindications
  - Significant spinal deformities (spondylolisthesis >grade I, scoliosis >25 degrees)
  - Bony ankylosis
  - Severe osteoporosis
  - Critical stenosis/cauda equina syndrome
- The X-Stop spacer (Medtronic, Memphis, TN) is FDA-approved for use at one or two levels of the lumbar spine (**Fig. 59.1**).

III. Technique
- Preoperative planning
  - Radiographs: evaluate for presence of spinal deformity (scoliosis on anteroposterior (AP), spondylolisthesis on lateral) and anklyosis (no segmental motion on flexion/extension views).

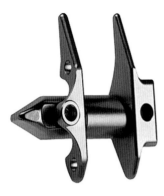

Fig. 59.1 Photograph of X-Stop device, Medtronic Spine, LCC, Memphis, TN. (© Medtronic Spine LLC).

- CT/MRI: confirm diagnosis of stenosis.
- Dual x-ray absorptiometry (DEXA): assess risk for osteoporotic fractures.
– Anesthesia: general, monitored anesthesia care (MAC), or local
– Positioning: lateral decubitus or supine on a radiolucent table; make sure that the lumbar spine is maintained in flexion
– A vertical midline incision centered over the affected segment(s) is made through the skin and fascia, with care taken to avoid attenuating the supraspinous/interspinous ligaments.
– After the levels are confirmed using fluoroscopy or intraoperative x-rays, a subperiosteal exposure of the spinous processes and laminae is performed without disrupting the facet capsules.
– The interspinous space is distracted so that the ISD may be inserted between two adjacent spinous processes (depending on the surgical protocol for each specific implant).
– May also be combined with a microdecompression (e.g., laminotomies)
– The wound is closed in layers, and a drain may or may not be used.

IV. Complications

– Intraoperative
  - Spinous process (SP) fracture
  - Malpositioning of implant
  - Inability to safely place the implant (e.g., attenuation of ligaments, excessively small interspinous space secondary to "kissing" SP or facet hypertrophy)
– Postoperative
  - SP fracture

- Device migration/dislocation
- Persistent/recurrent symptoms (same- versus adjacent-segment degeneration)
– In the series of Barbagallo et al, the incidence of complications was 10.1% (primarily spinous process fractures and device dislocations) with a reoperation rate of 7.2%.[2]

V. Postoperative Care

– May be performed in ambulatory setting as opposed to inpatient admission
– Immediate postoperative ambulation
– No bracing typically required
– Gradual return to normal activities

VI. Outcomes

– Kuchta et al published the 2-year results of 175 consecutive X-Stop procedures performed at a single center.[3]
- X-Stop brought significant improvement in clinical outcome measures.
- Reoperation rate of 4.6% (removal of implant with posterior decompression)
– Zucherman et al reported the results of a multicenter, prospective, randomized trial comparing X-Stop and nonoperative modalities for spinal stenosis (191 patients).[4]
- At 2 years, clinical outcomes of patients receiving X-Stop were significantly improved compared with those undergoing conservative treatments.
- No device-related complications, but 6% of X-Stop cohort required subsequent laminectomy
– There continues to be a paucity of data on other ISDs.

VII. Surgical Pearls

– Appropriate candidates for this technique should experience clear relief of their claudicatory symptoms with lumbar flexion or sitting.
– Flexion-extension lateral x-rays may identify the presence of bony ankylosis at the stenotic level(s), which may preclude the implantation of an ISD.
– The lumbar spine should be maintained in flexion to facilitate intraoperative distraction of the stenotic segments

- Hypertrophic facet joints may need to be partially excised to allow successful placement of the ISD.
- Care must be taken when inserting the ISD in osteoporotic patients, who may be at greater risk for spinous process fractures.

Common Clinical Questions

1. Which of the following patients is best suited for placement of an ISD?
   A. Patient with severe low back pain and minimal extremity symptoms
   B. Patient with claudication secondary to moderate stenosis and a grade II spondylolisthesis at L4-L5
   C. Patient with moderate stenosis at L3-L4 whose symptoms improve with sitting
   D. Patient with severe stenosis between L2 and L5 who complains of perianal numbness and bladder dysfunction

2. What is the primary mechanism by which ISD relieves claudicatory symptoms?
   A. Decreases facet joint forces
   B. Unloads posterior disc tissue
   C. Eliminates redundant ligamentum flavum and other compressive lesions
   D. Increases the dimensions of the spinal canal

3. Which is not a typical characteristic of neurogenic claudication?
   A. Pain is worse when walking uphill
   B. Symptoms improve with sitting
   C. Pain/numbness is worse with lumbar extension
   D. Symptoms do not change when riding a bicycle

References

1. Bono CM, Vaccaro AR. Interspinous process devices in the lumbar spine. J Spinal Disord Tech 2007;20(3):255–261
2. Barbagallo GM, Olindo G, Corbino L, Albanese V. Analysis of complications in patients treated with the X-Stop Interspinous Process Decompression System: proposal for a novel anatomic scoring system for patient selection and review of the literature. Neurosurgery 2009;65(1):111–119, discussion 119–120
3. Kuchta J, Sobottke R, Eysel P, Simons P. Two-year results of interspinous spacer (X-Stop) implantation in 175 patients with neurologic intermittent claudication due to lumbar spinal stenosis. Eur Spine J 2009;18(6):823–829
4. Zucherman JF, Hsu KY, Hartjen CA, et al. A multicenter, prospective, randomized trial evaluating the X STOP interspinous process decompression system for the treatment of neurogenic intermittent claudication: two-year follow-up results. Spine (Phila Pa 1976) 2005;30(12):1351–1358

Answers to Common Clinical Questions

1. C
2. D
3. A

60 Lumbar Arthroplasty

Ishaq Y. Syed, Barrett I. Woods, and Joon Y. Lee

I. Key Points

- Lumbar arthroplasty has recently been approved in the United States as an alternative treatment strategy to spinal arthrodesis in the treatment of refractory symptomatic discogenic back pain.
- Etiology of low back pain remains unclear, with numerous possible pain generators.
- Goals: preserve physiologic spinal motion, prevent facet arthropathy, prevent adjacent-segment disease, restore disc height, and provide long-term pain relief[1]
- The prosthesis should approximate the size and motion of the physiologic disc, avoid distracting the facet joints, and, ideally, reproduce the normal biomechanics (**Fig. 60.1**).
- No independent long-term, randomized, prospective study on any artificial disc has been published to date that clearly delineates the safety and efficacy of lumbar arthroplasty.

II. Indications

- Patient refractory to a minimum of 6 months of conservative, nonoperative treatment
- One- or two-level symptomatic degenerative disc disease in patients of age 18 to 60 years
- Correlative objective radiographic findings including disc desiccation, vacuum disc, high-intensity zone signal, and Medic signal changes

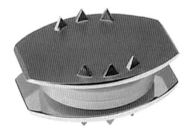

Fig. 60.1 Photograph of the Charite artificial disc (with permission from DePuy Spine, Inc.).

- Postdiscectomy axial back pain or juxtafusion disc degeneration
- Absence of central or lateral recess stenosis that may require posterior decompression to address concomitant radicular leg pain
- Provocative discography may demonstrate concordant pain reproduction and confirm diagnosis.

III. Contraindications

- Compromised structural integrity of bone
  - Tumor, osteoporosis (T-score <–2.5), osteomalacia, acute fracture
- Potential compromise of stability or alignment of implant
  - Scoliosis, spondylolysis, spondylolisthesis (>grade I), incompetent posterior elements
- Conditions that may compromise clinical outcome of disc replacement
  - Significant facet arthrosis, disc herniation with predominant radicular symptoms, central or lateral recess stenosis, disc height less than 5 mm
- Miscellaneous
  - Obesity (BMI >40), local or systemic presence of tumor or infection, pregnancy, intraspinal neoplasm

IV. Technique[2]

- Positioning
  - The patient is placed in the supine position on a radiolucent table with all bony prominences padded after institution of general anesthesia and Foley insertion to decompress the bladder.
  - C-arm fluoroscopy is used to identify the approach angle and location of the disc space and to verify that clear anteroposterior and lateral images can be attained.
- Standard sterile preparation and draping are performed and prophylactic intravenous antibiotics are administered.
- Exposure
  - The majority of prostheses are implanted by means of an open anterior approach similar to that used for anterior lumbar interbody fusion (ALIF).
  - A general or vascular surgeon can obtain access to the spine through either an anterior retroperitoneal approach (most preferred) or a midline transperitoneal approach.

- A left-sided approach is preferred between L3 and L5 due to the relative resilience of the aorta and ease of mobility compared with the vena cava.
- In accessing L5-S1 in male patients a right-sided approach is recommended to reduce the rate of injury of the superior hypogastric plexus, which can cause retrograde ejaculation.
- The retroperitoneal space is entered deep to the rectus sheath and the peritoneum, with the ureter retracted medially.
- Blunt dissection reveals the lateral edge of the psoas, and vascular structures are carefully mobilized and elevated off the anterior spine.
- Procedure
  - Fluoroscopic images are used to confirm the disc level and identify the midline.
  - A subtotal discectomy is performed by excising the anterior longitudinal ligament, annulus, and nucleus pulposus, leaving the lateral portion of the annulus intact.
  - The cartilaginous end plate is debrided from the osseous end plate. The integrity of the end plate is preserved to ensure implant fixation and avoid subsidence.
  - If necessary, the posterior longitudinal ligament (PLL) is released and posterior osteophytes debrided.
  - Special instruments are used to measure the footprint, lordotic angle, and core height.
  - Based on preoperative templating and intraoperative sizing, the appropriate trial is inserted.
  - The appropriately sized prosthesis is implanted after device-specific preparation of the end plate.
  - If the device has a polyethylene core, it is trialed and inserted after confirming on lateral fluoroscopy the restoration of desired disc height and lordosis.
- Fluoroscopy confirms the central position of the implant on the anteroposterior view. Ideally, the center of rotation of the device is 2 mm posterior to the sagittal midline of the vertebral body on the lateral view.
- Final confirmatory radiographs are obtained and the wound is closed in routine fashion.
- The approach varies according to the lumbar level accessed as well as device-specific modifications to the general technique.

V. Complications

- Approach-related complications (10 to 13%): vascular injury, phlebitis, pulmonary embolism, sexual dysfunction, and retrograde ejaculation.
- Postoperative retroperitoneal scarring makes revision surgery more difficult.
- Failure of the prosthesis primarily involves facet joint degeneration, subsidence, device migration, and adjacent-level disease.
- Cases of vertebral body fractures have been reported.
- Heterotopic ossification has been reported in varying degrees in 1.4 to 15.2% of patients.
- A prospective, randomized, multicenter Food and Drug Administration (FDA)–regulated clinical trial reported on complications of 589 patients.[3]
  - The disc replacement group was found to have an 8.8% reoperation rate, compared with 10.1% in the lumbar fusion control group. Mean time to reoperation was 9.7 months.
  - The primary reason for removal of the implant was device migration (75%).
  - A higher incidence of vascular injury occurred in the reoperation group (16.7%) compared with the primary group (3.4%).
  - Fourteen patients required posterior instrumented fusion for persistent low back pain (2.4%).

VI. Postoperative Care

- Patients bear weight as tolerated and are mobilized on the first postoperative day.
- A brace is typically not needed.
- Standing radiographs are obtained as soon as feasible postoperatively to document the position of the implant in the weight-bearing position.
- A gentle low back and abdominal strengthening program is implemented starting with the first postoperative day.
- The patient is given postoperative restrictions including avoidance of substantial extension, bending, twisting, or heavy lifting for the first 6 weeks.
- Progressive unrestricted activity is allowed after 6 weeks.

VII. Outcomes

- Results of a prospective, randomized, multicenter FDA-regulated trial conducted to assess the safety and efficacy of the procedure were recently published.[4]
  - The study reported on 160 patients who completed 5-year follow-up.
  - Patients were randomized to total disc replacement (TDR) or anterior interbody fusion using Bagby and Kuslich (BAK) cages with iliac crest autograft.
  - Overall success was 57.8% in the TDR group versus 51.2% in the BAK group.
  - Oswestry Disability Index (ODI), Visual Analogue Scale (VAS) pain scores, patient satisfaction, and SF-36 questionnaires were similar across the two groups.
  - The mean range at the index level was 6 degrees for the TDR patients and 1 degree for the BAK patients. Changes in disc height were similar for the two.
  - The authors concluded there is no statistical difference in clinical outcomes between the groups.
  - The TDR patients did reach a statistically higher rate of employment and lower rate of long-term disability compared with the BAK patients.
- The clinical efficacy, long-term durability, and potential complications need to be more clearly elucidated with the use of unbiased prospective randomized studies with long-term follow-up.

VIII. Surgical Pearls

- The lumbar spine is positioned in the neutral position to minimize tension on retroperioteneal vessels.
- Sympathetic and parasympathetic nerves must be carefully preserved to prevent erectile dysfunction and retrograde ejaculation in male patients.
- The integrity of end plates must be preserved to ensure good implant fixation and avoid subsidence.
- The implant must restore appropriate lordosis, have adequate end plate coverage, and avoid distraction of more than 3 mm to apply proper tension to the posterior ligaments.

Common Clinical Questions

1. All of the following are contraindications to total disc arthroplasty *except*:
   A. The presence of significant lateral recess stenosis
   B. Facet arthrosis
   C. Degenerative spondylolisthesis
   D. Smoking
   E. Obesity (BMI >40)

2. Which of the following statements is true with regard to total disc arthroplasty?
   A. Randomized prospective control trials have illustrated the efficacy of lumbar disc arthroplasty, establishing that it preserves normal biomechanics and reduces the incidence of adjacent-segment degeneration.
   B. A right-sided approach to the L5/S1 disc space is recommended in male patients undergoing total disc arthroplasty.
   C. The PLL is essential to the appropriate tensioning of the disc replacement and should not be excised.
   D. Heterotopic ossification is not a confirmed potential complication of total disc arthroplasty.
   E. A significant portion of the cranial and caudal end plate must be removed prior to placement of the implant for proper setting of the prosthesis.

References

1. Gamradt SC, Wang JC. Lumbar disc arthroplasty. Spine J 2005;5(1):95–103
2. Tropiano P, Huang RC, Girardi FP, Cammisa FP Jr, Marnay T. Lumbar total disc replacement. Surgical technique. J Bone Joint Surg Am 2006;88(Suppl 1 Pt 1):50–64
3. McAfee PC, Geisler FH, Saiedy SS, et al. Revisability of the CHARITE artificial disc replacement: analysis of 688 patients enrolled in the U.S. IDE study of the CHARITE Artificial Disc. Spine (Phila Pa 1976) 2006;31(11):1217–1226
4. Guyer RD, McAfee PC, Banco RJ, et al. Prospective, randomized, multicenter Food and Drug Administration investigational device exemption study of lumbar total disc replacement with the CHARITE artificial disc versus lumbar fusion: five-year follow-up. Spine J 2009;9(5):374–386

Answers to Common Clinical Questions

1. D
2. B

61 Lumbosacroiliac Fixation

Amit R. Patel, Alexander R. Vaccaro, and Ravi K. Ponnappan

I. Key Points

- Lumbosacroiliac (LSI) fixation provides the strongest biomechanical construct for sacral fractures and lumbopelvic dissociations.[1]
- The construct spans the sacrum and allows for relatively normal load transfer from the lumbar spine through the sacroiliac (SI) joints to the pelvis, permitting early post-op weight bearing.
- In long constructs, including L5-S1, iliac (pelvic) fixation improves fusion rates of vertebrae.[2]
- Iliac screws must remain in bone throughout their length to prevent injury to pelvic viscera and neurovascular structures.[3]
- Sacropelvic relationships should be measured and taken into account in performing long-segment fixation extending into the sacrum/ilium (**Table 61.1** and **Fig. 61.1**).

II. Indications

- Complex sacral fractures with or without pelvic discontinuity
- Adult scoliosis patients with L5-S1 spondylolisthesis

Table 61.1 Commonly Measured Pelvic Parameters

Sacral slope	An angle subtended by a horizontal reference line and the sacral end plate
	Normal around 40 degrees (varies with patient's position)
Pelvic tilt	Angle formed by a vertical line from the center of the femoral heads and the line from the femoral heads to the middle of S1 end plate
	Measures 11.9 to 10.3 degrees (varies with patient's position)
Pelvic incidence	Angle between a line drawn perpendicular to the sacral plate at its midpoint and a line connecting the midpoint of the middle axis of the femoral heads
	Mean normal value is 48 to 53 degrees
	Low: flattened lumbar lordosis, low shear stress at lumbosacral junction, low risk of progression of spondylolisthesis
	High: high sacral slope, high pelvic tilt, increased lordosis, high shear stress at lumbosacral junction, high risk of progression of spondylolisthesis

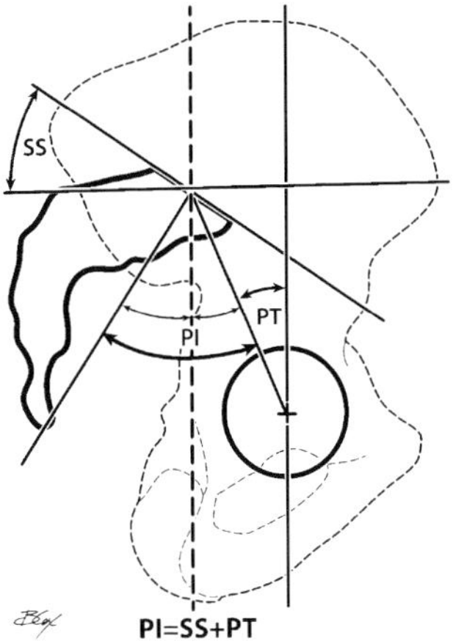

Fig. 61.1 Sacropelvic radiographic measurements.

PI=SS+PT

- Revision lumbosacral fusion
- Adult isthmic spondylolisthesis
- High-grade dysplastic spondylolisthesis

III. Technique

- A subperiosteal dissection is made to the lumbar transverse processes, sacral ala, and posterior superior iliac spine (PSIS).[3]
  - While exposing the sacrum, stay extraperiosteal and avoid falling into the dorsal sacral foramina.
- Using blunt and sharp elevators, lift the musculature off of the inner and outer aspects of both iliac wings to help establish the direction for iliac screw placement.
- S1 pedicle screw: Placement begins by identifying the region where the ala and lateral S1 facet meet; a high-speed bur can be used to mark the starting point (**Fig. 61.2**).[3]
  - This point is typically 1 cm cephalad to and slightly lateral to the S1 foramen.
- S2 pedicle screw: Placement begins by identifying the inferior medial aspect of the dorsal S1 foramen and the superior medial aspect of the dorsal S2 foramen; the starting point is the middle of an imaginary line connecting the two points, which can be marked with a high-speed bur (**Fig. 61.2**).[3]
- Use a gearshift probe to create a path from this starting point to the anterior cortex of the sacrum; gently tap the gearshift with a mallet to perforate the anterior cortex.[3]

- S1 screw: typically 6.5 mm in diameter and 40 to 45 mm in length; should be aimed medially for the sacral promontory
- S2 screw: typically 6.5 mm in diameter and 50 to 60 mm in length; should aim 30 to 35 degrees laterally and tilt cephalad 15 to 20 degrees (parallel to the SI joint)
  - Iliac (pelvic) screw: placement begins by identifying the inferiomedial aspect of the PSIS (**Fig. 61.2**)
  - Using a high-speed bur or a rongeur at the PSIS, find cancellous bone and then use the gearshift probe to develop a screw path that runs between the inner and outer cortex of the ilium.
  - The path, directed toward the anterior inferior iliac spine (AIIS), should not be forced and should be produced easily; if resistance is met, consider a larger soft-tissue exposure and/or the use of fluoroscopy to guide the gearshift along a more appropriate path.[3]
    - The combination obturator-outlet view best shows the proper starting point and path of the iliac screw.[1]
    - The combination obturator-inlet view confirms that the screw has not violated the inner or outer iliac cortex (**Fig. 61.3**).[1]
    - A true lateral oblique view of the pelvis or iliac ensures that there is no sciatic notch or acetabular encroachment of the iliac screws and confirms full accommodation of the screw length (**Fig. 61.4**).
    - A simplified method of iliac screw insertion is to place one's finger within the sciatic notch along the outer table of the ilium and use this landmark as a guide in probe and screw insertion, without the need for intraoperative fluoroscopy or Kirschner wire (K-wire) guidance.

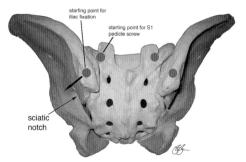

Fig. 61.2 Posterior view of pelvis. Note starting points for the sacral and iliac screws.

61 Lumbosacroiliac Fixation

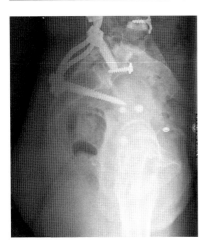

Fig. 61.3 Lateral lumbopelvic x-ray demonstrating appropriately positioned pelvic fixation. Note position of pelvic screws in relation to the sciatic notch.

- Using a K-wire and tap, the final iliac screw is placed; it is typically 7.5 to 8 mm in diameter and 65 to 90 mm in length.
  - In revision cases where iliac crest bone was harvested for grafting for the index procedure, iliac screw placement can be more challenging and longer screws may be used.[3]
  - Iliac screws must stay entirely within bone given the proximity of various pelvic structures.
- A rod is used to connect the sacral screw, the iliac screw, and the construct.

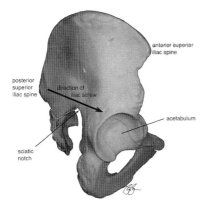

Fig. 61.4 Lateral view of pelvis showing anatomic landmarks and direction of safe placement of the iliac screws.

IV. Complications

- Infection and wound rates approach 20%.[4]
- Symptomatic hardware requiring removal[3]
- A formal SI joint arthrodesis is generally not performed; as a consequence, the implant may fracture due to fatigue failure.[4]
- Superior gluteal artery injury from sciatic notch violation[4]
- Wound breakdown due to disruption of the distal erector spinae musculature attachment. When elevating the posterior paraspinal muscles to expose the medial border of the ilium, be careful not to disrupt the distal attachment of the erector spinae muscles as that may lead to wound problems.

V. Postoperative Care

- Early patient mobilization
- External orthosis (if utilized) must include leg extension (to immobilize hip).[1]

VI. Outcomes

- L5-S1 fusion rates approach 92% with utilization of sacropelvic fixation.[4]
- Iliac screw placement is possible in revision cases; in one series, 34 of 36 patients had successfully placed iliac screws despite previous iliac crest graft harvesting.[4]
- Iliac screw loosening is reportedly as high as 52%, although this did not correlate with pseudarthrosis; the rate of iliac screw breakage is considerably lower (5.3%).[2]
- Nearly half of patients report being able to feel their instrumentation.[2]
- The infection rate is reported at 3.7%.[4]

VII. Surgical Pearls

- The site of iliac crest bone grafting should be made more superiorly along the crest to maintain adequate bone stock for iliac/pelvic bolt fixation.[3]
- LSI fixation can be combined with iliosacral screws (triangular osteosynthesis) to stabilize the weight-bearing axis and the pelvic ring.[5]
- In the placement of bicortical S1 screws, medial screw angulation is necessary to avoid traversing the L5 nerve root.[1]
- Separate (accessory) incisions can be utilized for iliac fixation with the use of subcutaneous tunneling to connect to lumbosacral fixation.[3]

Common Clinical Questions

1. Which pelvic view best confirms that the iliac screw has not violated the inner or outer cortex of the ilium?
   A. Lateral
   B. Anteroposterior
   C. Iliac oblique
   D. Obturator-inlet
   E. Obturator-outlet

References

1. Schildhauer TA, Bellabarba C, Nork SE, Barei DP, Routt ML Jr, Chapman JR. Decompression and lumbopelvic fixation for sacral fracture-dislocations with spino-pelvic dissociation. J Orthop Trauma 2006;20(7):447–457
2. Kuklo TR, Bridwell KH, Lewis SJ, et al. Minimum 2-year analysis of sacropelvic fixation and L5-S1 fusion using S1 and iliac screws. Spine (Phila Pa 1976) 2001;26(18):1976–1983
3. Bradford DS, Zdeblick TA. Master Techniques in Orthopaedic Surgery: The Spine. 2nd ed. Philadelphia, PA: Lippincott; 2004:336–345
4. Herkowitz HH, Garfin SR, Eismont FJ, et al. The Spine. 5th ed. Philadelphia, PA: Elsevier; 2006:1180–1183.
5. Kim JH, Horton W, Hamasaki T, Freedman B, Whitesides TE Jr, Hutton WC. Spinal instrumentation for sacral-pelvic fixation: a biomechanical comparison between constructs ending with either S2 bicortical, bitriangulated screws or iliac screws. J Spinal Disord Tech 2010;23(8):506–512

Answers to Common Clinical Questions

1. D. Refer to **Fig. 61.3**. The obturator-inlet view best confirms that the iliac screw has remained intracortical, which is of critical importance given the proximity of the pelvic contents to the ilia. The obturator-oblique view is used to confirm the chosen starting point and the iliac screw path. The lateral view can show if a screw has violated the sciatic notch. The iliac oblique view confirms that the screw has not advanced into the acetabulum. The anteroposterior view does not have a significant role in iliac screw placement.

62 Sacrectomy

Ioannis Papanastassiou, Mohammad Eleraky, and Frank D. Vrionis

I. Key Points

- A posterior and combined approach to and instrumentation for total sacrectomy are feasible.
- Try to obtain wide margins and consider the use of intraoperative adjuvants (cryotherapy, phenol, brachytherapy, etc.).
- Use adjuvant radiation therapy (preferably intensity-modulated radiation therapy (IMRT) or proton beam) for contaminated margins.

II. Indications

- Aggressive benign tumors of the sacrum (giant cell tumors, osteoblastoma)
- Malignant primary sacral tumors (chordoma, Ewing's sarcoma/primitive neuroepithelial tumor [PNET], osteosarcoma, etc.)
- Selected cases of metastatic tumors/multiple myeloma (frequently located in the sacrum)
- Pelvic tumors invading sacroiliac joint and sacrum (chondrosarcoma, Ewing sarcoma, osteosarcoma, etc.)

III. Technique

- Sacrectomy can be total or subtotal, a stand-alone operation or performed in the context of more complex sacropelvic resections (extended internal/external hemipelvectomies).
- Subtotal resections can be categorized according to the resection plane.
- Transverse/axial resection: usually done between sacral segments (S1/S2, S2/S3, below S3)
- Sagittal resection: can be in the midline (hemisacrectomy) or located more laterally (e.g., through or lateral to the neuroforamens)[1,2]
- Approach: depending on the location and tumor type, the approach could be posterior (longitudinal or transverse) or combined anteroposterior.

Posterior Approach

- It is generally accepted that sacrectomies at the S2/S3 level and not extending to the rectum can be performed via a posterior-only approach. For S1/S2 resections controversy exists; for total sacrectomies (L5-S1 level), most authorities recommend a combined approach, although there are reports describing total sacrectomy through a posterior approach alone.
- The type of posterior (transverse or longitudinal) incision may be indicated from a previous biopsy or from the tumor location. A longitudinal approach is typically employed, sometimes with a transverse component (T-type, **Fig. 62.1**): after the skin incision (with the biopsy tract incorporated), the gluteus maximus is dissected laterally and the erector spinae are detached from the midline and posterolateral aspect of the sacrum and flaps elevated in an upward fashion; this maneuver greatly facilitates surgical exposure.
- Subsequently, a laminectomy is done in the desired level and the cauda equina is ligated with double silk sutures and cut in the axilla of the most caudal nerve roots to be preserved (**Fig. 62.2**).
- The sacrum is freed from its attachment to surrounding structures (pelvic floor–anococcygeal ligament, sacrotuberous/sacrospinous ligaments, piriformis muscles). Piriformis resection should be as wide as possible as this has been found to decrease local recurrence.
- Finally, sacrectomy is completed using osteotomes; caution is recommended to the whole surgical team at this point because massive hemorrhage may commence.

Combined Approach (Anteroposterior)

- Typically, the anterior resection comes first. The surgery is preferably performed in a staged fashion (anterior → supine, posterior → prone) with an interval of 2 to 3 days between stages; this is believed to reduce morbidity. However, there are advocates of a single-stage operations either in the lateral position or in the supine/prone position.
- The anterior approach could be open, laparoscopic, intraperitoneal, or extraperitoneal. Involvement of the rectum makes the anterior intraperitoneal approach mandatory (typically by a general surgeon); if there is a clear plane between rectum and tumor, especially if the tumor is located eccentrically, a retroperitoneal approach may be used.[1,2]

IV Surgical Techniques

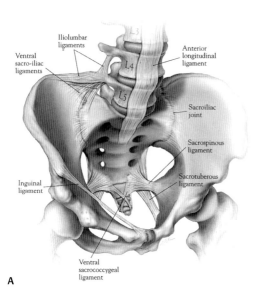

A

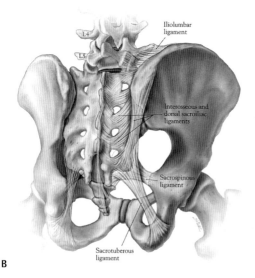

B

Fig. 62.1 Ligamentous anatomy of the lower lumbar spine, sacrum, and pelvis. **(A)** Ventral sacrum. **(B)** Dorsal sacrum. (From Dickman, Fehlings, Gokaslan, Spinal Cord and Spinal Column Tumors, Thieme; pg. 634, Fig. 44-1A,B.)

62 Sacrectomy

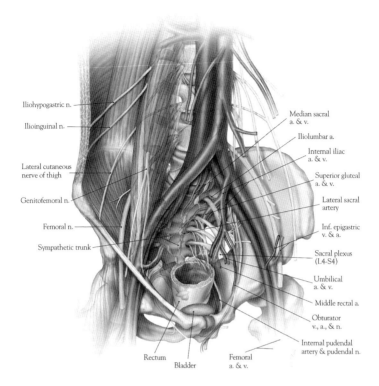

Fig. 62.2 Relationship of the ventral surface of the sacrum to the major pelvic structures, arteries, veins, and neural structures. (From Dickman, Fehlings, Gokaslan, Spinal Cord and Spinal Column Tumors, Thieme; pg. 635, Fig. 44-2.)

- At the end of the anterior stage, complete mobilization of the rectum is accomplished or a colostomy is performed; ligation of the internal iliac vessels is done with discectomy or osteotomy at the desired level and anterior osteotomy of the sacroiliac (SI) joints (or more laterally if needed). A radiopaque marker may be left at the discectomy/osteotomy level to facilitate localization at the second stage.
- It is widely believed that the use of a vertical rectus abdominis myocutaneous flap reduces the risk of wound infection/breakdown. This should be done at the first stage and the flap left in the wound to be utilized at the end of the posterior operation.

Reconstruction
- If the sacrectomy is performed below the S1/S2 level, reconstruction in general is not needed; however, a higher chance of sacral insufficiency fractures has been reported. Indications for instrumentation include total sacrectomy, partial sacrectomy involving more than 50% of SI joints, or sagittal hemisacrectomy that obliterates the SI joint unilaterally or bilaterally. However, even for total sacrectomies, some authorities believe that any stabilization is unwarranted, since this typically prolongs the operation and increases morbidity and risk of infection. Total sacrectomy is believed to create a flail axial skeleton, leading to pain or mechanical kinking of neurovascular structures or viscera and significantly affecting ambulation, a set of conditions favoring reconstruction.
- Reconstruction began in the 1980s with Harrington rods, moved to the Galveston-Luque wire technique in the 1990s, and now consists of a two-to-four-rod construct interconnected with sacral bars; pedicle screws are placed from L2-L3 caudally and the pelvis is anchored with long iliac screws (two to four).
- Cortical strut grafts (e.g., fibular or femoral diaphysis) can be used to bridge the osseous gap between the SI joints or iliac wings. They provide a more biologic fixation and the ability to form an osseous bridge and maintain continuity with the disrupted ring. This may prove very important in long-term survivors.[1,2]
- A newer and more technically challenging technique has been described by the Mayo group. Two fibular grafts are placed between L5 and the supra-acetabular region bilaterally along the force transmission lines, providing triangulation and increasing resistance to failure by two times.[3] Experience indicates that it may be easier to insert the strut grafts in the posterior inferior iliac spine.

IV. Complications

- Hemorrhage (injury of internal iliac, iliolumbar, and median sacral vessels, eg), which may be life threatening
- Visceral damage (rectum, ureters)
- Wound healing problems/infection (may be as high as 50%)
- Sensorimotor, bowel, bladder, and sexual dysfunction. The higher the resection level, the greater the morbidity. As a general rule, preservation of at least one S3 nerve leads to the preservation of function in two-thirds of patients, unilateral sacrectomy

has good results in 90%, and S1/S2 resections or total sacrectomies result universally in loss of function (**Table 62.1**).[4] Saddle anesthesia is common; motor loss is encountered only in cases of S1 root resection.
- Sacral insufficiency fractures
- General medical complications (pneumonia, ileus, deep vein thrombosis (DVT), etc.). Generally, the morbidity and mortality are high (5% perioperative deaths in Sloan Kettering series).[5]

V. Postoperative Care

- Stabilization of the patient is crucial in the first postoperative days (typically in the intensive care unit).
- Ambulation may be commenced immediately for low resections, or in a delayed fashion, depending on the level of stability and fixation quality, with walking aids.
- Keep wound clean, with frequent dressing changes to prevent contamination from rectum.
- Give stool softeners and high-volume food supplements. Patients may need to manually disimpact stools. Gradually attempt bladder training, with the possible need for patients to self-catheterize.

VI. Outcomes

- Survival is greatly dependent on the type of the tumor, previous operations, and tumor location. For sacral chordomas, which are the most common tumors warranting sacrectomy, 5-year and 10-year survival are 68% and 40%, respectively (SEER database). Local recurrence occurs in about 40% (28% for wide versus 64% for intralesional in one series of 64 chordomas). Distant metastasis occurs in one-third of patients.[5]

Table 62.1 Bladder and Bowel Function after Sacrectomy

Resection level	Spared nerve roots	Normal bowel	Normal bladder
S1/S2	Both S1	0%	0%
S2/S3	Both S2	40%	25%
S3/S4	Both S3	100%	69%
Variable	Unilateral	67%	60%
Hemisacrectomy	Unilateral S1 to S5	87%	89%

VII. Surgical Pearls

- The posterior-only approach is useful for S1/S2 resections and the combined anteroposterior approach (in a staged fashion) is practiced for higher resections.
- Use of the rectus abdominis flap in combined procedures reduces wound complications.
- Anticipate and prepare the surgical team for blood loss when initiating a posterior osteotomy (ensure good hydration, give aminocaproic acid, make PRBCs and FFPs available).
- For total sacrectomies use a two- (or four-) rod construct with interconnecting sacral bars. Strut allografts (either transverse or in a triangular fashion) are desirable to promote fusion.
- Wide resection is crucial to prevent local recurrence and significantly affects survival. Try to obtain negative margins in the sacrospinal canal and wide surgical margins posteriorly, by excising parts of the piriformis, gluteus maximus, and sacroiliac joints.

Common Clinical Questions

1. Which nerve roots are critical for bladder/bowel function and should be preserved if possible?
2. What is the incidence of local recurrence after wide and intralesional resection of sacral chordomas? Does it affect survival?
3. Which level of resection can be performed safely via a posterior approach only, and when is a combined approach mandated?

References

1. Mavrogenis AF, Patapis P, Kostopanagiotou G, Papagelopoulos PJ. Tumors of the sacrum. Orthopedics 2009;32(5):342
2. Fourney DR, Rhines LD, Hentschel SJ, et al. En bloc resection of primary sacral tumors: classification of surgical approaches and outcome. J Neurosurg Spine 2005;3(2):111–122
3. Dickey ID, Hugate RR Jr, Fuchs B, Yaszemski MJ, Sim FH. Reconstruction after total sacrectomy: early experience with a new surgical technique. Clin Orthop Relat Res 2005; 438:42–50
4. Todd LT Jr, Yaszemski MJ, Currier BL, Fuchs B, Kim CW, Sim FH. Bowel and bladder function after major sacral resection. Clin Orthop Relat Res 2002;(397):36–39
5. Schwab JH, Healey JH, Rose P, Casas-Ganem J, Boland PJ. The surgical management of sacral chordomas. Spine (Phila Pa 1976) 2009;34(24):2700–2704

Answers to Common Clinical Questions

1. At least one S3 root should be preserved if possible, which is associated with good function in approximately two-thirds of patients.
2. 28% and 64%, respectively; local recurrence has a significant negative impact on survival
3. Resection below S2 may be safely performed posteriorly only; for S1/S2 controversy exists, while above S1 (total sacrectomy) a combined-approach, staged operation should be undertaken.

63 Vertebral Body Augmentation

Mohammed Eleraky and Frank D. Vrionis

I. Key Points

- Vertebral augmentation is commonly employed in treating compression fractures in patients with osteoporosis or spine tumors.
- Two different percutaneous vertebral augmentation methods for cement application into the vertebral body have been documented: vertebroplasty and kyphoplasty.
- In vertebroplasty, polymethylmethacrylate (PMMA) cement is injected percutaneously into the collapsed vertebral body.
- Kyphoplasty involves placing inflatable bone tamps percutaneously into a vertebral body. The inflation of the bone tamp allows some restoration of vertebral height. After deflation, the cavity that has been produced is filled by injection of PMMA.
- Two randomized clinical trials showed that improvement in patients with painful osteoporotic vertebral fractures was similar between those treated with vertebroplasty and those treated with a simulated procedure, at one month follow-up.[1,2]
- Compared with nonsurgical management, balloon kyphoplasty resulted in improvements in quality of life and disability measures and reduction of back pain in patients with acute painful vertebral fractures.[2]

II. Indications

- Severe pain or progressive collapse due to vertebral body compression fractures in patients with osteoporosis (primary or secondary).
- Severe pain or progressive collapse due to vertebral body metastasis or multiple myeloma. Treatment algorithm for painful thoracic or lumbar vertebral body fractures in cancer patients (**Fig. 63.1**).
- Contraindications to vertebral augmentation include asymptomatic lesions, patients who are improving on conservative care, ongoing local or systemic infection, retropulsed bone fragment or epidural tumor causing myelopathy, and allergy to bone cement.

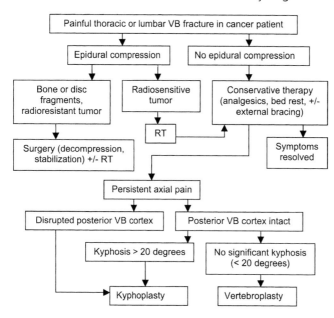

Fig. 63.1 Treatment algorithm for painful thoracic or lumbar vertebral body fractures in cancer patients. See text for details. VB = vertebral body; RT = radiation therapy. (Reproduced with permission from Fourney DR, Schomer DF, Nader R, Chlan-Fourney J, Suki D, Rhines LD, Ahrar K, Gokaslan ZL. Percutaneous vertebroplasty and kyphoplasty for painful vertebral body fractures in cancer patients. SCSCT; pg. 624, Fig. 43-3.)

Diagnosis
- Magnetic resonance imaging (MRI) scan of the spine (T1 and short T1 inversion recovery [STIR] sequences) to detect vertebral body edema and associated impending fractures
- Computed tomography (CT) scan of the fractured vertebral body with sagittal reconstruction to evaluate posterior vertebral wall integrity
- Bone scan in some cases to assess acuity of fracture and exclude metastasis in different levels

III. Technique
- Procedures can be performed under general or local anesthesia.
- Patient is placed in prone position on Jackson radiolucent table, with postural reduction of kyphosis if present.

- Biplanar fluoroscopy is used.
- Both techniques start with the percutaneous insertion of (11 gauge) Jamshidi needle or guide pin into the fractured vertebra and end with the injection of PMMA.
- This can be achieved through a transpedicular approach in nearly every case.
- In the thoracic spine the needle can be inserted extrapedicularly, between the rib head and lateral aspect of the pedicle (**Fig. 63.2**).
- Single or bilateral injection can be performed (it is important to fill the center of the vertebral body).

Vertebroplasty
- After correct positioning of the needle, the inner stylet is removed.
- Contrast material is then injected to ensure that the needle is not positioned in the venous flow path (optional).
- Cement, in thin liquid form, is injected into the vertebra using multiple small syringes.
- The flow of the cement should be followed on the image intensifier.

Kyphoplasty
- After proper needle positioning, a series of tools (drill, curette) are used to create a working channel. Once inserted, the balloons are inflated using volume and pressure controls (digital manometer) to create a cavity within the vertebra.
- Once this has been achieved, the balloons are deflated and removed.
- Thick cement can be fed through the cannula under low pressure to fill the cavity created by the balloon tamp.
- In cases involving the upper thoracic spine, the shoulders can interfere with the lateral view, so a stack of pillows of appropriate height should be placed under the chest to lower both shoulders. Alternatively, the arm and the shoulder are left hanging down parallel to the trunk.

IV. Complications
- Procedure-related: cement leakage can result from fracture clefts or improper instrument position and can occur in the spinal canal, neuroforamen, or disc space.
- Medical: pulmonary embolism, hemo- or pneumothorax, soft-tissue hematomas

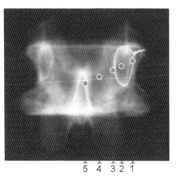
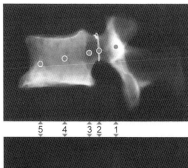
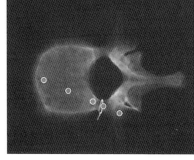

Fig. 63.2 Entry points and trajectories for the transpedicular approach during kyphoplasty. (Courtesy of Medtronic.)

- New adjacent vertebral fracture due to leakage of cement into the disc
- Pedicle fracture

V. Postoperative Care

- Mobilize early with no need for bracing.
- Clinical evaluation and plain spinal radiographs
- Discharge home when patient meets discharge criteria (usually same day or on postoperative day 1).

VI. Outcomes

- All studies reported significant improvements in pain score and functional outcome.[1,3]
- The risk of neurologic sequelae ranges from 0.4 to 4.0% according to various reports.[2–4]
- The complication rate is considerably higher for spinal metastasis due to lytic areas involving the vertebral cortex.

- A recent study by Kallmes et al,[1] however, showed that improvements in pain and pain-related disability associated with osteoporotic compression fractures in patients treated with vertebroplasty were similar to those for the control group, without treatment.

VII. Surgical Pearls

- The possibility of cement leakage can be overcome through the use of high-quality imaging and slow application of PMMA in a viscous state.
- In cases of focal kyphosis due to index fracture, the levels above and below the fracture should also be considered in the treatment plan. No more than three levels should be treated at one setting. This policy minimizes the risk of microembolization (cement and fat emboli).[4]

Common Clinical Questions

1. Contraindications to vertebral augmentation include all of the following *except*:
   A. Asymptomatic lesions
   B. Retropulsed bone fragment
   C. Epidural tumor causing myelopathy
   D. Severe pain due to vertebral body compression fractures in patients with osteoporosis

2. Procedure-related complications include all of the following *except*:
   A. Cement leakage
   B. Pulmonary embolism, hemo- or pneumothorax
   C. New adjacent vertebral fracture
   D. Three levels attempted at one setting

References

1. Kallmes DF, Comstock BA, Heagerty PJ, et al. A randomized trial of vertebroplasty for osteoporotic spinal fractures. N Engl J Med 2009;361(6):569–579
2. Wardlaw D, Cummings SR, Van Meirhaeghe J, et al. Efficacy and safety of balloon kyphoplasty compared with non-surgical care for vertebral compression fracture (FREE): a randomised controlled trial. Lancet 2009;373(9668):1016–1024
3. Lee MJ, Dumonski M, Cahill P, Stanley T, Park D, Singh K. Percutaneous treatment of vertebral compression fractures: a meta-analysis of complications. Spine (Phila Pa 1976) 2009;34(11):1228–1232
4. Mendel E, Bourekas E, Gerszten P, Golan JD. Percutaneous techniques in the treatment of spine tumors: what are the diagnostic and therapeutic indications and outcomes? Spine (Phila Pa 1976) 2009;34(22, Suppl):S93–S100

Answers to Common Clinical Questions

1. D
2. D

64 Spinal Cord Tumor Resection

Michelle J. Clarke and Timothy F. Witham

I. Key Points

- Intradural tumor resection has the potential for significant neurologic morbidity.[1]
- Prognosis and outcome are highly variable and dependent on pathology.[1,2]

II. Indications

- Diagnosis or treatment of a contrast-enhancing intradural lesion in a symptomatic patient
  - Sensory or motor deficits and sphincter dysfunction
  - Localized pain, especially nonmechanical pain exacerbated by recumbency
  - Not indicated for transverse myelitis, multiple sclerosis, or drop metastases
  - In malignant lesions, consider biopsy and adjuvant therapy to avoid neurologic morbidity.

III. Technique

- Place patient in prone position with Mayfield clamp (Integra LifeSciences, Plainsboro, NJ).
- Preoperative corticosteroids and broad-spectrum antibiotics are routinely administered.
- Neuromonitoring is required.
  - Continuous somatosensory evoked potentials (SSEPs)
  - Pre-positioning motor evoked potentials (MEPs) provide a baseline that can be used throughout the case.
- Standard midline incision with subperiosteal dissection of the paraspinal muscles.
- Laminectomy or laminoplasty is performed one level above and one level below the rostral and caudal poles of the tumor.
  - Immaculate hemostasis and placement of moist Cottonoids (Saramall, Tandil, Argentina) in the epidural space will prevent the accumulation of blood in the operative cavity.
- Midline durotomy is performed just rostral to the tumor and extended caudal to the tumor (**Fig. 64.1**).
  - Ultrasound prior to the dural opening may help define the location of the tumor.

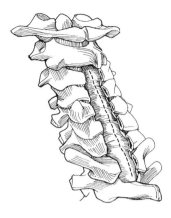

Fig. 64.1 The durotomy is completed and the arachnoid is incised. (From Vaccaro AR, Albert TJ, Spine Surgery: Tricks of the Trade 2nd ed, Thieme; Fig. 4.2.)

- Use tack-up sutures to tent the dura laterally to the paraspinal muscles.
- The arachnoid is preserved and opened separately under microscopic guidance.
- The arachnoid can be clipped to the dural edges using small vascular clips.
- Locate midline to minimize neurologic morbidity.
  - The tumor may distort the cord; thus, the posterior median sulcus may be estimated by inspecting the bilateral dorsal root entry zones or identifying the convergence of small vessels in the midline.
  - Dorsal column mapping by monitoring SSEPs and directly stimulating the cord may be helpful.
- A midline myelotomy is started in the area of maximum cord enlargement.
  - Extend the incision superiorly and inferiorly to expose the tumor in its entirety.
- Begin dissecting the tumor at the area of maximal enlargement (**Fig. 64.2**).
  - Carefully spread the posterior columns with a micro-dissector.
  - Pial sutures may be used at the edge of the incision to provide gentle traction.
- Once the tumor is exposed, send a specimen for frozen section pathology.
  - High-grade tumors are debulked; postoperative adjuvant therapy is required.
  - Low-grade glial tumors and ependymomas are more aggressively approached
- En bloc resection is recommended when possible.[2]
  - Reduces tumor spillage

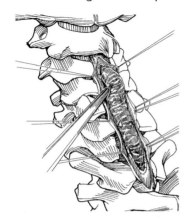

Fig. 64.2 Tumor dissection is initiated in the middle portion of the tumor, which is the bulkiest. (From Vaccaro AR, Albert TJ, Spine Surgery: Tricks of the Trade 2nd ed, Thieme; Fig. 4.3.)

- Reduces intralesional bleeding and maintains a better surgical plane
– Large tumors may require piecemeal resection.
– To resect, gently push the spinal cord away from the lesion using micro-instruments.
  - Minimize movement of the intact spinal cord to prevent injury.
  - An ultrasonic aspirator may be useful.
– Note: dissection/resection along the median raphe may be difficult.
  - Beware of coagulating the anterior spinal artery or its branches.
– Post-resection ultrasound may be valuable in determining the extent of resection.
– Irrigate inside the thecal sac to remove all blood products.
– Immaculate watertight dural closure is needed.
  - Consideration can be given to dural patches/grafts to enlarge the diameter of the thecal sac in patients with expansible lesions and local swelling.
– Dural sealant should be considered.
– If a laminoplasty is called for, replace the lamina using pre-drilled mini-plates.
  - This may decrease the incidence of cerebrospinal fluid (CSF) leak.
– Irrigate and close the incision in a watertight fashion.

IV. Complications

- Neurologic injury
  - Significant motor morbidity
  - Significant proprioceptive morbidity
  - Sphincter dysfunction (can be minimized if the conus is avoided)
- CSF leak
- Wound infection
  - Increases with adjuvant cytotoxic agents
- Post-laminectomy kyphosis
  - Greatest risk: children <3 years, patients with preoperative deformity, patients with preoperative neurologic deficit
  - Laminoplasty may reduce this risk.

V. Postoperative Care

- Place patient supine and require bed rest for 24 to 48 hours as a CSF leak precaution.
- Patient can be weaned from steroids over 2 to 4 weeks.
- Consider postoperative magnetic resonance imaging (MRI) with and without contrast within 48 hours of surgery.
  - Consider reoperation for residual tumor (depending on pathology and neurologic status).
- Gradually mobilize the patient with the assistance of physical therapy.
  - Most patients will have sensory changes that will make ambulation difficult.
- Leave Foley catheter in place until patient is ambulatory.
  - Straight catheterization is needed for sphincter dysfunction.
- Patient can be discharged to home or rehab facility depending on functional status once discharge criteria are met (typically, tolerating diet, having adequate pain control on oral medications, and, depending on functional status, voiding and ambulating).
- Depending on the pathologic findings, the patient should have a consultation with radiation oncology and neurologic oncology personnel to discuss adjuvant therapy.
  - No radiation or chemotherapy should be given until the wound is healed, which typically requires 3 to 4 weeks.

VI. Outcomes

- Highly dependent on tumor pathology and the availability of adjuvant therapies
- A large proportion of patients require inpatient rehabilitation.
- In the event of recurrence, consider further surgery.

VII. Surgical Pearls

- Detailed preoperative discussion of risks is mandatory.
  - Postoperative neurologic deficit is common and unpredictable.
  - Dorsal column dysfunction is expected.
- Neurologic monitoring is mandatory.
  - Epidural MEPs can help prevent neurologic injury.
- Laminoplasty may decrease the risk of postoperative CSF leak and kyphosis.
  - Place mini-plates on lamina and drill pilot holes before performing the laminectomy to ease repair.
- Begin dissection at the midpoint of the lesion, where it is the bulkiest, to reduce injury.
- In lesions with associated cysts, the laminectomy need not extend beyond the solid tumor.
  - Cyst walls are typically nonneoplastic, and complete tumor resection results in cyst resolution.

Common Clinical Questions

1. Where and in what direction should the myelotomy be performed?
2. If the tumor has a cystic component, does this need to be resected?
3. What type of neuromonitoring is appropriate?

References

1. Constatini S, Siomin V, Epstein F. Surgical management of intramedullary spinal cord tumors. In Fessler RG and Sekhar L, eds. Atlas of Neurosurgical Techniques: Spine and Peripheral Nerves. New York: Thieme; 2006
2. Hanbali F, Fourney DR, Marmor E, et al. Spinal cord ependymoma: radical surgical resection and outcome. Neurosurgery 2002;51(5):1162–1172, discussion 1172–1174
3. Yang S, Yang X, Hong G. Surgical treatment of one hundred seventy-four intramedullary spinal cord tumors. Spine (Phila Pa 1976) 2009;34(24):2705–2710

Answers to Common Clinical Questions

1. Longitudinally in the midline of the spinal cord. With splitting of the dorsal columns, proprioceptive deficit is minimized.
2. No. The cyst wall is usually nonneoplastic and the cyst will resolve.
3. Continuous intraoperative SSEPs and MEPs are required.

65 Surgical Resection of Spinal Vascular Lesions

Timothy D. Uschold, Alim P. Mitha, and Steve W. Chang

I. Key Points

- The natural history of spinal vascular lesions is usually malignant. Given the eloquence of local tissue, early definitive treatment is favored whenever feasible.
- All arteriovenous (AV) lesions require preoperative spinal angiography.
- Preservation of the anterior spinal artery (ASA) is paramount during attempts at surgical treatment or embolization.
- The optimal trajectory for the resection of spinal cavernous malformations is determined by the two-point method. A line connecting the center of the lesion with its most accessible margin determines the approach. Some lesions without pial contact may still be resected.
- Timing of surgical intervention after hemorrhage is controversial, although the presence of acute hemorrhage may aid in early resection of some cavernomas.

II. Indications

- Cavernous malformations: Surgery is recommended for all accessible lesions that reach a pial surface. Small, deep-seated asymptomatic lesions can be followed. Deep lesions with evidence of repeated hemorrhage or expansion should be considered for surgery.[1]
- Extradural-intradural AV malformations (AVMs): Palliative attempts at flow reduction and/or selective targeting of high-risk features are appropriate in the setting of progressive symptoms related to steal, repeated hemorrhage, mass effect, or congestion.
- Intramedullary and conus AVMs: Surgical resection, typically with preoperative embolization, is recommended if gross total excision can be achieved. Embolization alone for cure has been demonstrated but remains more controversial.
- Intradural-dorsal and intradural-ventral AV fistula (AVF): all require definitive treatment with either surgery or nonparticulate embolization. If clinical history and imaging findings suggest an intradural-dorsal AVF despite a negative angiogram, surgical exploration is warranted.
- Extradural AVF: all require definitive treatment; endovascular intervention is favored.

III. Technique

- Posterior or posterolateral approach via laminectomy or laminoplasty
  - Added costotransversectomy or facetectomy may allow further lateral exposure.
  - The dura is opened in a linear fashion and the arachnoid is tacked to the dura.
  - If additional anterolateral visualization is necessary, the dentate ligaments may be transected and tacked contralaterally with 6-0 Prolene suture to facilitate gentle rotation of the spinal cord. This may be done across several levels for maximum effect (**Fig. 65.1**).
- Cavernous malformations
  - When necessary, myelotomy is made sharply with a linear pial opening. Appropriate zones for entry into the cord include the dorsal midline and the lateral dorsal sulcus at the dorsal root entry zone. This trajectory enters the substantia gelatinosa. A third entry option is the lateral trajectory behind the dentate ligaments and between the dorsal and ventral spinocerebellar tracts (**Fig. 65.2**).
  - The lesion is dissected circumferentially. Coagulation of the cavernoma may be necessary to shrink and debulk the lesion's

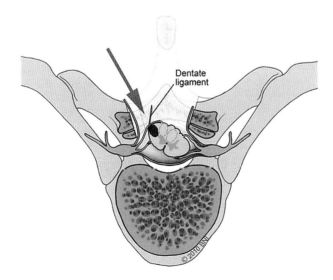

Fig. 65.1 Gentle spinal cord rotation is facilitated by retraction of dentate ligament(s) (used with permission from Barrow Neurological Institute).

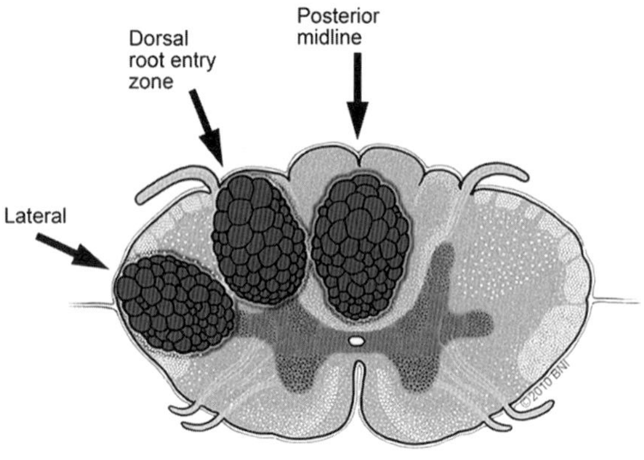

Fig. 65.2 Alternative posterior and posterolateral zones of entry for myelotomy (used with permission from Barrow Neurological Institute).

interior. The associated venous anomaly should be preserved. Surrounding hemosiderin-stained spinal cord is not taken.[1]
- Intradural-dorsal AVFs: Following dural opening, the arterialized vein is followed to its intradural interface along the root sleeve, where the radicular artery pierces the dura. The intradural fistulous connection is clipped, bipolared, and transected.
- Extradural AVF: transarterial endovascular coil embolization is typically the preferred modality of treatment, although transvenous routes have been described.
- Intradural-ventral AVFs: Anterior and posterolateral trajectories have been described. The fistula is bipolared and transected such that arterial supply to the ASA and normal venous drainage is preserved. Venous varices can be further excised. Nonparticulate embolization may be useful in selected cases, although surgery remains the gold standard.
- Intramedullary spinal AVMs: Arterial rather than venous feeders should be sharply dissected circumferentially, cauterized, and transected first. The largest draining vein is typically cauterized and transected last for removal of the specimen.
- Extradural-intradural AVMs: Embolization may be the primary palliative modality for the setting of symptomatic steal, repeated hemorrhage, or vascular congestion. Surgery is typically reserved for relief of persistent, symptomatic mass effect.

IV. Complications

- Cerebrospinal fluid leak, wound complications.
- Delayed or acute neurologic decline: May be attributable to progressive venous thrombosis, especially in the setting of embolization for intradural-dorsal AVFs. Routine postprocedural heparinization is considered in these patients. Blood pressure control is strict, and judicious use of steroids is advised before intervention.

V. Postoperative Care

- Postprocedural angiography and/or magnetic resonance imaging (MRI) is essential to verify treatment effect, especially in the setting of new neurologic deficits.

VI. Outcomes

- Cavernous malformations: Subtotal resection offers nominal benefit. Initial postoperative deterioration has been reported in 24 to 50%, but long-term follow-up data suggest improved neurologic function in as many 46 to 58%.
- Intradural-dorsal AVFs: The primary benefit of surgery over endovascular treatment remains risk of recurrence (as high as 98% initial success for surgery vs. 46 to 85% for embolization).[2] Endovascular abilities are improving. Motor improvements have been reported in approximately 60% of patients compared with 40% showing improvements in sphincter dysfunction (Aminoff-Logue [AL] Scale, **Table 65.1**), irrespective of treatment modality. Numerically, improvements in AL scores are typically modest (about one point).
- Intradural-ventral AVFs: Available series are mostly small, but neurologic improvement or stabilization following surgery has been reported to range from 87.5 to 95%. Preoperative embolization may be useful in limiting flow rate (and in some cases for cure), but incomplete occlusion has resulted in more modest improvements compared with surgery.[3]
- Extradural AVFs: Outcomes reported in numerous case reports have been favorable in terms of fistula obliteration and clinical improvement. In the setting of acute hematoma, surgical evacuation within 12 hours is an important prognostic.
- Extradural-intradural AVMs: Most multimodality attempts are purely palliative. Rare cases may be amenable to embolization followed by operative resection.

Table 65.1 Aminoff-Logue Scale

Gait dysfunction
1. Leg weakness or gait change without significant activity impairment
2. Restricted walking but no DME assist required
3. Cane for ambulation
4. Crutches or walker for ambulation
5. Bed-bound, does not stand, confined to wheelchair
Urinary dysfunction
1. Hesitancy, urgency, and/or frequency
2. Intermittent incontinence or retention
3. Full incontinence or retention

Abbreviation: DME, durable medical equipment.

Source: Modified from Aminoff MJ and Logue V. The Prognosis of Patients with Spinal Vascular Malformations. Brain 1974;(97):211–218.

- Intramedullary AVMs: Clinical improvement rates of 33 to 67% have been reported for surgery, compared with rates of 8 to 20% for clinical decline. Rates of postsurgical angiographic cure have ranged from 59 to 100%. Further endovascular data using Onyx is anticipated. The most appropriate and definitive strategy remains preoperative embolization (when technically appropriate) followed by microsurgical excision.
- Conus AVMs: Little published experience. Aggressive multimodality treatment can result in clinical improvement or stabilization in addition to angiographic cure.

VII. Surgical Pearls

- Intraoperative electrophysiologic monitoring of somatosensory evoked potentials (SSEPs) and motor evoked potentials (MEPs) is essential for all cases. In the setting of AV lesions, serial indocyanine green angiography (ICG) and/or intraoperative spinal angiographic runs before and during resection are often useful.
- Anterior or anterolateral approaches to the resection of spinal vascular lesions are seldom advised due to the risk of ASA compromise and poor dural closure.[4]
- Sharp rather than blunt dissection is favored when possible.
- If required, myelotomy should expose the entire cranial-caudal extent of the lesion to minimize parenchymal retraction and aid in visualizing feeding pedicles.

– Pressure measurements in the arterialized veins of intradural dorsal AVFs can be transduced using a small-gauge needle. Pressure should more closely approximate central venous pressure following fistula obliteration.

Common Clinical Questions

1. Name the primary advantage of surgery (in terms of outcome) over embolization for intradural-dorsal AVFs.
2. Name three zones of entry for myelotomy from a posterior approach.
3. Name three intraoperative tools or strategies useful in guiding and confirming treatment for AVMs and AVFs.

References

1. Vishteh AG, Sankhla S, Anson JA, Zabramski JM, Spetzler RF. Surgical resection of intramedullary spinal cord cavernous malformations: delayed complications, long-term outcomes, and association with cryptic venous malformations. Neurosurgery 1997;41(5):1094–1100, discussion 1100–1101
2. Steinmetz MP, Chow MM, Krishnaney AA, et al. Outcome after the treatment of spinal dural arteriovenous fistulae: a contemporary single-institution series and meta-analysis. Neurosurgery 2004;55(1):77–87, discussion 87–88
3. Cho KT, Lee DY, Chung CK, Han MH, Kim HJ. Treatment of spinal cord perimedullary arteriovenous fistula: embolization versus surgery. Neurosurgery 2005;56(2):232–241
4. Connolly ES Jr, Zubay GP, McCormick PC, Stein BM. The posterior approach to a series of glomus (Type II) intramedullary spinal cord arteriovenous malformations. Neurosurgery 1998;42(4):774–785, discussion 785–786

Answers to Common Clinical Questions

1. Decreased risk of recurrence with surgery
2. Dorsal midline, dorsal lateral sulcus, lateral between the nerve roots
3. Intraoperative monitoring, ICG, intraoperative spinal angiography, intravascular pressure transduction

Appendices

Positioning

Tien V. Le, Juan S. Uribe, and Fernando L. Vale

Topic	Positioning
Prone positioning on Mizuho OSI "Jackson" Spinal Table	• Patient initially supine on radiolucent imaging top of the Jackson table • Pad bony prominences appropriately (see below). • Temporarily tuck arms with thin sheet. • Place the Jackson Spinal Surgery Table Top over patient and temporarily hold in place with pins for adjustment of pads. • Position rigid plastic head rest directly over Prone View headrest or other soft head rest. • Thoracic pad to be positioned between sternal notch and xyphoid • Center the hip and thigh pads for appropriate support. • Leg pads centered over rest of legs, leaving room for both feet once turned prone • Place a bed sheet folded to width of ~2 feet and centered over the lower half of the arms for later use in tucking. • Attach four seatbelts, one for upper thorax, one at hips, one at thigh, and one at lower leg. • Remove pin and compress Jackson frame until there is some resistance at caudal end, then replace pin in new slot. • Remove pin and compress Jackson frame until there is firm resistance rostrally, then replace pin in new slot • Refasten all four seatbelts tightly. • Count for four seatbelts and four pins both rostrally and caudally. • Loosen resistance at head of bed. • Discuss which side to turn patient with partner at caudal end and the anesthesiologist. • Turn in brisk, smooth fashion 180° into prone position. • Remove seatbelts and remove pins securing the posterior bed and remove the posterior bed. • Double-check positioning of all padding and confirm adequacy. • Check foley position and be sure genitals in males are free of compression. • Abdomen should be decompressed, allowing for diaphragmatic excursion. • Check for neutral position of cervical spine and reposition Prone View as needed.

Topic	Positioning
Padding and prophylaxis	• Pad all bony prominences to prevent postoperative neuropathies. • May use egg-crate foam padding or any other soft material such as gel pads or Tempur-Pedic foam. • Wrists should be padded to decrease risk of median neuropathy. • Elbows should be padded to decrease risk of ulnar neuropathy. • Knees/fibular head should be padded to decrease risk of common peroneal neuropathy. • The pelvis anterior superior iliac spine should be padded to decrease risk of lateral femoral cutaneous neuropathy. • An axillary roll can be placed at the upper chest wall when in a lateral decubitus position to decrease risk of brachial plexopathy. • Eye goggles and slight reverse trendelenburg position may help decrease undo pressure on eyes when in prone position, which decreases risk of postoperative blindness.
Anterior cervical approach	• Supine position • Place intrascapular shoulder roll. • Head midline placed in chin strap and with 5–10 lbs of traction • Neck in neutral position • Pad all bony prominences appropriately. • Tape shoulders with 3" silk tape and pull to caudal end of operating table to maximize view of caudal cervical spine. • Tuck arms to side in secure fashion, make sure thumbs point up. • May use soft wrist ties using unrolled KERLIX roll for later use by circulator for more visualization of caudal levels in extreme cases • Slight reverse trendelenburg
Posterior cervical approach	• Place in prone position using Jackson spinal table as above. • Gardner-Wells tongs may be placed in neutral position (3–4 cm directly above the pinna and inferior to superior temporal line) prior to flipping for additional axial cervical traction and reduction if needed. • Likewise, some may opt to use a Mayfield skull clamp for rigid fixation for certain cases (e.g., severe kyphotic deformities). • Tuck arms using preplaced sheet by wrapping sheet around the arms and onto the thoracolumbar region. • Secure with multiple towel clamps. • Be sure thumbs are facing down. • Tape shoulders with 3" silk tape and tape to caudal end of Jackson table. • Tape the skin overlying the trapezius with 3" silk tape bilaterally, and tape to caudal end of Jackson table until posterior skin of neck is taught. • Place in slight reverse trendelenburg.

Topic	Positioning
Posterior cervical approach for occipital cervical fusion	• Place in prone position using Jackson table as above. • Gardner-Wells tongs may be placed in neutral position (3–4 cm directly above the pinna and inferior to superior temporal line) prior to flipping for additional axial cervical traction and reduction if needed. • Likewise, some may opt to use a Mayfield skull clamp for rigid fixation prior to fusion. • Tuck arms using preplaced sheet by wrapping sheet around the arms and onto the thoracolumbar region. Secure with multiple towel clamps. • Be sure thumbs are facing down. • Tape shoulders with 3" silk tape and tape to caudal end of Jackson table. • Tape the skin overlying the trapezius with 3" silk tape bilaterally and tape to caudal end of Jackson table until posterior skin of neck is taught. • Place in slight reverse trendelenburg. • Slightly flex the cervical spine and place chin in military tuck position to allow for better exposure of occiput and occipital-cervical junction, keeping the neck neutral.
Posterior lumbar approach	• For unstable fractures or when manipulation of lumbar spine is to be kept to a minimum, position patient with Jackson table as above. • For operations without instability (e.g., microdiskectomy), may use a "Wilson frame" or positioning on two large parallel, longitudinally oriented gel rolls with enough room to allow for diaphragmatic excursion and abdominal decompression. • Failure to allow for abdominal decompression leads to increased pressure transmitted to epidural veins, complicating surgery with increased bleeding. • For kyphoplasty/vertebroplasty, may use two large gel rolls, with one spanning the width of the chest and one spanning the width of the pelvis. • Regardless of specific procedure, for lumbar operations, arms should be abducted and forearms forward, resting on a soft pillow which is positioned on top of an armrest. • The arms should not be abducted more than 90° and the elbows should not have any direct pressure on them to minimize ulnar neuropathy. • Axillary padding should be used to minimize brachial plexus injuries. • Keep patient in slight reverse trendelenburg.

Topic	Positioning
Anterior lumbar approach	• Patient is supine on an operating table with arms tucked to the side. • All bony prominences appropriately padded • May use additional roll in lumbosacral region for increased lordosis.
Lateral transpsoas approach	• C-Max table or other table capable of flexion/extension at the hip to be used • Patient is placed in lateral decubitus position depending on which side is approached for procedure. • An axillary roll should be placed. • The superior iliac crest should be positioned just past the "break" in the table. • A moderately sized roll may then be placed at the break, especially for an L4/5 disc space, this is not as important if operating at L2/3 or higher. • Hips are flexed with knees bent, allowing for more relaxed iliopsoas muscles. • Fluoroscopy is used to establish a "true" AP view with the C-arm in its most neutral position. • Once established, 3" silk tape is used to secure the patient at the iliac spines. • More tape is used to secure the thoracic cavity. Be sure to protect the nipples with foam when applying the tape. • The legs must be taped down to secure the patient in this fixed position. • An arm board is used to support the lower arm. • An additional arm board is used to support the upper arm, or stacked pillows may be used to support the upper arm.
Lateral thoracic approach	• The same basic positioning is done for transpsoas approach, but be sure to leave enough room for operating at the appropriate thoracic level(s).

II Selected Spinal Orthoses[1,2]

Tien V. Le, Juan S. Uribe, and Fernando L. Vale

Class	Example	Benefits	Limitations	Uses
Cervical: Cervical orthoses (CO)	Soft collar	• Light • Inexpensive • Comfortable • High compliance	• Minimal purchase of occiput & mandible • Still permits up to 80% of motion	• Cervical sprains • Post-op support • Proprioceptive reminder limiting extremes of neck movement • Not for patients with bony instability
Cervical: Occipital-mandibular cervical orhoses (OMC)	Thomas collar	• More rigid than CO • Better purchase of occiput & mandible • Better restriction of flexion-extension	• No caudal fixation • Poor lateral bending & rotation control • Still no significant restriction of motion	• Temporary immobilizer in acute trauma • Not for patients with bony instability

Class	Example	Benefits	Limitations	Uses
Cervical: Occipital-mandibular high thoracic orthoses (OMHT) or High thoracic cervico-thoracic orthoses (CTO) • More effective at upper cervical spine (C0–C3) versus mid & lower segments • Primarily restricts flexion-extension • Poor restriction of lateral bending & rotation • Occipital-mandibular & better upper thoracic purchase (above sternum anteriorly & above T3 spinous process posteriorly)	Miami J collar	• Most effective of high thoracic CTO's in stabilizing all planes (73% flexion/extension, 51% lateral bending, 65% rotation) • Relatively low occipital & mandibular skin pressure, reduces risk of skin ulceration	• Parallelogram effect	• Long term immobilizer for severely unstable injury • Postop support

Class	Example	Benefits	Limitations	Uses
	Aspen collar	• Less restricting than Miami J but more so than Philadelphia • Relatively low skin pressure, reduces risk of skin ulceration • Cleanable and replaceable liners • Large anterior and posterior openings for better airflow	• Parallelogram effect	• Long term immobilizer for cervical instabilities • Postop support
	Philadelphia collar	• Most popular • Comfortable	• Parallelogram effect • Higher skin contact increases risk of skin ulcerations • Plastazote foam can be very hot and is less rigid than other high thoracic CTO's	• Cervical sprains • Mild cervical injuries and minor instabilities • Temporary immobilizer in acute trauma • Post-op support
	NecLoc collar	• Ease of use • Application with minimal manipulation of c-spine	• Parallelogram effect	• Temporary immobilizer in acute trauma • "Extrication collar"

Class	Example	Benefits	Limitations	Uses
Cervical: Occipital-mandibular low thoracic orthoses (OMLT) or Low thoracic CTO • Mid to lower cervical segments involved as well • Adds three-point bending moment • Most restrictive of motion of cervical orthoses due to longer length and better thoracic purchase • Better control of rotation & sagittal motion • Limited control in lateral bending • No sufficient control of motion at O-C1 • Extends past sternum anteriorly and past T3 spinous process posteriorly	Yale brace (modified Philadelphia)	• Very good restriction of combined flexion-extension (86% motion restriciton) • More effective than SOMI in limiting flexion-extension at C2/3 and C3-T1 • Comfortable • Good compliance	• Less effective than SOMI in limiting flex-ext at C1/2	• Cervical injuries including mid and lower levels • Upper thoracic injuries

II Selected Spinal Orthoses

Class	Example	Benefits	Limitations	Uses
	SOMI brace	• Effective for C1–C5, especially in flexion-extension • Comfortable • Well tolerated	Not as effective in controlling extension	• Cervical injuries including mid and lower levels • Upper cervical fx that are unstable in sagittal plane • Upper thoracic injuries
	Minerva brace	• Best of cervical orthoses in limiting axial rotation (88% motion restriction) • Least pronounced "Snaking effect" • Occipital support & forehead strap for better immobilization of the head • Adequate immobilization from C1–C7 • Better C1/2 immobilization	• Custom molded more effective than "off-the-shelf" version	• Cervical injuries including mid and lower levels • May be an option when Halo is considered. One study indicated it had stabilizing characteristics comparable to Halo vest • Upper thoracic injuries
	Aspen CTO	• Incorporates the Aspen collar • Give the option to "step-down" the level of motion restriction		• Cervical injuries including mid and lower levels • Upper thoracic injuries

Class	Example	Benefits	Limitations	Uses
Thoraco-lumbar spinal orthoses (TLSO) • Thoracolumbar & upper lumbar injuries • Limited effect on segmental motion • Three-point bending forces at the upper thorax & pelvis with midportion of brace at thoracolumbar junction to control gross-body movement • Best for control of gross body motion • Not as effective for low lumbar and sacral segments	Jewett hyper-extension brace	• Three-point fixation to sternum, pubis, & thoracolumbar junction • Lightweight • Easily adjustable for flexion-extension restriction	• Not effective for preventing deformity • Pressure-sensitive areas may develop • May not fit appropriately if kyphotic deformity exists already or in cases of scoliosis	• Control flexion motion

Class	Example	Benefits	Limitations	Uses
	Full-contact TLSO	• Most effective for nonoperative management of thoracolumbar fractures • Distributes force over wide surface area • Improved fixation of pelvis and thorax • Better control of lateral bending and axial rotation • Good compliance	• May get hot due to full contact • Bulk • Expensive	• Instabilities in more than one plane • Impaired skin sensation • Multiple osteoporotic compression fractures • Morbidly obese or noncompliant patients

Class	Example	Benefits	Limitations	Uses
Lumbosacral orthoses (LSO) • Lumbar spine difficult to brace because of limited caudal fixation points & physiologic hypermobility • Questionable effectiveness • Braces are primarily a reminder to restrict gross trunk movements • LSO & TLSO do not adequately stabilize segmental motion in lower lumbar spine and lumbosacral junction • Extending with thigh spica reduces gross pelvic motion, but segmental translation with axial loading not affected & patients do not tolerate this because of severe limitations in walking and sitting	Lumbosacral corset	• Very comfortable • Low profile • Inexpensive	• Little effect on intersegmental spinal motion or loads • No stabilizing effect on sagittal, axial, or transverse intervertebral translation • Paradoxical increase in motion at L5/S1	• Diminish pain • Decrease lumbar spine mobility • Support the paraspinal muscles

Class	Example	Benefits	Limitations	Uses
	Full-contact LSO	• More rigid	• May get hot due to full contact • May not adequately stabilize segmental motion in lower lumbar spine and lumbosacral junction • Bulk	• Diminish pain • Decrease lumbar spine mobility • Support the paraspinal muscles • Post-op support

References

1. Benzel EC. Spine Surgery: Techniques, Complication Avoidance, and Management. Second edition. Philadelphia: Elsevier, 2005, Vol 2, pp 1915–1921
2. Browner J, Levine T. Skeletal Trauma: Basic Science, Management, and Reconstruction. Third edition. Philadelphia: W.B. Saunders Co., 2003, Vol. 1, pp 751–756

III Scales and Outcomes

Mark S. Greenberg

Description

Numerous grading scales are available for initial assessment of spine-related disorders, as well as for outcome measurement to determine effectiveness of treatment. This appendix presents some of the more widely used scales. For copyright protection purposes, questionnaires are not reproduced herein.

Modified Japanese Orthopedic Association Score

Table 1 Modified JOA Score for Cervical Myelopathy[1]*

Score	Description
Upper Extremity (UE) motor dysfunction	
0	Unable to feed self
1	Unable to use knife and fork; can eat with spoon
2	Can use knife and fork with much difficulty
3	Can use knife and fork with slight difficulty
4	None (normal)
Lower Extremity (LE) motor dysfunction	
0	Unable to walk
1	Can walk on flat surface with walking aid
2	Can walk up and or down stairs with handrail
3	Lack of smooth and stable gait
4	None (normal)
Sensory Deficit	
Upper Extremity	
0	Severe sensory loss or pain
1	Mild sensory loss
2	None (normal)
Lower Extremity	
0	Severe sensory loss and pain
1	Mild sensory loss
2	None (normal)

Score	Description
Trunk	
0	Sever sensory loss or pain
1	Mild sensory loss
2	None (normal)
Sphincter Dysfunction	
0	Unable to void
1	Marked voiding difficulty
2	Some voiding diffuculty (urgency or hesitation)
3	None (normal)

- Total score ranges from 0 to 17 (normal).

Functional Independence Measure (FIM)

The Functional Independence Measure (FIM)[2] was developed to provide uniform evaluation of disability for spinal cord injuries. It rates 18 items shown in **Table 2** (13 motor, 5 cognitive) on the 7 level scale shown in **Table 3**. The FIM has high internal consistency and is a good indicator of burden of care

Table 2 The Functional Independency Measure (FIM)

Classification	Item
Motor	
Self-care	Eating
	Grooming
	Bathing
	Dressing - upper body
	Dressing - lower body
	Toileting
Sphincter control	Bladder management
	Bowel management
Mobility	Bed, chair, wheelchair
	Toilet
	Tub, shower
Locomotion	Walk or wheelchair
	Stairs

Classification	Item
Cognitive	
Communication	Comprehension
	Expression
Social Cognition	Social Interaction
	Problem Solving
	Memory

Table 3 The 7 FIM Rating Levels of Disability

Degree of Dependency	Level of Function	Score
No helper	Complete independence	7
	Modified independence	6
Modified dependent on a helper	Supervision	5
	Minimal assist (≥ 75% independent)	4
	Moderate assist (≥ 50% independent)	3
Complete dependent on a helper	Maximal assist (≥ 25% independent)	2
	Total assist (< 25% independent)	1

Table 4 Nurick Grade of Disability from Cervical Spondylosis[3]

Grade	Description
0	signs or symptoms of root involvement without myelopathy
1	myelopathy, but no difficulty in walking
2	slight difficulty in walking, able to work
3	difficulty in walking but not needing assistance, unable to work full-time
4	able to walk only with assistance or walker
5	chairbound or bedridden

Oswestry Disability Index (ODI)

A ten-question survey, each response is graded 0 to 5 (0 indicates no disability).[4] The score is then converted to a percentage; 0% would be no disability, and 100% would be the highest disability.

Neck Disabillty Index (NDI)

Neck Disability Index[5]: a ten-question survey similar to the Oswestry Disability Index for the lumbar spine. Mild disability is defined as a score of 10–28%; moderate, 30–48%; sever, 50–68%; complete, 72%.

36-Item Short Form Health Survey (SF-36)

The Medical Outcomes Study Short Form 36[6] is a 36-item self-administered questionnaire used to measure health status and outcome from the patient's perspective. Although this has been widely used for health policy and for some research, it is not specific enough for many spine-related issues. See reference 5 for the original publication. It produces an 8-scale measure of functional health and wellbeing. Permission to use the instrument must be obtained from the Medical Outcomes Trust (www.sf-36.com).

Zurich Claudication Questionnaire (ZCQ)

The ZCQ is a validated questionnaire[7] that evolved from the Swiss Spinal Stenosis Questionnaire (SSS) and consists of eighteen questions that pertain to symptom severity, level of function, and patient satisfaction. It is oriented toward patients with lumbar spinal stenosis. The final score is calculated as an unweighted mean of all answered questions and ranges from 1 to 5 (5 being more severe). While not a statistically valid calculation, the questionnaire demonstrated good reproducibility, internal consistency, and validity.

References

1. Chiles BW III, Leonard MA, Choudhri HF, Cooper PR. Cervical spondylotic myelopathy: patterns of neurological deficit and recovery after anterior cervical decompression. Neurosurgery 1999;44(4):762–769
2. Forer S, Granger C, et al. Functional independence measure. The Buffalo General Hospital, State University of New York at Buffalo, Buffalo, NY, 1987
3. Nurick S. The pathogenesis of the spinal cord disorder associated with cervical spondylosis. Brain 1972;95(1):87–100
4. Fairbank JC, Couper J, Davies JB, O'Brien JP. The Oswestry low back pain disability questionnaire. Physiotherapy 1980;66(8):271–273
5. Vernon H, Mior S. The Neck Disability Index: a study of reliability and validity. J Manipulative Physiol Ther 1991;14(7):409–415
6. Ware JE Jr, Sherbourne CD. The MOS 36-item short-form health survey (SF-36). I. Conceptual framework and item selection. Med Care 1992;30(6):473–483
7. Stucki G, Daltroy L, Liang MH, Lipson SJ, Fossel AH, Katz JN. Measurement properties of a self-administered outcome measure in lumbar spinal stenosis. Spine (Phila Pa 1976) 1996;21(7):796–803

Index

Note: Page numbers followed by *f* and *t* indicate figures and tables, respectively.

A

AAS. *See* Atlantoaxial subluxation (AAS)
ABC (mnemonic), of trauma management, 114
Abdominal aorta, 36
Abducens palsy, with lumbar puncture/drain, 80
ABI. *See* Ankle-brachial index (ABI)
Abscess, spinal, 129*f*, 131–132
   drainage, costotransversectomy for, 300–303
   epidural. *See* Spinal epidural abscess (SEA)
Accessory atlantoaxial ligament, 13*t*
ACDF. *See* Anterior cervical discectomy and fusion (ACDF)
Acetaminophen (APAP), 66
   and opioids, combinations, 67
Adam forward bending test, 163, 165
ADI. *See* Atlantodental interval (ADI)
Airway management, in anterior cervical techniques, 232, 235–236
Alar ligament, 13*t*
Alar plates, 5, 6*f*
ALIF. *See* Anterior lumbar interbody fusion (ALIF)
ALL. *See* Anterior longitudinal ligament (ALL)
American Spinal Injury Association (ASIA) scoring system, 114, 115*t*
Aminoff-Logue Scale, 413, 414*t*
Analgesics
   nonopioid, 66
   opioid, 67
Anesthesia, depth of, monitoring, 59–60
Aneurysmal bone cyst, spinal, 139
Angiography
   spinal, 172
      of arteriovenous lesions, 177
      for lateral extracavitary approach, 291
      with vascular pathology, 410
      with surgical resection of vascular lesions
         intraoperative, 414
         postoperative, 413
Angle of trunk rotation, 165
Ankle-brachial index (ABI), 155
Ankle clonus, testing for, 45
Ankylosing spondylitis (AS), 154, 180
   seronegative arthropathy, 180–182
   thoracic pedicle technique for, 285
Annulus fibrosus, 27
   embryology of, 4
   tears in, 146
Ansa cervicalis, 17
Anterior atlantooccipital membrane, 13*t*
Anterior cervical corpectomy, 232–237, 234*f*
Anterior cervical discectomy and fusion (ACDF), 227, 230, 238–242
Anterior cervical foraminotomy, 243–247, 244*f*–245*f*
Anterior costotransverse ligament, 24*t*
Anterior longitudinal ligament (ALL), 11, 13*t*, 18, 24*t*, 31*t*
Anterior lumbar interbody fusion (ALIF), 359–363
Anterior sacroiliac ligament, 37
Anterior spinal artery (ASA), 18, 23
   and arteriovenous lesions, 174–178
   preservation, in surgery for vascular lesions, 410
Anticoagulation
   prophylactic, 66–67
   therapy with
      for deep vein thrombosis, 67
      for pulmonary embolism, 67
Antinuclear antibody(ies) (ANA), 180
Apical ligament, 13*t*
Arcuate foramen, 11
Arteriovenous fistulas (AVFs), 172
   extradural, 174, 175*t*, 177–178
      surgical resection of, 410, 412
      outcomes with, 413

Arteriovenous fistulas (AVFs) (*continued*)
    intradural-dorsal, 173–174, 175*t*, 177
      surgical resection of, 410, 412
        outcomes with, 413
    intradural-ventral, 174, 175*t*, 177–178
      surgical resection of, 410, 412
        outcomes with, 413
    preoperative angiography of, 410
    Spetzler classification of, 172, 175*t*
Arteriovenous malformations (AVMs), 172
    conus, 174, 176*t*, 177–178
      surgical resection of, 410
        outcomes with, 414
    extradural-intradural, 174, 176*t*, 178
      surgical resection of, 410, 412
        outcomes with, 413
    intramedullary, 174, 176*t*, 177–178
      surgical resection of, 410, 412
        outcomes with, 414
    preoperative angiography of, 410
    Spetzler classification of, 172, 176*t*
Artery of Adamkiewicz, 23
    injury to, 23
Arthritis
    enteropathic, 180
    psoriatic, 180
    rheumatoid. *See* Rheumatoid arthritis (RA)
Articular capsule, 28
AS. *See* Ankylosing spondylitis (AS)
ASA. *See* Anterior spinal artery (ASA)
Astrocytomas, 143–144
    high-grade, 143–144
    low-grade, 143–144
Atlantoaxial joint, fracture of, 215
Atlantoaxial subluxation (AAS), in rheumatoid arthritis, 180, 183
Atlantodental interval (ADI), 180, 183, 215
Atlanto-occipital condyle distance, 116
Atlanto-occipital dissociation, 116–117
Atlas (C1), 9. *See also* Cervical spine, C1-C2
    anatomy of, 10–11, 10*f*
    anterior tubercle, 10*f*, 11
    embryology of, 4
    fracture of, 117
    groove for vertebral artery, 10*f*, 11
AVFs. *See* Arteriovenous fistulas (AVFs)
AVMs. *See* Arteriovenous malformations (AVMs)
Axial lumbar interbody fusion (AxiaLIF), 364–367, 365*f*
Axis (C2), 9. *See also* Cervical spine, C1-C2
    anatomy of, 10–12, 11*f*, 217*f*
    congenital malformations, 215
    dens fracture, 119–120, 119*f*
    embryology of, 4
    fracture of, 117–118, 118*f*
      classification of, 118, 118*f*
    odontoid process, 11–12
    ossification centers, fusion of, 6
    pars interarticularis, 11, 11*f*
    pedicles, 11, 11*f*
    spinous process, 11, 11*f*
    traumatic spondylolisthesis of, 117–118

B

Babinski sign, 45, 48, 141, 150, 204
Back pain, 71–72, 154, 165. *See also* Low back pain, in adults
    axial
      from facet joint disease, 157–158
      from intervertebral disc disease (without deformity), 156–157
    with spinal epidural abscess, 193
Balloon kyphoplasty, 398
Bamboo spine, 181, 182*f*
Basal plates, 5, 6*f*
Basion, 10
Bedside procedures, 76–82
Biceps brachii muscle, 45*t*
Biceps femoris muscle, 45*t*
Biologics, spinal, 94–98
Bispectral index, 60
Bladder function, after sacrectomy, 394–395, 395*t*
Bone graft(s), 94
    allograft for, 95*t*, 96
    autograft for, 94–96, 95*t*
    characteristics of, 94, 95*t*
    demineralized bone matrix for, 95*t*, 96
    extenders, 95*t*, 96–97

mechanical stability of, 94
osteoconduction by, 94, 95t
osteogenesis by, 94, 95t
osteoinduction by, 94, 95t
surgical pearls, 97
Bone morphogenetic protein(s) (BMP), 95t, 96–97
Bone scintigraphy, 55
in ankylosing spondylitis, 181
of spinal infections, 128
for vertebral body augmentation, 399
Boston brace, 167
Bowel function, after sacrectomy, 394–395, 395t
Bowel prep, for axial lumbar interbody fusion, 364–365
Brachial plexus, 17
Brachioradialis muscle, 45t
Breast cancer, spinal metastases, 136–139
Brown-Sequard syndrome, 141, 143
BRYAN Cervical Disc, 229f, 229t, 230
Bulbocavernosus reflex, 33
Burst fractures, 121, 122f
thoracic, transpedicular approach for, 296–299

C

Cancer, spinal metastases. *See also* Metastatic disease
epidemiology, 83
Capsular ligament, 13t
Carisoprodol, 69
Carotid sheath, 18, 19f
Carotid triangle, 18
Cauda equina, 28, 35
formation of, 6, 7f
Cauda equina syndrome, 181, 192–193, 325
Caudal cell mass, anomalies of, 106–110
Cavernous malformations, 172–173
surgical resection of, 410
outcomes with, 413
technique for, 411–412
Central cord syndrome, 147–148
Ceramics, as bone graft extenders, 95t, 97
Cerebrospinal fluid (CSF) leak, 206, 211, 235, 251, 273–274, 299, 344, 407

Cervical arthroplasty, 227–231, 229f
devices for, 228, 229f, 229t
revision of, 228
Cervical bar, 147
Cervical laminectomy
manual, 249
with or without fusion, 248–252
posterior, technique for, 249
Cervical lateral mass fixation, 249–251, 249f–250f
Cervical nerve roots, 12, 14, 17
compression, neuroforaminal, posterior cervical foraminotomy for, 259–264
decompression, posterior cervical foraminotomy for, 259–264
injury, intraoperative, 251
Cervical plexus, 17
Cervical spine, 19f
age-related changes in, 54
anatomy of, 73f
anterior exposure, 238–239, 239f
anterolisthesis, 265
bony anatomy of, 16–17, 16f
C1-C2. *See also* Atlas (C1); Axis (C2)
congenital malformations, 215
degenerative disease of, 215
inflammatory disease of, 215
ligamentous instability, 215
surgical techniques, 215–220
traumatic fractures, 215
wiring technique for, 218
C1-C2 transarticular screws, technique for, 218
C1 lateral mass screw
with C2 pars, pedicle, or translaminar screws, 216–218
technique for, 216
congenital vertebral fusion, 110–111
corpectomy. *See* Anterior cervical corpectomy
C2 pars screw, technique for, 216
C2 pedicle screws, technique for, 217
C2 translaminar screws, technique for, 217
degenerative disease, 146, 215
discectomy, anterior approach, 278, 279f

Cervical spine *(continued)*
  disc herniation, 17, 146–147
    central, 147
    lateral, 146–147
  facet dislocations, 265
  flexion/compression injury, 265
  flexion/distraction injury, 265
  foraminotomy
    anterior. *See* Anterior cervical foraminotomy
    posterior, 259–264, 261*f*
  jumped facet
    bilateral, 265
    unilateral, 265
  laminoforaminotomy, 259–264, 261*f*
  laminoplasty, 253–258, 254*f*–255*f*
  ligamentous anatomy of, 18
  lordotic curvature of, 16–17
  mobility of, 17
  muscular anatomy of, 18
  neural anatomy of, 17
  open reduction techniques, 265–270
    anterior approach, 265–267, 267*f*, 269
    posterior approach, 265, 267–268, 268*f*, 269
  physical examination of, 46
  posterior instrumentation of, 16
  spondylitic myelopathy, 147–150, 149*f*
  spondylosis, laminoplasty for, 253–258
  subaxial, 16
    lateral masses of, 16–17
    trauma, 120–121
      imaging of, 120
      mechanism of injury in, 120
  surgery, monitoring during, 63–64
  surgical pearls, 19–20
  trauma, 116–121
  vascular anatomy of, 17–18
Cervical-thoracic junction (CTJ)
  anatomy of, 276
  biomechanics of, 276
  deformity, 277
  fractures of, 277
  infection, 277
  neoplasms of, 277
  pathology of, 276
  reconstruction and fixation at, 276
    anterior approach, 277–278
      suprasternal, 277
      transclavicular, 277
      transmanubrial/sternal splitting, 277–278, 278*f*, 280–281
    anterolateral (transthoracic) approach, 278–279
    posterior approaches, 279–280, 283
Chance fracture, 121, 122*f*
Charite artificial disc, 378*f*
Charleston brace, 167
Chassaignac tubercle, 16
Chiari I
  clinical features of, 204
  decompression, 204–208, 205*f*
Chiari II, with myelomeningocele, 106
Chin-on-chest deformity, 277
Chondrification, 3
Chondrosarcoma
  sacral involvement in, 390
  spinal, 139–141
Chordoma
  sacral, 390
  spinal, 139–141
Chyle leak, 274
Chylothorax, 274
Clonus, 141, 150
Cobb angle, 160, 166, 166*f*
Coccyx, 33
Codeine, 67
Collagen, 95*t*, 97
Common iliac artery, 36
Complex regional pain syndrome, percutaneous lead spinal cord stimulation for, 74
Compound motor action potential (CMAP), 59
Compression fracture(s)
  osteoporotic, 398
  tumor-related, 398
Compression fractures, thoracolumbar, 121, 122*f*
Computed tomography (CT), 51–52, 52*f*
  for axial lumbar interbody fusion, 364
  of C1-C2, 215
  of cervical disc herniation, 147

of cervical-thoracic junction, 276
of congenital anomalies, 101–102
in diffuse idiopathic skeletal hyperostosis, 185
of epidural spinal metastases, 138
indications for, preoperative, 14, 25
for lateral extracavitary approach, 291
of lumbar stenosis, 374
of ossification of posterior longitudinal ligament, 185
of primary epidural spinal tumors, 140
of screw placement, in thoracic pedicle technique, 287
of spinal infections, 128
of surgical site infection, 133
of thoracic disc herniation, 151
in trauma patient, 114
for vertebral body augmentation, 399
Congenital anomalies, 101–113
of caudal cell mass, 106–110
of dysjunction, 103–106
of notochord formation, 102–103
of segmentation, 110–111
Congenital block vertebrae, 110–111
Conus, ascension of, 6, 7f
Conus medullaris, 28
Conus syndrome, 192–193, 325
Corpectomy
anterior cervical, 232–237, 234f
thoracoscopic approach to, 304
Costotransversectomy, 300–303, 301f
Costovertebral joint pain, thoracoscopic approach to, 304
Costovertebral ligament, 24t
Coup de poignard. *See* Cavernous malformations
Coxal (innominate) bones, 35
Craniovertebral junction (CVJ), 9
bony anatomy of, 10–12, 10f–11f
ligamentous structures of, 9, 9f, 12, 13t
muscular anatomy of, 12–14
neural anatomy of, 12
vascular anatomy of, 12
Craniovertebral stability, Powers ratio for, 116, 116f
Crankshaft phenomenon, 163

Cruciate ligament, 13t, 14
CT. *See* Computed tomography (CT)
CT angiography
of cervical-thoracic junction, 276
in cervical trauma patient, 117
preoperative, 14
CT myelography, 52
of cervical disc herniation, 147
of cervical spondylotic myelopathy, 148
of congenital anomalies, 101–102
of intramedullary spinal cord tumors, 144
of spinal tumors, 142
of thoracic disc herniation, 151
Cutaneous nerve(s), of posterior head and neck, 17
Cyclobenzaprine, 69

D

Deep tendon reflex(es), grading, 46t
Deep vein thrombosis (DVT)
prophylaxis, 66–67
treatment of, 67
Deformity, spinal, 163–171. *See also* Kyphosis; Scoliosis
nonfixed, requiring 5 to 10 degrees of correction per segment, 309–313
thoracic pedicle technique for, 285
thoracoscopic approach to, 304
Degenerative spinal disease
of C1-C2, 215
cervical, 146, 215
kyphoscoliosis caused by, 277
kyphosis caused by, 160–161
lumbar, 154–162, 359, 364
radiculopathy with, 154–155
magnetic resonance imaging of, 54, 146
scoliosis in, 160–161
thoracic, 146
Deltoid muscle, 45t
Dens fracture (C2), 119–120, 119f
Dermal sinus tract, 101f
dorsal, 105
Dermatome(s), 44f
sacral nerve supply to, 35, 35f
thoracic, 23
Dermomyotomes, 3

Diagnostic procedures, 71–73
pearls, 74
Diastematomyelia, 101*f,* 102–103
Diazepam, 69
Diclofenac, 66
Diffuse idiopathic skeletal hyperostosis (DISH), 180, 184–185, 184*f*
Digastric muscle, 18
Direct lateral lumbar interbody fusion (DLIF), 354–358
Disc degeneration. *See also* Degenerative spinal disease
magnetic resonance imaging of, 54
Discectomy, thoracoscopic, 304–305, 307
Disc herniation
cervical, 17, 146–147
central, 147
lateral, 146–147
extruded, 54
imaging of, 147, 151
lumbar, 27–29. *See also* Cauda equina syndrome; Conus syndrome
surgical pearls, 31
magnetic resonance imaging of, 54
nomenclature for, 54
protrusion, 54
sequestered, 54
thoracic, 150–152
central, 150
centrolateral, 150
costotransversectomy for, 300–303
lateral, 150
lateral extracavitary approach to, 291–295
transpedicular approach for, 296–299
Discitis, 127–129, 129*f*
of cervical-thoracic junction, 277
and spinal epidural abscess, 193–194
thoracoscopic approach to, 304
transthoracic approach to, 314–317
Discography, provocation, 71, 72*f*
Disc stimulation, 71, 72*f*
single-needle technique, 71, 72*f*
DLIF. *See* Direct lateral lumbar interbody fusion (DLIF)

Dual-energy x-ray absorptiometry (DEXA), 374
Durotomy, unintended
in thoracoscopy, 306
in transpedicular approach to thoracic spine, 298–299
Dysphagia, 184–185

E
Ectoderm, 4
Ehlers-Danlos syndrome, 166
Electroencephalography, intraoperative, 59
Electromyography (EMG)
in cervical laminoplasty, 253
spontaneous (sEMG), 57, 60–61
advantages and disadvantages of, 61
applications of, 63–64
technical pearls, 62
technique for, 61
triggered (tEMG), 57
advantages and disadvantages of, 62–63
applications of, 63–64
technical pearls, 63
technique for, 62
in thoracic pedicle technique, 287
Embryology
spinal, 3–7
spinal cord, and congenital anomalies, 101–102, 101*f*
Endoderm, 4
Enteropathic arthritis, 180
Enthesitis, 180
Enthesopathy, in ankylosing spondylitis, 181
Eosinophilic granuloma, spinal, 139
Ependymomas, 143–144
Epiblast, 4
Erector spinae muscle(s), 23, 30, 38*t*
Esophageal injury, intraoperative, 274
Ewing sarcoma
sacral, 390
spinal, 139–141
Extensor carpi radialis muscle, 45*t*
Extensor hallucis longus muscle, 45*t*
External costal muscle(s), 23
Extreme lateral interbody fusion (XLIF), 354–358

F

FABER (acronym), 47
FABERE test, 181
Facet capsule ligament, 24*t*
Facet screw fixation/fusion, 368–372, 370*f*
FADIR (acronym), 47–48
Femoral stretch test, 47
Filum terminale. *See also* Tight filum terminale syndrome
   fibrolipomas of, 104–105, 109
   formation of, 6, 7*f*
Flexor digitorum profundus I and II muscles, 45*t*
Fluoroscopy
   in axial lumbar interbody fusion, 365–366
   in cervical open reduction techniques, 266
   intraoperative
      in odontoid screw fixation, 221–222, 222*f*–223*f*
      with thoracic disc herniation, 151–152
   in lumbar arthroplasty, 380
   of screw placement, in thoracic pedicle technique, 287
Foramen magnum, anatomy of, 10
Foraminotomy, lumbar, minimally invasive technique for, 330–332
Fortin finger test, 47
Fracture(s)
   of atlantoaxial joint, 215
   of atlas (C1), 117
   of axis (C2), 117–118, 118*f*
      classification of, 118, 118*f*
   burst, 121, 122*f*, 296–299
   C1-C2, traumatic, 215
   of cervical-thoracic junction, 277
   Chance, 121, 122*f*
   compression
      osteoporotic, 398
      thoracolumbar, 121, 122*f*
      tumor-related, 398
   dens, of axis, 119–120, 119*f*
   hangman's, 117–118, 118*f*
   imaging of, 117, 122, 124
   Jefferson, 215
   odontoid
      anterior oblique dens fracture, 224
      direct fixation of, 221–226
      type 2, 215
      type 3, 215
   sacral, 123–124
      classification of, 123, 124*f*
   thoracic
      lateral extracavitary approach to, 291–295
      traumatic, thoracic pedicle technique for, 285
      vertebral burst, transpedicular approach for, 296–299
   thoracolumbar, 121–123, 122*f*
   vertebral body, in cancer patients, 398, 399*f*
Fungal infection, spinal, 130–131

G

Gait
   assessment of, 46
   ataxic, 150
Gardner-Wells tongs, 77–78, 78*f*
Gastrocnemius muscle, 45*t*
Gastrulation, 4
Giant cell tumor, spinal, 139
Globus, 184
Gluteus maximus muscle, 38*t*
Gluteus medius muscle, 38*t*
Gluteus minimus muscle, 38*t*
Greater occipital nerve, 12
Grisel's syndrome, 12

H

Halo orthosis and traction
   complications of, 79
   contraindications to, 76
   indications for, 76
   outcomes with, 81
   post-procedure care for, 80
   surgical pearls, 81
   technique for, 76–78, 78*f*
Halo rings, 77–78
Hangman's fracture, 117–118, 118*f*
Headache, post-LP, 80
Hemangioma, spinal, 139
Hematoma
   intracranial subdural, with lumbar puncture/drain, 80
   spinal, 190–192, 191*f*
      epidural, 190
         with lumbar puncture/drain, 80

Hematoma *(continued)*
   subarachnoid, 190
   subdural, 190
Hemorrhage
   intramedullary, 190. *See also* Arteriovenous malformations (AVMs); Cavernous malformations
   of vascular lesions, surgical intervention after, 410
Heparin
   low-dose, 67
   low-molecular-weight, 67
   prophylactic, 67
   therapeutic, 67
High-intensity zone (HIZ), on MRI, 54
Hip pain, assessment of, 47
Hoffmann sign, 45, 48
HOX genes, 3–4
Hydrocodone, 67
Hydromorphone, 67
Hygroma, intracranial subdural, with lumbar puncture/drain, 80
Hyperreflexia, 141, 204
   lower extremity, 150
Hypoblast, 4

I

Iliac artery(ies), 36
Iliac crest, 33
Iliacus muscle, 38*t*
Iliac vein(s), 36
Iliocostalis muscle, 23, 30
Iliolumbar ligament, 34*f*, 36
Iliopsoas muscle, 45*t*
Image navigation, in lumbar facet screw fixation/fusion, 368–372, 370*f*
Imaging
   in ankylosing spondylitis, 181
   of atlas fracture, 117
   for axial lumbar interbody fusion, 364
   in cauda equina syndrome, 193
   of cavernous malformations, 173
   of cervical disc herniation, 147
   of cervical spondylitic myelopathy, 148–149, 149*f*
   of cervical-thoracic junction, 276
   of cervical trauma patient, 116–120
   of congenital anomalies of segmentation, 111
   in conus syndrome, 193
   of diastematomyelia, 102
   in diffuse idiopathic skeletal hyperostosis, 185
   of discitis, 128
   of dorsal dermal sinus, 105
   of epidural infection, 132
   of epidural spinal metastases, 138
   of fibrolipomas of filum terminale, 109
   of granulomatous infections, 131
   of intramedullary spinal cord tumors, 143–144
   for lateral extracavitary approach, 291
   with myelocele/myelomeningocele repair, 106
   of ossification of posterior longitudinal ligament, 185
   postoperative, with surgical resection of vascular lesions, 413
   of pyogenic vertebral osteomyelitis, 128
   in rheumatoid arthritis, 183
   of sacral fractures, 124
   of Scheuermann kyphosis, 169, 169*f*
   spinal, 51–55. *See also specific modality*
     surgical pearls, 56
   of spinal epidural abscess, 194
   of spinal hematoma, 191, 191*f*
   of spinal lipomas, 104
   of spinal tumors, 142
   of split notochord syndrome, 103
   of spondylolisthesis, 158
   of surgical site infection, 133
   in syndrome of caudal regression, 110
   of thoracic disc herniation, 150–151
   of thoracolumbar fractures, 122
   in tight filum terminale syndrome, 109
   in trauma patient, 114–115
   of tuberculous infections, 131
Imbalance
   coronal, 309, 359
   sagittal, 309, 359
Immobilization, spinal, 114
IMRT. *See* Intensity-modulated radiation therapy (IMRT)

Indocyanine green (ICG) angiography, 178
Infection(s)
 of cervical-thoracic junction, 277
 with lumbar puncture/drain, 80
 magnetic resonance imaging of, 53
 spinal, 127–135
  drainage, costotransversectomy for, 300–303
  epidural, 131–132
  granulomatous, 127, 130–131
  hematogenous, 127
  postoperative, 127, 132–134
  pyogenic, 127–129, 129f
 surgical site, 132–134
 thoracic pedicle technique for, 285
 transthoracic approach to, 314–317
Inferior gluteal nerve, 36
Inferior oblique muscle, 12, 14f
Inferior vena cava, 36
Infuse®, 97
Intensity-modulated radiation therapy (IMRT), 84, 390
Intermediate horn, 5, 6f
Internal iliac artery, 36
Internal iliac vein, 36
Interosseous ligament, 37
Interspinous devices (ISDs), 373–376
Interspinous ligament, 18, 24t, 31t
Interspinous process decompression, 373–377
Intervertebral foramen, 28, 28t
ISDs. See Interspinous devices (ISDs)

J
Jefferson fracture, 215
Joint position sense, assessment of, 43

K
Kambin's triangle, 343, 343f
Ketorolac tromethamine, 66
Kyphoplasty, 398
 technique for, 400, 401f
Kyphoscoliosis
 degenerative, 277
 uncompensated, correction, 309–313
Kyphosis. See also Scheuermann kyphosis
 of cervical-thoracic junction, post-laminectomy, 277

 correction
  costotransversectomy for, 300–303
  thoracic pedicle technique for, 285
 degenerative, 160–161
 fixed, requiring more than 30 degrees of correction, 309–313
 normal thoracic, 164
 post-laminectomy, 277, 359, 407
 posttraumatic, 277
 in Scheuermann kyphosis, 169, 169f

L
Laminectomy
 cervical
  manual, 249
  with or without fusion, 248–252
  posterior, technique for, 249
 lumbar, 333–335, 334f
 thoracic, 23
Laminoplasty
 cervical, 253–258, 254f–255f
 definition of, 253
Laségue sign, 47
Lateral retroperitoneal trans-psoas interbody fusion, minimally invasive, 354–358
Lateral sacral artery(ies), 36
Latissimus dorsi muscle, 23
Lesser occipital nerve, 12
Levatores costarum longus and brevis, 23
Ligamentum flavum, 24t, 31t
Ligamentum nuchae, 18
Lipoma(s)
 intradural, 103–105
 spinal, 101f, 103–105
Lipomyelocele, 101f, 103–105
Lipomyelomeningocele, 101f, 103–105
Longissimus capitis muscle, 14
Longissimus muscle, 23, 30
Long tract signs, 150
 assessment for, 45
Longus colli muscle(s), 11, 18, 19f
Lordosis, normal lumbar, 164
Lortab, 67
Low back pain, in adults, 373, 378
 axial, 354
 mechanical, 359
 steroids for, 68

LP. *See* Lumbar puncture
LSI. *See* Lumbosacroiliac (LSI)
Lumbar artery(ies), 30
Lumbar arthroplasty, 378–383
  prosthesis for, 378, 378f
Lumbar drain
  complications of, 80
  contraindications to, 76
  indications for, 76
  post-procedure care for, 80
  surgical pearls, 81
  technique for, 78–79
Lumbar interbody fusion
  anterior (ALIF), 359–363
  axial (AxiaLIF), 364–367, 365f
  direct lateral (DLIF), 354–358
  extreme lateral (XLIF), 354–358
  lateral retroperitoneal trans-psoas, minimally invasive, 354–358
  posterior (PLIF), 336, 338–340, 339f
  transforaminal (TLIF), 336–340
    minimally invasive, 341–347
Lumbar nerve roots, 28–29
Lumbar plexus, 29f, 355, 355f
Lumbar puncture
  complications of, 80
  contraindications to, 76
  indications for, 76
  outcomes with, 81
  post-procedure care for, 80
  surgical pearls, 81
  technique for, 78–79
Lumbar spine. *See also* Thoracolumbar spine
  age-related changes in, 54
  anatomy of, 72f
  anterior interbody fusion using Bagby and Kuslich (BAK) cages, 382
  bony anatomy of, 27–28, 27t
  degenerative disease of, 154–162, 359, 364
  disc herniation, 27–29. *See also* Cauda equina syndrome; Conus syndrome
  surgical pearls, 31
  facet joint, 28
  facet screw fixation/fusion, 368–372, 370f
  foraminotomy, minimally invasive technique for, 330–332
  herniated nucleus pulposus, 325
  interspinous process decompression, 373–377
  laminectomy, 333–335, 334f
  lateral extracavitary approach to, 291–295, 293f
  ligamentous anatomy of, 30, 31t
  microdiscectomy, 325–329
  muscular anatomy of, 30
  neural anatomy of, 28–30, 39f
  open anterior (transperitoneal) approaches to, 318, 322
  physical examination of, 46–47
  postdiscectomy collapse with neural foraminal stenosis, 359
  retroperitoneal approaches to, 318–324
  surgery, monitoring during, 64
  surgical pearls, 31
  three-column model of, 26–27, 26f
  total disc replacement, 382
  vascular anatomy of, 30, 321
  venous plexuses, 30
  vertebral body augmentation, 398–403
Lumbar stenosis, 373
Lumbosacral plexus, 35
Lumbosacral spine, retroperitoneal approach to, 319, 320f
Lumbosacroiliac (LSI) fusion, 384–389, 386f–387f
Lung cancer, spinal metastases, 136–139

M
Magerl technique, 19
Magnetic resonance angiography (MRA)
  of arteriovenous lesions, 177
  in cervical trauma patient, 117
Magnetic resonance imaging (MRI), 52–54, 53f
  of adolescent idiopathic scoliosis, 167
  in ankylosing spondylitis, 181
  of arteriovenous lesions, 177
  artifacts, 54
  for axial lumbar interbody fusion, 364

Index

in cauda equina syndrome, 193
of cavernous malformations, 173
of cervical disc herniation, 147
of cervical spondylotic myelopathy, 148, 149f
of cervical-thoracic junction, 276
in cervical trauma patient, 117
of Chiari I, 204
contraindications to, 54
in conus syndrome, 193
of degenerative spinal disease, 146
of disc degeneration, 54
of disc herniation, 54
of discitis, 128
of epidural infection, 132
of epidural spinal metastases, 138
gadolinium contrast for, 53
of herniated nucleus pulposus, 190
high-intensity zone (HIZ), 54
of infection, 53
of intramedullary spinal cord tumors, 143–144
for lateral extracavitary approach, 291
of lumbar stenosis, 374
of Modic end plate changes, 54
of ossification of posterior longitudinal ligament, 185
postoperative, with surgical resection of vascular lesions, 413
of primary epidural spinal tumors, 140
in rheumatoid arthritis, 183
of Scheuermann kyphosis, 169
of scoliosis, 163
of spinal cord injury, 53–54
of spinal dysraphism, 101
of spinal epidural abscess, 190, 194
of spinal hematoma, 190–191, 191f
of spinal tumors, 136, 142
of spondylolisthesis, 158
of surgical site infection, 133
of thoracic disc herniation, 150–151
in trauma patient, 115
of tumors, 53
T1-weighted, 53
T2-weighted, 53
for vertebral body augmentation, 399
Mantle layer, 5, 6f
Marfan syndrome, 166
Marginal layer, 6, 6f
Marie-Strümpell disease, 180
Medial branch block, 71–72
Median sacral artery, 36
Mediastinum, superior, 277
Meningioma, 141–143
Meningopleural fistula, 273–274
MEPs. *See* Motor evoked potentials (MEPs)
Mesoderm, 4
Metastatic disease
 sacral, 390
 spinal, 142
  epidemiology, 83
  epidural, 136–139
  radiation therapy for, 83
  vertebral body, 398
Metastatic epidural spinal cord compression (MESCC), 137
Microdiscectomy
 lumbar, 325–329
  minimally invasive technique for, 327
  open technique for, 325–326, 326f
 thoracoscopic, 304
Milwaukee brace, 167
Modic end plate changes, magnetic resonance imaging of, 54
Monitoring, neurophysiologic, 57–65
 in cervical laminoplasty, 253
 in cervical open reduction techniques, 266
 in cervical spinal surgery, 63–64
 intraoperative, 144, 152
 in surgical resection of vascular lesions, 414
 multiple modalities used in, 63–64
 in occipitocervical fusion, 199
 in spinal cord tumor resection, 404, 408
 in transoral odontoidectomy, 211
Morphine, 67
Motor evoked potentials (MEPs), 57
 advantages and disadvantages of, 59–60
 applications of, 63–64, 144, 152
 in cervical laminoplasty, 253
 in cervical open reduction techniques, 266

Motor evoked potentials (MEPs) *(continued)*
   intraoperative, in surgical resection of vascular lesions, 414
   in occipitocervical fusion, 199
   in spinal cord tumor resection, 404, 408
   technical pearls, 60
   technique for, 59
   in transoral odontoidectomy, 211
Motor function, evaluation, 43
Motor horn, 5, 6*f*
MRA. *See* Magnetic resonance angiography (MRA)
MRI. *See* Magnetic resonance imaging (MRI)
Multifidus muscle, 23, 30, 38*t*
Multiple myeloma, 140, 398
   sacral involvement in, 390
Muscle(s), survey groups, 43, 45*t*
Muscle relaxants, 68–69
Muscle strength, grading system for, 43, 44*t*
Muscle stretch reflex(es), 47*t*
   grading, 45, 46*t*
Myelocele, 105–106, 107*f*–108*f*
   multilayer closure of, 106, 107*f*–108*f*
Myelocystocele, terminal, 6
Myelography, 52, 52*f*
Myelomeningocele, 101*f,* 105–106, 107*f*–108*f*
   multilayer closure of, 106, 107*f*–108*f*
Myelopathy, cervical, 227
Myelotomy, in surgical resection of vascular lesions, 411, 412*f,* 414
Myotomes, 3

N

Naproxen, 66
Narcotics. *See* Opioid(s)
Navigation, spinal
   advantages of, 90, 92
   applications of, 92
   surgical pearls, 92
   systems/technology for, 90–91, 91*f*
Nerve root tension signs, 46
Nerve sheath tumor
   paraspinal, costotransversectomy for, 300–303
   thoracoscopic approach to, 304

Neural arches, 4
Neural folds, 5, 5*f*
Neural tube, 4–5, 5*f*
Neuroblasts, 5
Neuroenteric fistula, 101*f*
Neurofibromas, 141–143
Neurogenic claudication, 155–156, 373
Neurogenic shock, 114
Neuromonitoring, 57–65. *See also specific modality*
Neuroorthopedic syndrome, 104
Neuropore, 3
Nonsteroidal anti-inflammatory drugs, 66
Notochord, 3–4, 6
   formation of, anomalies related to, 102–103
Nucleus pulposus, 27–28
   age-related changes in, 146, 154
   embryology of, 4, 6
   herniated, 190
      lumbar, 325
      thoracic, 277
         transthoracic approach to, 314–317

O

Occipital condyles, 9–10
Occipital condyle screw fixation, 201
Occipital fixation, 200, 200*f*
Occipital plate and rod system, 200–201, 200*f*
Occipitocervical fusion, 199–203, 200*f*
Occiput, 9–10
Odontoid agenesis, 215
Odontoidectomy, transoral, 209–214
Odontoid fracture
   anterior oblique dens fracture, 224
   direct fixation of, 221–226
   type 2, 215
   type 3, 215
Odontoid screw fixation, 221–226, 222*f*–223*f,* 225*f*
Omohyoid muscle, 18
Opioid(s)
   for pain, 67
      adjuncts to, 66
   weak, 67
Opisthion, 10

Os odontoideum, 215
Ossification, 3
Ossification centers
  spinal, 6
  vertebral, 4
Ossification of posterior longitudinal ligament (OPLL), 150, 180, 185–186
  cervical laminoplasty for, 253–258
  transthoracic approach to, 314–317
Osteoblastomas, spinal, 139
Osteoconduction
  by bone grafts, 94, 95*t*
  definition of, 94
Osteogenesis
  by bone grafts, 94, 95*t*
  definition of, 94
Osteoid osteomas, spinal, 139
Osteoinduction
  by bone grafts, 94, 95*t*
  definition of, 94
Osteomyelitis
  of cervical-thoracic junction, 277
  and spinal epidural abscess, 193
  thoracic, lateral extracavitary approach to, 291–295
  thoracoscopic approach to, 304
  transthoracic approach to, 314–317
  vertebral, 127–129
Osteoporosis, vertebral body compression fractures in, 398
Osteosarcoma
  sacral, 390
  spinal, 139–141
Oxycodone, with acetaminophen, 67

P

PADI. *See* Posterior atlantodental interval (PADI)
Pain
  axial, 146
  back. *See* Back pain
  with cervical disc herniation, 146
  of Chiari I, 204
  discogenic mediated
    diagnosis of, 71, 72*f*
    treatment of, 73
  hip joint, 154
  with intramedullary spinal cord tumors, 143
  neck, 71–72
  nonoperative/interventional procedures for, 71–74
  radicular, 146
    with lumbar degenerative disease, 154–155
    with lumbar puncture/drain, 80
  sacral, assessment of, 47
  sacroiliac, 72, 154
  with thoracic disc herniation, 150
  tumor-related, 398
Pain medication
  clinical pearls, 69
  dosage and administration of, 66
Palmar hyperhidrosis, sympathectomy for, 304–305, 307
Pancoast tumor(s), resection of, 271–275
Paragangliomas, 141–143
Paraplegia, with thoracic disc herniation, 150
Parasites, granulomatous spinal infection caused by, 130–131
Patient-controlled analgesia (PCA), 67
Patrick test, 47, 181
Pedal pulse(s), palpation for, 48
Pedicle screw, percutaneous placement of, 348–353, 349*f*–351*f*
Pedicle subtraction osteotomy (PSO), 309–313
  technique for, 309–310, 310*f*
Pelvic incidence, 384*t*, 385*f*
Pelvic tilt, 384*t*, 385*f*
Percocet™, 67
Percutaneous lead spinal cord stimulation, 74
Percutaneous medial branch radiofrequency neurotomy, 73–74
Percutaneous pedicle screw placement, 348–353
  AP-based targeting method, 348–353, 349*f*–351*f*
Peripheral nerves, sensory distribution of, 44*f*
Peripheral neuropathy, percutaneous lead spinal cord stimulation for, 74
Phrenic nerve, 17
Physical examination
  clinical pearls, 48

Physical examination *(continued)*
spinal
individualization of, 43
main components of, 43–48
mechanical, 46
motor, 43
reflex, 45–46
sensory, 43
Pinprick testing, 43
Plain radiographs, 51
of adolescent idiopathic scoliosis, 166–167, 166f
in ankylosing spondylitis, 181
of cervical disc herniation, 147
in cervical open reduction techniques, 266
of cervical spondylotic myelopathy, 148
of cervical-thoracic junction, 276
of discitis, 194
of intramedullary spinal cord tumors, 144
for lateral extracavitary approach, 291
of lumbar spine, 373
in rheumatoid arthritis, 183
of Scheuermann kyphosis, 169, 169f
of screw placement, in thoracic pedicle technique, 287
of spinal infections, 128
of thoracic disc herniation, 151
Plasmacytoma, spinal, 139–141
Pleural effusion, 294
PLIF. *See* Posterior lumbar interbody fusion (PLIF)
PLL. *See* Posterior longitudinal ligament (PLL)
Pneumonia, postoperative, prevention of, 294
Polymethylmethacrylate (PMMA) cement, for vertebroplasty, 398
Polyradiculopathy, selective spinal nerve block for, 72–73
Positron emission tomography, of primary epidural spinal tumors, 140
Posterior atlantodental interval (PADI), 180, 183
Posterior atlantooccipital membrane, 13t

Posterior cervical foraminotomy, 259–264, 261f
classical procedure, 260
minimally invasive procedure, 260–261
Posterior costotransverse ligament, 24t
Posterior inferior cerebellar artery, 18
Posterior longitudinal ligament (PLL), 18, 24t, 31t
continuation at CVJ, 13
ossified, 150
tears in, 146
Posterior lumbar interbody fusion (PLIF), 336, 338–340, 339f
Posterior sacroiliac ligament, 34f, 37
Posterior spinal artery (PSA), 18, 23
and arteriovenous lesions, 174–178
Post-laminectomy syndrome
percutaneous lead spinal cord stimulation for, 74
selective spinal nerve block for, 72–73
treatment of, 73
Pott's disease, 130
of cervical-thoracic junction, 277
Powers ratio, 116, 116f
PRESTIGE ST Cervical Disc System, 229f, 229t, 230
Priapism, 46t
Primitive groove, 3–4
Primitive neuroectodermal tumors, sacral, 390
Primitive node, 4
Primitive streak, 4
ProDisc-C, 229f, 229t, 230
Proprioception, assessment of, 43
Pseudarthrosis
posterior, 359
revision/repair for, 364, 368
Pseudomeningocele, 206
PSO. *See* Pedicle subtraction osteotomy (PSO)
Psoas muscle, 38t
Psoriatic arthritis, 180
Pudendal nerve, 36
Pulmonary embolism, treatment of, 67

Q
Quadriceps femoris muscle, 45t

R

RA. *See* Rheumatoid arthritis (RA)
Radiate ligament, 24t
Radiation therapy, 390. *See also* Intensity-modulated radiation therapy (IMRT); Radiosurgery
  conventional fractionated, 83–86
  surgical pearls, 87
  spinal, 83–89
Radicular artery(ies), 23, 30
Radiculopathy, 28–29, 47, 364
  acute, steroids for, 68
  cervical, 48
    one-level, 227
  chronic, percutaneous lead spinal cord stimulation for, 74
  with lumbar degenerative disease, 154–155
  with lumbar herniated nucleus pulposus, 325
  selective spinal nerve block for, 72–73
  treatment of, 73
Radiography. *See also* Imaging; Plain radiographs
  in trauma patient, 114
Radiosurgery, spinal, 83–84, 86
  candidate lesions for, 87
  indications for, 86–87
  stereotactic, 83–84, 84f–85f
  surgical pearls, 87
  target immobilization for, 86
  target localization for, 86
Rectus capitis posterior major muscle, 14, 14f
Rectus capitis posterior minor muscle, 14, 14f
Recurrent laryngeal nerve
  anatomy of, 241
  intraoperative management of, 241
Reflex(es), testing, 45–46
Reiter syndrome, 180
Retrograde ejaculation, after ALIF, 361
Retroperitoneal approaches, to thoracolumbar spine, 318–324
  conventional open access, 318–322, 320f
  left-sided, 318, 321
  right-sided, 318, 321

Retroperitoneum, anterior structures in, 360, 360f
Retropharyngeal anatomy, 210, 210f
Reverse straight-leg raising, 47
Rheumatoid arthritis (RA), 154, 180, 182–184
Rheumatoid factor (RF), 180
Rhombois muscle, 23
Rib(s), 21–22
Risser method, 166
Romberg test, 46, 150
Rotatores longus and brevis, 23, 30

S

Sacral fractures, 123–124
  classification of, 123, 124f
Sacral nerve roots, 35–36, 35f
Sacral pain, assessment of, 47
Sacral slope, 384t, 385f
Sacrectomy, 390–397
  bowel and bladder function after, 394–395, 395t
  combined approach for (anteroposterior), 391–393
  posterior approach for, 390–391, 392f–393f
  reconstruction in, 394
Sacroiliac joint, 33, 35. *See also* Lumbosacroiliac (LSI) fusion
Sacroiliac joint block, 72
Sacroiliac spine, 33
  bony anatomy of, 33–35, 34f
  ligamentous anatomy of, 36–37
  muscular anatomy of, 38t
  neural anatomy of, 35–36, 35f
  surgical pearls, 37
  vascular anatomy of, 36
Sacropelvic radiographic measurements, 384t, 385f
Sacrospinous ligament, 34f, 37
Sacrotuberous ligament, 34f, 37
Sacrum, 33, 34f
  articulations, 33
Scheuermann kyphosis, 163, 168–170, 169f
Schmorl nodes, 168–169
Schwannoma, 141–143
Sciatic nerve, 35–36
Scintigraphy. *See also* Bone scintigraphy
  of spinal infections, 128

Sclerotomes, 3–4
Scoliosis
  adolescent idiopathic, 163–168
  curves, structural *versus* nonstructural, 164
  definition of, 163
  degenerative, 160–161
  etiology of, 163
  idiopathic
    classification of, 163
    definition of, 163
    Lenke classification of, 164*f*
    major curve of, 163, 164*f*
    minor curve of, 163, 164*f*
    pathophysiology of, 164–165
    thoracic pedicle technique for, 285
    three-dimensional characteristics of, 163
Seatbelt injury, 121
Segmental medullary artery(ies), 18, 30
sEMG. *See* Electromyography (EMG), spontaneous
Semispinalis capitis muscle, 14, 14*f*
Semispinalis thoracis muscle, 23
Sensory horn, 5, 6*f*
Serratus posterior inferior muscle, 23
Serratus posterior superior muscle, 23
Shear test, 47
Shock, neurogenic, 114
Shoulder pain, 46
Smith-Peterson osteotomy (SPO), 309–313
  technique for, 310–311, 311*f*
Somatosensory evoked potentials (SSEPs), 57
  advantages and disadvantages of, 58
  applications of, 63–64, 144, 152, 186
  in cervical laminoplasty, 253
  in cervical open reduction techniques, 266
  intraoperative, in surgical resection of vascular lesions, 414
  in occipitocervical fusion, 199
  in spinal cord tumor resection, 404
  technical pearls, 58–59
  technique for, 58
  in transoral odontoidectomy, 211
Somites, 3, 5, 5*f*

Spinal canal, cervical, 16
  congenital stenosis, laminoplasty for, 253–258
  stenosis, 147
Spinal cord
  cervical, 17
    venous plexuses, 18
  compression
    with cervical disc herniation, 146
    metastatic epidural, 137
    with thoracic disc herniation, 150–152
    by tumor, steroids for, 68
  congenital anomalies of, 101–102, 101*f*
  embryology of, 5–6, 6*f*
    and congenital anomalies, 101–102, 101*f*
  gray matter, formation of, 5
  thoracic, 23
    compression, transthoracic approach to, 314–317
    tumors. *See also* Tumor(s)
      intramedullary, surgery for, monitoring during, 64
    resection, 404–409, 405*f*–406*f*
  white matter, formation of, 6
Spinal cord injury. *See also* Trauma
  complete, 114
  incomplete, 114, 115*t*
  magnetic resonance imaging of, 53–54
  steroids for, 66, 68, 115
  surgical timing in, 115
  in transpedicular approach to thoracic spine, 298
Spinal emergency(ies), 190–195
Spinal epidural abscess (SEA), 190, 193–194
  thoracoscopic approach to, 304
Spinalis muscle, 30
Spinal nerve block, selective, 72–73
Spinal stenosis, treatment of, 73
Spinal thoracis muscle, 23
Spirochetes, granulomatous spinal infection caused by, 130–131
Splenius cervicis muscle, 23
Split notochord syndrome, 103
SPO. *See* Smith-Peterson osteotomy (SPO)

Spondyloarthropathy(ies), 180–189
  seronegative, 180
  seropositive, 180
Spondylolisthesis, 158–160, 159f, 359, 364
  isthmic, 28
Spondylolysis, 28
Spondylosis
  cervical
    medial branch block for, 71–72
    percutaneous medial branch radiofrequency neurotomy for, 73–74
  lumbar
    medial branch block for, 71–72
    percutaneous medial branch radiofrequency neurotomy for, 73–74
  thoracic
    medial branch block for, 71–72
    percutaneous medial branch radiofrequency neurotomy for, 73–74
Sprengel deformity, 110–111
Spurling maneuver, 46
SSEPs. See Somatosensory evoked potentials (SSEPs)
Stereotactic radiosurgery, spinal, 83–84, 84f–85f
Sternal splitting approach, to cervicalthoracic junction, 277–278, 278f, 280–281
Sternocleidomastoid muscle, 18
Steroid(s)
  epidural, 68
    applications of, 73
    injection technique for, 73
    purpose of, 73
  indications for, 68
    for low back pain, 68
    in pain management, 68
    for spinal cord injury, 66, 68, 115
Straight-leg raising, 47
Strength evaluation, 43, 44t
Suboccipital nerve, 12
Suboccipital triangle, muscles of, 12–14, 14f
Sulcus limitans, 5–6
Superior gluteal nerve, 36
Superior oblique muscle, 12, 14f
Supraspinous ligament, 18, 24t, 30, 31t
Surgical site infection(s) (SSI), 132–134
Sympathectomy, thoracoscopic, 304–305
Syndrome of caudal regression, 109–110
Syringomyelia, 204

T

Tandem gait, assessment of, 46
Tectorial membrane, 13t
tEMG. See Electromyography (EMG), triggered
Temperature sense, assessment of, 43
Tethered spinal cord, surgery for, monitoring during, 64
Therapeutic procedures, nonoperative/interventional, 73–74
Thoracic duct injury, 274
Thoracic nerve roots, 23
Thoracic pedicle technique, 285–290, 286f
  salvage techniques, 287
Thoracic spine, 21
  anatomy of, 305, 306f
  bony anatomy of, 21–22, 21f–22f
  degenerative disease, 146
  disc herniation, 150–152
    central, 150
    centrolateral, 150
    costotransversectomy for, 300–303
    lateral, 150
    lateral extracavitary approach to, 291–295
    transpedicular approach for, 296–299
  fractures
    lateral extracavitary approach to, 291–295
    traumatic, thoracic pedicle technique for, 285
  herniated nucleus pulposus, transthoracic approach to, 314–317
  intravertebral/intrapedicular lesions, transpedicular approach for, 296–299
  kyphosis, 21
    progressive, 23
    laminectomy of, 23
    lateral extracavitary approach to, 291–295, 293f

Thoracic spine *(continued)*
  ligamentous anatomy of, 23, 24t
  motion of, 21
  neural anatomy of, 23
  osteophytes, lateral extracavitary approach to, 291–295
  spinal canal stenosis, transthoracic approach to, 314–317
  surgery, monitoring during, 64
  surgical pearls, 23–25
  thoracoscopic approach to, 304–308
  transpedicular approach to, 296–299, 297f
  transthoracic approach to, 314–317
  tumor, spinal canal decompression for, transpedicular approach for, 296–299
  vascular anatomy of, 23
  vertebral body augmentation, 398–403
  vertebral burst fracture, transpedicular approach for, 296–299
Thoracolumbar fascia, 30
Thoracolumbar fractures, 121–123, 122f
Thoracolumbar injury classification and severity score (TLIC-SS), 121
Thoracolumbar spine
  retroperitoneal approaches to, 318–324
  thoracoabdominal approach to, 319–321
  vascular anatomy of, 321
Thoracoscopy, 304–308
Thoracotomy, open, 304, 307
Three-column model, of lumbar spine, 26–27, 26f
Tibialis anterior muscle, 45t
Tight filum terminale syndrome, 106–109
Tizanidine, 69
TLIF. *See* Transforaminal lumbar interbody fusion (TLIF)
Tonsillar herniation, with lumbar puncture/drain, 80
Tonsillar pole, inferior, location of, relative to foramen magnum, variation with age, 207t
Transforaminal lumbar interbody fusion (TLIF), 336–340
  minimally invasive, 341–347
Transpedicular screws, percutaneous placement of, 348–353, 349f–351f
Transthoracic approach, 314–317
Transverse foramen, 10f, 18
Trapezius muscle, 23
Trauma, 114–126. *See also* Spinal cord injury
  cervical, 116–121
  classification of, 114, 115t
  field management of, 114
  thoracic, transthoracic approach to, 314–317
Triceps brachii muscle, 45t
Trigger point injection, 74
Tuberculoma, spinal. *See* Pott's disease
Tuberculosis, spinal, 130–131
Tumor(s)
  of cervical-thoracic junction, 277
  epidermoid, with lumbar puncture/drain, 80
  magnetic resonance imaging of, 53
  sacral, 390
  spinal, 136–145
    costotransversectomy for, 300–303
    epidemiology, 83
    epidural
      metastatic, 136–139
      primary, 139–141
    extradural, 136, 137f
    intradural, 404
    intradural extramedullary, 136, 137f, 141–143
    intradural intramedullary, 136, 137f, 141
    intramedullary, 143–144
    radiation therapy for, 83
    vertebral body collapse with, 398
  spinal cord
    compression by, steroids for, 68
    intramedullary, surgery for, monitoring during, 64
    resection, 404–409, 405f–406f
  thoracic
    lateral extracavitary approach to, 291–295

spinal canal decompression for, transpedicular approach for, 296–299
transthoracic approach to, 314–317
thoracic pedicle technique for, 285

U

Ultrasound
  prenatal, 101–102
  renal, 102
Uncovertebral joints, 19

V

Vascular claudication, 155
Vascular pathology, spinal, 172–179
  surgical resection of, 410–415
Vena cava filter, 66–67
Ventriculus terminalis, 5
Vertebrae
  biopsy, thoracoscopic approach to, 304
  cervical, 16, 16*f*
    congenital fusion, 110–111
  embryology of, 3–4
  lumbar, 27–28, 27*t*
    pars interarticularis (isthmus), 28
    transverse process, 28
  reconstruction, thoracoscopic approach to, 304
  thoracic, 21–22, 21*f*–22*f*

Vertebral arches, 4
Vertebral artery(ies), 12, 19*f*
  cervical, 17–18
  injury, intraoperative, 211–212, 218, 235, 251
Vertebral body
  augmentation, 398–403
  fractures, in cancer patients, 398, 399*f*
  metastatic disease in, 398
Vertebral column, lumbar, bony borders of, 27*t*
Vertebral osteomyelitis, pyogenic, 127–129
Vertebroplasty, 398
  technique for, 400
Vibratory sense, assessment of, 43
Vicodin™, 67
Vicoprofen™, 67

W

Wackenheim line, 116
Warfarin, 67
Wildervanck syndrome, 110–111
Wilmington brace, 167
Wiltse plane, modified, 342, 342*f*
Wolf's law, 234–235

X

XLIF. *See* Extreme lateral interbody fusion (XLIF)
X-Stop spacer, 373, 374*f,* 375